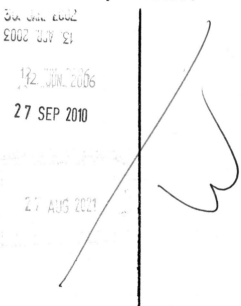

Benefits and Hazards of Exercise

Benefits and Hazards of Exercise

Edited by

DOMHNALL MACAULEY

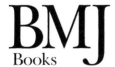
BMJ Books

© BMJ Books 1999
BMJ Books is an imprint of the BMJ Publishing Group

First published in 1999
by BMJ Books, BMA House, Tavistock Square,
London WC1H 9JR

www.bmjbooks.com

British Library Cataloguing in Publication Data

A catalogue record for this book is available from the British Library

ISBN 0-7279-1412-X

Typeset by Apek Typesetters, Nailsea, Bristol
Printed and bound by Latimer Trend, Plymouth

Contents

Contributors

F Conconi, *Department of Applied Biochemistry, University of Ferrara, Italy*

D M Bailey, *School of Applied Sciences, University of Glamorgan, Wales, UK*

K L Bennell, *School of Physiotherapy, University of Melbourne, Australia*

H J N Bethell, *Cardiac Rehabilitation Centre, Hampshire, England, UK*

P D Brukner, *Olympic Park Sports Medicine Centre, Melbourne, Australia*

R Budgett, *British Olympic Centre, Middlesex, England, UK*

B Davies, *School of Applied Sciences, University of Glamorgan, Wales, UK*

M Donelly, *Division of Community Geriatrics, Department of Family Practice, University of British Columbia, Vancouver, BC, Canada*

K Dudgeon, *School of Psychology, Queens University of Belfast, Northern Ireland, UK*

A L Dunn, *Cooper Institute for Aerobics Research, Dallas, Texas, USA*

C B Eaton, *Brown University School of Medicine, Memorial Hospital of Rhode Island, RI, USA*

J Elliot, *Short Term Assessment and Treatment Unit, Vancouver General Hospital, Vancouver, BC, Canada*

C Fersini, *Department of Internal Medicine, University of Ferrara, Italy*

C Foster, *Department of Public Health, Institute of Health Sciences, University of Oxford, England, UK*

R Graham, *School of Psychology, Queens University of Belfast, Northern Ireland, UK*

A E Hardman, *Department of Physical Education, Sports Science and Recreation Management, Loughborough University, England, UK*

M Hillsdon, *London School of Hygiene and Tropical Medicine, London, UK*

J Kremer, *School of Psychology, Queens University of Belfast, Northern Ireland, UK*

J B Leiper, *University Medical School, Aberdeen, Scotland, UK*

C R Madeley, *Department of Virology, University of Newcastle upon Tyne, England, UK*

S A Malcolm, *School of Human Biosciences, La Trobe University, Melbourne, Australia*

F Manfredini, *Post Graduate School of Sports Medicine, University of Ferrara, Italy*

R Manfredini, *Department of Clinical and Experimental Medicine, University of Ferrara, Italy*

A D Martin, *School of Human Kinetics, University of British Columbia, Vancouver, BC, Canada*

R J Maughan, *University Medical School, Aberdeen, Scotland, UK*

W J McKenna, *Department of Cardiovascular Sciences, St George's Hospital, London, UK*

M M Meade, *School of Leisure and Tourism, University of Ulster at Jordanstown, Northern Ireland, UK*

L M Menard, *Brown University School of Medicine, Memorial Hospital of Rhode Island, RI, USA*

N S Peirce, *Centre for Sports and Metabolism and Nutrition Unit, Nottingham, UK*

E C Rhodes, *School of Human Kinetics, University of British Columbia, Vancouver, BC, Canada*

R E Rhodes, *Faculty of Physical Education and Recreation, University of Alberta, Edmonton, AB, Canada*

D Scully, *School of Leisure and Tourism, University of Ulster at Jordanstown, Northern Ireland, UK*

S Sharma, *Department of Cardiovascular Sciences, St George's Hospital, London, UK*

R J Shephard, *School of Physical and Health Education, University of Toronto, Canada*

S M Shirreffs, *University Medical School, Aberdeen, Scotland, UK*

J E Taunton, *Allan McGavin Sports Medicine Centre, Department of Family Practice and School of Human Kinetics, University of British Columbia, Vancouver, BC, Canada*

M Thorogood, *London School of Hygiene and Tropical Medicine, London, UK*

M A van Baak, *Department of Human Biology, University of Maastricht, The Netherlands*

G Whyte, *Department of Cardiovascular Sciences, St George's Hospital, London, UK*

L A Wolski, *School of Human Kinetics, University of British Columbia, Canada*

Introduction

Exercise is a major industry. Leisure centres promote it, doctors endorse it, and the general public are enthusiastic. Suddenly health has become exciting, trendy, and enjoyable. But how much exercise is good for you, how often, how hard and for how long? And what are the hazards? How can we prevent over-training and ensure that those who exercise can deal with viral illness, manage diabetes, or cope with international travel? The answers to these questions and many others are to be found in this book, a must for all of us who are involved in promoting physical activity and advising people who are interested in exercise.

We take you through the latest evidence on the benefits of exercise. There is very strong epidemiological evidence of the benefits of physical activity but this book tells us much more about the quantity and quality required to gain these benefits, and addresses further evidence that cumulative periods of exercise throughout the day are also of value. Putting theory into practice is not always easy, so we explore the most effective methods of getting people active and staying active.

Illness is no exclusion to exercise and, indeed, exercise has long been an integral part of rehabilitation from heart disease. We bring together the latest evidence on exercise and cardiac rehabilitation. Exercise also has a role in the treatment of chronic illnesses such as diabetes and hypertension, and in keeping older people fit and active. There may be hazards with physical activity, however, and as sudden death associated with sport always has a major impact, we address this issue in particular. Over-training and viral illness are two other important problems that sports physicians and general practitioners often meet in their consulting rooms. The diagnosis and treatment of these two very difficult problems is still evolving but we bring you the latest findings.

If you look after international athletes or patients going abroad on holiday, you may be asked about the effects of altitude, time zones, or the need for fluid replacement. So, we include chapters addressing all these issues. If you exercise too much you may suffer over use injuries or stress fractures, another condition where diagnosis or treatment is not easy. And we could not publish this book without including a discussion of the psychological effects of exercise.

Modern educational theory suggests that we should not be passive recipients of information. To aid those who may be preparing for examinations or those who wish to test their self learning the authors have included some multiple choice questions at the end of each chapter. I hope you enjoy the challenge.

This book is the combined work of some of the most outstanding figures in international research and brings together chapters covering some of the most important aspects of sport and exercise medicine. We have enjoyed putting it together and we hope that you enjoy reading it and find it useful.

D MacAuley

1 What is the optimal type of physical activity to enhance health?

R J Shephard

Summary

This chapter examines the potential of active daily living as a means of gaining the cardiovascular and health rewards previously sought through vigorous aerobic fitness programmes. Cross sectional studies of occupational and leisure activity show encouraging associations between such activity and good health; in workers, the gross intensity of effort needed for health benefits is 20 kJ/min. There has been less unanimity on the threshold intensity needed in leisure activities, but various recent "position statements" have decreased the recommendation to 50% of an individual's maximum oxygen intake, sustained for 30 minutes on most days of the week. Lifestyle activities such as walking seem likely to reach this intensity in older individuals but are unlikely to do so in young adults. A growing number of controlled longitudinal studies of brisk walking programmes have shown gains in aerobic fitness, modest reductions in blood pressure, improvements in lipid profile, increased bone density, and enhanced mood state, with less consistent reductions of body fat. Gains have been greatest, however, in elderly, sedentary, and obese people. The main component of active living – fast walking – seems likely to enhance health in such populations, but it is unlikely to be effective in young adults who are in good initial health.

Introduction

A number of governments, including those of the United States and Canada, are currently changing the emphasis of their health promotional programmes from the advocacy of vigorous aerobic exercise to the concept of "active living" – that is, the incorporation of moderate physical activity into everyday living. It is thus important to review the effectiveness of this tactic relative to the structured exercise classes of traditional fitness programmes.

Activity pattern and health benefits

It is now well accepted that the habit of regular physical activity reduces an individual's age-adjusted risk of mortality from all causes and cardiovascular disease.[1-13] A number of recent reports[1-9] and reviews[1,2,8-10] have further suggested that the largest gain in prognosis is realised as a person progresses from the lowest to the next lowest level of physical activity or physical fitness. Occasional dissenting reports still suggest a need for vigorous physical activity.[14-17] Nevertheless, many policy makers now argue that the health of sedentary late 20th century adults can be improved through the adoption of quite low levels of leisure activity, possibly of insufficient intensity to augment traditional markers of physical fitness such as the maximal oxygen intake.

If such expectations prove well founded then there is justification in shifting the emphasis of health promotion programmes from costly "high-tech" structured and supervised classes of aerobic exercise, with their inherent problems of limited recruitment and high drop out rates,[18-19] to the encouragement of an activity daily lifestyle, including such pursuits as walking, cycling, and gardening.

Activity patterns and psychosocial issues

The impact of the recommended activity pattern on recruitment, adherence, and programme costs will not be explored in any detail. Nevertheless, we may note that it is easier for a person who is currently sedentary to adopt and to maintain modest lifestyle activities such as walking than to participate in a structured programme of vigorous aerobic exercise.

Moreover, if a person elects the vigorous pursuit of daily activities rather than attendance at a specific exercise class then the costs of special equipment, clothing, and facilities are largely avoided and the time demands are also much reduced. Many of those who currently fail to exercise regularly claim that a lack of time, a lack of facilities, and cost are major reasons why they remain sedentary.[20] In consequence, programmes that emphasise unsupervised activity such as daily walking can sometimes be more effective than supervised structured exercise classes.[19,21] Indeed, simple local interventions such as posters recommending use of the stairs[22,23] or a programme that advocates commuting by bicycle or on foot[24] sometimes augment daily physical activity by a substantial amount, although attempts to incorporate a less specific vision of "active living" into a broader community-wide health promotion campaign have had only limited success.[25]

Current issues regarding activity patterns and health

Taking as our criterion of programme effectiveness a reduction in cardiovascular risk factors rather than an increase in aerobic fitness, the choice between moderate lifestyle activities and a more intensive and formal exercise programme raises several important research issues.

- Is adoption of the currently recommended "active daily lifestyle" correlated with indicators of future good health? If so, can issues of selection bias be excluded by appropriate longitudinal experiments?
- What is the minimum weekly amount of physical activity needed to yield clinically significant health benefits? Is this minimum "dose" of exercise consistent for various types of physical activity and for population groups that differ in age, sex, socioeconomic status, and ethnic background?
- What weekly quantity of physical activity is likely to be generated through employment in a "heavy" occupation or the encouragement of active living?

Box 1.1   Current controversies concerning exercise and health

- Can "active daily living" meet health objectives?
- What is the minimum weekly activity needed for health benefits?
- Is this minimum consistent across types of exercise and types of population?
- How much activity is generated by "heavy work" or "active living"?
- Is an "active living" approach as effective as structured exercise?

• How do community gains in health related fitness compare between programmes that have focused on encouraging an overall active lifestyle and other initiatives that have emphasised participation in formal structured exercise programmes?

Associations between an overall active lifestyle and health indicators

Cross sectional studies of occupation and leisure have provided many encouraging reports of associations between an active lifestyle and the maintenance of good cardiovascular health. Longitudinal studies generally support the inferences drawn from the cross sectional data, and in particular a growing number of reports indicate health benefits from the adoption of rapid walking.

Occupational studies

Cross sectional comparisons between physically demanding and sedentary occupations have almost without exception shown an association between the physical demands of employment and protection against ischaemic heart disease.[26] Such observations, however, are open to the important objection that the staff engaged to perform "heavy" work are either recruited by management[27] or self selected[28] in terms of personal health and interest in an active lifestyle.

Brunner and Manelis claimed that the problem of self selection was overcome in their study of an Israeli kibbutz, where residents were given little choice in their assigned duties.[29] But even in this special situation it is difficult to believe that the management committee took no account of physique and physical abilities when deciding what work any given person should undertake.

Studies of active leisure

Many reports show a positive association between self reported leisure activity and cardiac health.[1,2,26,30] In general, the stronger the study design, the larger the gradient in risks of all cause and cardiac death.[26]

The well documented impact of self selected exercise on cardiac risk factors[31–34] can be illustrated (table 1.1).[35] Participants were questioned about the frequency with which they engaged in demanding physical activity, the intensity of their active leisure

Table 1.1   Gradients of established cardiac risk factors with self reported physical activity (based on data from Shephard and Bouchard)[35]

Risk factor	Perceived intensity			Perceived frequency		
	Low	Medium	High	Low	Medium	High
Men						
Total skinfolds (mm)	114	104	98	104	96	101
HDL cholesterol (mmol/l)	1.19	1.14	1.19	1.11	1.21	1.15
PWC 150 (watts/kg)	1.69	1.73	1.95	1.79	1.73	1.79
Resting heart rate (beats/min)	58	59	56	63	57	53
Women						
Total skinfolds (mm)	168	148	141	150	131	126
HDL cholesterol (mmol/l)	1.35	1.46	1.43	1.36	1.53	1.56
PCW 150 (watts/kg)	1.15	1.23	1.36	1.20	1.28	1.49
Resting heart rate (beats/min)	67	62	63	65	61	61

HDL=high density lipoprotein

pursuits, their perceived level of fitness, and their perceived level of physical activity relative to their peers. On each of these measures, differences between the least active quarter or third and the most active in terms of average skinfold thickness, high density lipoprotein (HDL), cholesterol, serum triglycerides, PWC 150, and resting heart rate (table 1.1) were as large as or larger than would have been expected in response to most structured exercise programmes. The problem remains, however, that active leisure was self selected, so that at least a part of the observed gradient in cardiac risk factors could have a constitutional origin.

Randomised longitudinal studies

There are fewer problems of initial subject selection in longitudinal studies where participants are assigned randomly to a control group or a programme of enhanced physical activity.

Nevertheless, the volunteers for such experiments do tend to be young, relatively fit non-smokers of high socioeconomic status. Even the findings for this subgroup of the population can be invalidated by a high drop out rate of unfit people from the experimental group or a defection of fit subjects from the control group, or both.

One randomised controlled trial of lifestyle activity found a 4.5% increase in aerobic power, a 10.3% increase in treadmill endurance time, and a 5% increase in HDL cholesterol in those who had been assigned to a 10 week active commuting programme of walking or cycling.[24]

Box 1.2   Is walking an adequate stimulus?

- Commonest form of "active living"
- Health benefit most likely in sedentary, obese, and elderly people
- Self selected pace may provide inadequate stimulus in young adults
- Fast walking reaches training heart rate in most adults >50 years
- Walking does not augment muscle strength but enhances functional capacity concerning exercise and health in elderly people

---

Reported responses to walking

The major component of an active lifestyle is usually rapid walking.[20] Many studies have shown that walking programmes have a beneficial influence on various indicators of good health (table 1.2).

Those likely to benefit from such an approach have tended to be sedentary,[47,55,56,63,77] obese,[37,48] and elderly.[39,46,52,54,57,59,60,65,68,69] In such people even a period of deliberate walking in a shopping mall may demand 70–80% of maximum oxygen intake.[39] Porcari *et al.* noted that 95% of women and 83% of men over the age of 50 years reached a training heart rate while carrying out unpaced walking "as fast as possible".[78]

Walking does not usually increase muscle strength.[45] Nevertheless, it seems to yield important functional gains in frail elderly people. Specifically, an association has been noted between a regular daily 30 minute walk and the ability to climb stairs.[75]

Amount of activity required for cardiovascular health

If an exercise programme is very intense then quite short sessions may be sufficient to enhance cardiovascular health. With more moderate, lifestyle programmes, however, a substantial total volume of physical activity is required for benefit. Recent position statements have been developed from both occupational and leisure studies.

Occupational studies

An early review of occupational data suggested that a daily work site energy expenditure of 1.7–3.8 MJ (400–900 kcal) was needed

Table 1.2 Influence of walking programmes on various measures of health status

Health indicator	Sample	Programme	Design	Health improved	Reference
Blood pressure	107M aged 40–60	14wk, 70–75% HR_{MAX}	Lc	Yes	36
	65M, 297F aged 47	21wk, 10 000 steps/day	L	Yes	37
	24M aged 40–56	20wk, 63–76% HR_{MAX}	Lc	Yes	38
	34F aged 61–81	8wk, 70–80% HR_{MAX}	Lc	Yes	39
	46F aged 20–40	24wk, 56%, 67% or 86% HR_{MAX}	Lc	Not at low intensity	40
	56F aged 61.3	24wk, 60% $\dot{V}O_{2\ PEAK}$	Lr	Yes	41
	33M&F aged 64	37wk, 60% $\dot{V}O_{2,\ MAX}$	Lc	Yes	42
	34M&F aged 61	58wk, 47%, 57% HR_{RES}	Lc	Yes	43
	M&F aged 60–69	4wk, 50% $\dot{V}O_{2\ MAX}$	L	Yes	44
	25M, 31F aged 70–79	26wk, 75–85% $\dot{V}O_{2\ MAX}$	Lc	Yes	45
HDL cholesterol	80F aged 60–70	26wk, 2/wk 16–45 min	Lc	No	46
	107M aged 40–60	14wk, 70–75% HR_{MAX}	Lc	Yes	36
	34F aged 61–81	8wk, 70–80% HR_{MAX}	Lc	Yes	39
	46F aged 20–40	24wk, 56%, 67% or 86% HR_{MAX}	Lc	Yes	40
	28F aged 44.9	52wk, 60% HR_{MAX}	Lc	Yes	47
	10M aged 19–31	16wk, 5.1 km/h	L	Yes	48
	35M aged 47.0	Postal carriers	C	Yes	49
	3621 adults (65% F)		C	Yes (high, moderate but not low duration)	50
	107M aged 30–35	52wk, 70–85% $\dot{V}O_{2\ MAX}$	Lc	Yes	51
	17F	11wk, 71% HR_{MAX}	L	No	52
	255F post-menopause	52wk, 6.4–7.2 km/h	L	No	53

Table 1.2 Continued

Health indicator	Sample	Programme	Design	Health improved	Reference
Body fat/body mass	65M, 297F aged 47	21wk 10 000 steps/day	L	Yes	37
	26M aged 40–56	20wk, 63–76% HR$_{MAX}$	Lc	Yes	38
	107M aged 40–60	14wk, 70–75% HR$_{MAX}$	Lc	No	36
	46F aged 20–40	24wk, 56%, 67% or 86% MAX	Lc	Not low intensity	40
	80F aged 60–70	26wk, 2wk 16–45 min	Lc	No	46
	6M aged 19–31	16wk, 5.1 km/h	L	Yes	48
	81M aged 30–55	52wk, 70–85% capacity ($\dot{V}O_2$ MAX)	Lc	Yes	51
	17F aged 20–40	11wk, 71% HR$_{MAX}$	L	No	52
	44F aged 44.9	52wk, 6.5 km/h	Lc	No	55
	14M, 1F aged 16	13wk, 80% HR$_{MAX}$	L	Yes	56
	35F aged 25–45	15wk, 5/wk 45 min	Lc	No	58
	30M aged 52–88	6wk, mixed programme	L	Yes	59
	7M aged 52–88	42wk, mixed programme	L	No	59
	23F aged 57–79	12wk, mixed programme	Lc	No	60
Aerobic power	107M aged 40–60	14wk, 4wk	Lc	Yes	36
	65M, 297F aged 47	21wk, 10 000 steps/day	L	Yes	37
	46F aged 20–40	24wk, 56%, 67% or 86% HR$_{MAX}$	L	Yes	40
	17F aged 20–40	11wk 71% HR$_{MAX}$	Lc	Yes	52, 53
	24F, 8M aged 68	9wk, 57%, 70% $\dot{V}O_2$ MAX	Lc	Yes	57
	35F aged 25–45	15wk, brisk walk	Lc	No	58
	32M aged 52–88	6wk, mixed programme	L	Yes	59
	7M aged 52–88	42wk, mixed programme	L	Yes	59
	23F aged 52–79	13wk, mixed programme	L	Yes	60
	64M aged 40–60	12wk, 42–60% or 63–81% $\dot{V}O_2$ MAX	Lc	Yes	61
	44F aged 44.9	52wk, 6.5 km/h	L	Yes @ 2 mmol/lactate	62
	14M, 12F aged 35–53	12wk, 60% $\dot{V}O_2$ MAX	Lr	Yes	63
	44M aged 22	2wk, 10–30 km/day	L	Yes (submax)	64
	14F, 1M aged 16	11wk, 3wk	L	Yes	65
	24F aged 67–89	10wk, 40%, 60% HR$_{RES}$	L	Yes	66

Table 1.2 Continued

Health indicator	Sample	Programme	Design	Health improved	Reference
Osteoporosis	73F	Two intensities of walking, 40% and 60% HR reserve	Lc	No (wrist)	66
	17F aged 49–64	62% $\dot{V}O_2$ MAX 5/wk	Lc	No	67
	229F aged 50–60	Walk 11 km/wk 3 yr	Lc	No (wrist)	68
	36F aged 60.2	52wk, weighted belt	Lc	Yes with Ca^2	69
	280F, 120M	Case-control (femoral fractures)	C	Yes	70
	239 post menopause	12km/wk v < 1.6 km/wk	Lc	Yes	71
	F aged 30–60	52wk, 2.5h/wk	Lc	Yes	72
	33F aged 45–67	30wk, walking	L	Yes (> anaerobic threshold)	73
	162F	Aerobics + walking	C	Yes with Ca^{2+}	74
	619 aged 70	Daily 30 min walk	L	Yes	75
Mental health	35F aged 25–45	15wk, brisk walking	L	Yes	58
	19F, 17M aged 37	Single walk 55–72% $\dot{V}O_2$ MAX	C		76

C = cross sectional study; L = longitudinal study; Lc = longitudinal controlled study; Lr = randomised longitudinal controlled study; M = male; F = female; wk = weeks; HR = heart rate; max = maximum; res = reserve; HDL = high density lipoprotein.

to enhance health related fitness and reduce cardiovascular or overall mortality.[79] If such an energy expenditure had been distributed uniformly over an entire working day it would have boosted resting energy expenditure by an average of only 4–8 kJ/min (1–3 kcal/min).

In some jobs, health benefits have reflected periods of relatively high intensity effort, interspersed with relaxation breaks or rest pauses. But in other occupations, such as postal carriers,[80,81] the benefit seems to be due to several hours a day of moderate and relatively uniform activity at gross intensities of 20 kJ/min (95 kcal/min) or less.[82]

Studies of active leisure

The minimum intensity of effort required to improve cardiovascular health is likely to be greater in active leisure than at work because the duration of most active leisure pursuits is shorter than a normal eight-hour working day.

Traditionally, physiologists who were interested in developing cardiovascular fitness called for intensities of exercise near to the ventilatory threshold, a level of physical activity that is likely to boost the aerobic power of the average sedentary person by as much as 20%.[83,84] On the other hand, several recent papers have suggested that much of the desired increase in health related fitness can be attained by exercising at much lower intensities of effort, possibly insufficient to induce any increase in aerobic power.[3–13,85] Moreover, with the important exception of a study of British civil servants,[14] the largest gain in cardiovascular prognosis was seen in people in the lowest category of physical activity or aerobic fitness, as opposed to those in the next higher category.[65]

Additional health benefits associated with progression to much higher levels of physical activity or fitness have been disappointingly small. The activity related benefit was greater in two investigations where differences in habitual physical activity were inferred from measurements of aerobic fitness than in other studies where activity patterns were estimated from questionnaire responses.[85] Indeed, self reports of walking were not associated with any protection against hypertension.[86] Two studies compared cardiac risk factors with reported physical activity and physical fitness in the same participants;[87,88] in confirmation of the inferences from interstudy comparisons, the relation to cardiac risk factors was closer for fitness than for physical activity.

This does not necessarily mean that one must increase aerobic fitness to enhance health. It could also be that patterns of physical activity are indicated more precisely by the measurement of aerobic fitness than by activity questionnaires.

Recent position statements

Recent quasi-experimental data on the health benefits of moderate activity led the American College of Sports Medicine (ACSM) to modify an earlier "position stand", reducing the recommended minimum intensity of the aerobic component of an exercise prescription to 50% of aerobic power, practiced for 1-hour three to five times a week.[10,11] The revised recommendation is now supported by the American Heart Association,[89] the American Medical Association,[90] the United States Surgeon General,[12] Heart Canada, and the Canadian Society of Exercise Physiology.[91] In Canada the daily recommendation is graded from 20–30 minutes of vigorous effort, such as aerobics, to 30–60 minutes of moderate effort such as brisk walking, to 60 minutes of effort such as light walking.[91] In the United States the current call is for moderate physical activity on most days of the week.[12] In an average 75 kg middle aged man with an aerobic power of 35 ml/[kg.min], the revised standard implies that health needs will on average be satisfied by an energy expenditure of about 5 METS (27 kJ/min or 6.5 kcal/min) where 1 MET is an oxygen consumption of about 3.5 ml/[kg.min] at resting metabolic rate.

Because the peak aerobic power declines progressively with age, the intensity corresponding to 50% of aerobic power drops to around 3 METS (19 kJ/min or 4.5 kcal/min) in an elderly or an

---

Box 1.3   Current United States recommendation for aerobic fitness

- Minimum recommended effort is 50% of aerobic power for at least 30 minutes on most days of the week
- Required 30 minutes of exercise can be distributed over several sessions a day
- Intensity equivalent to 17.5 ml/[kg.min] (5 METS or 27 kJ/min or 6.5 kcal/min) in a middle aged man
- Intensity equivalent to 10.5 ml/[kg.min] (3 METS or 19 kJ/min or 4.5 kcal/min) in elderly or unfit people
- Unpaced walking more easily meets this requirement in elderly people

---

unfit individual. One corollary of this age differential is that elderly, sedentary, obese, and disabled individuals are the groups most likely to benefit from low intensity exercise programmes.

Although most studies have focused on the minimum intensity and duration of effort required for cardiovascular health, active living has the potential to enhance many other aspects of health (table 1.2). The key to obtaining some of these benefits, such as the control of body fat content, may be the absolute energy expenditure per week rather than the intensity of effort that is chosen.[92]

Activity generated by an active lifestyle

Even the currently advocated minimum intensity of activity for health (5 METS in middle aged adults) seems fairly demanding relative to the energy cost of commonly reported voluntary leisure pursuits such as walking and cycling.

Walking

The most commonly reported self imposed leisure activity is walking.[20] There is a general relation between the self selected walking pace and aerobic power ($r = 0.64$).[78] In part because of a waning aerobic power, many older people progressively decrease their walking speed.[98] By the 8th decade the typical woman regards 3.2 km/h (2 mph) as a comfortable walking speed. But if we assume that the average adult adopts a walking pace of 4.8 km/h, then the gross energy cost is likely to be around 19 kJ/min (12 ml/ [kg.min]/oxygen consumption) in a man of 75 kg.[95-97] This intensity of effort plainly meets the new ACSM standard[10] in the case of elderly people but is inadequate for young or middle aged individuals.

Morris and Hardman have maintained that a prescription of "brisk" walking is appropriate to maintain physical fitness.[98] In their experience such a recommendation generally yields a pace that is some 60% of aerobic power;[53,99] if asked to walk a mile (1.6 km) as fast as possible, two thirds of adult men and 90% of women attain a heart rate in the optimal training zone (70% or greater). People are unlikely to walk as fast as possible in the course of their ordinary leisure, but they might do so if the activity was a part of their normal journey to and from work.

The energy cost of rapid walking varies substantially from one person to another, and the average costs of common activities remain controversial.[100–102] One estimate suggests that to develop the targeted gross expenditure of 5 METS (a net energy expenditure of 4 METS or 14/ml/[kg.min]) a young or middle aged person would need to attain an unrealistically high walking pace of 140 m/min, 8.4 km/h (5.2 mph).[11] Other options for reaching the 5 MET standard include jogging or walking on soft or uneven terrain. Walking up a 5% gradient increases energy expenditure by 50% and descent of a hill demands almost as much energy as walking on the level; energy costs may also increase two to threefold for walking in snow.[97]

Cycling and other leisure activities

Cycling is another commonly reported lifestyle activity.[20] If the cyclist adopts a speed of 16 km/h (10 mph) the net energy cost is typically 29 kJ/min, an adequate intensity for maintenance of good health. Other activities of appropriate intensity include skiing at 4.0 km/h, swimming at 25 m/min, walking upstairs, the heaviest forms of gardening, sawing hardwood, and chopping wood.[97] Most recreational activities and domestic chores, however, fall below even the revised ACSM requirements.

Physiological responses

Table 1.2 summarises physiological responses to walking.

Duncan *et al.* compared strolling at 4.8 km/h, brisk walking at 6.4 km/h, and aerobic walking at 8 km/h.[40] The participants, women aged 20–40 years, were followed for 24 weeks. Gains of aerobic power increased with walking speed, but the threshold for benefit was the relatively rapid pace of 5.6 km/h (4 mph). In contrast, decreases in body fat and total cholesterol concentration were as large with moderate as with brisk exercise.

Hopkins *et al.* studied randomly selected adult New Zealanders.[94] They noted that "hard" physical activity (as assessed by either their own CORE questionnaire or the Stanford questionnaire) correlated relatively strongly with aerobic power ($r=0.40$), a decrease in skinfold ($r=0.22$), vital capacity ($r=0.19$), and protection against exercise induced myocardial ischaemia ($r=0.14$). Improvements in lipid profile, however, were seen only when participants walked a minimum of 13 km/week;[51] no protection was found in those reporting only "low" intensities of

13

physical activity.

DiPietro *et al.* examined adults aged 60–86 years.[105] In their study, vigorous leisure activity correlated with aerobic power; in contrast, leisure walking and the total leisure activity showed a modest correlation with body fat but not with aerobic power.

Commuting as a motivating force

Can the time pressures of commuting generate the sense of urgency that is needed to reach an appropriate intensity of physical activity when a person is walking or cycling?

Sallis *et al.* noted that such activities as getting off the bus early or parking some distance away from one's destination were associated with favourable cardiac risk factor profiles among 5930 participants in the Stanford five city trial.[106] But too often, potential commuter cyclists are deterred by the unpleasantness of cycling in traffic and the difficulty in finding a secure place to park bicycles.[107] Vuori *et al.* asked a small group of Tampere citizens who normally drove to work to adopt either walking or cycling as their method of commuting for a 10-week period.[24] Almost all of those who were contacted accepted the proposal for a 10-week trial. Commuting boosted physical activity by 30 minutes or more in each direction every day. The pace chosen by the cyclists corresponded to an oxygen consumption of 23–24 ml/[kg.min], in the range of 65–70% of aerobic power for a sedentary middle aged adult. The walking speed of 5.7 km/h was also relatively brisk but probably commanded an oxygen consumption of no more than 13 ml/[kg.min], only about 37% of aerobic power. The average heart rates during the journey were 131 and 121 beats/min, corresponding to 65% and 55% of aerobic power. Presumably, the heart rates of the walkers were augmented by a combination of heat, hills, and the carrying of a briefcase.

The chosen speed of habitual walkers may be somewhat higher than that of the sedentary volunteers who were recruited by Vuori *et al.*[24] Spelman *et al.* found an average walking speed of 6.4 km/h, corresponding to 52% of aerobic power (5.2 METS) in 22 women and seven men with a mean (SD) age 35 (9 years); the total mean (SD) increase in weekly energy expenditure due to walking was 4.7 (2.0) MJ. Unpublished personal observations suggest that even in an active group (a regular walking club for middle aged and older adults cover distances of 10–12 km each session) the average pace is only about 4 km/h.

Empirical response to structured and unstructured programmes

Weight loss

The Behavioural Risk Factor Surveillance System survey of 1989 provided data showing the impact of various types of physical activity on participants who were attempting to decrease their body mass.[109] Unfortunately, data on participation in aerobics programmes were included only for women. The loss of weight from unstructured running was as great, and that from unstructured cycling was almost as great, as that for formal aerobics programmes. In contrast, unstructured walking and gardening seemed to induce weight loss only in the older (and presumably the less fit) members of the group.

Worksite exercise programmes

Worksite exercise programmes provide much information on the response to structured physical activity, although the interpretation of results is complicated because most programmes have included a variety of health promotional options in addition to exercise.[110,111] Moreover, the random allocation of participants to experimental and control groups is rarely possible in the workplace, and many worksite studies have been uncontrolled. Finally, results are usually available only for a small residue of high adherents to the programme, so that any benefits tend to be exaggerated.[111]

Perhaps the best worksite study was that conducted at the Johnson & Johnson Corporation.[112] This averaged the response of all employees at the test locations. Over a 2-year period, a well financed and well organised structured programme of aerobic exercise yielded a 2% decrease in body fat, a 6% increase in aerobic power, a 7% decrease in serum cholesterol concentration, a 4 mm Hg decrease in systolic blood pressure, and a 1 mm Hg decrease in diastolic blood pressure. Such benefits are smaller than those seen among individuals who themselves select an active lifestyle but, at least in terms of aerobic power, are greater than what has been achieved by asking volunteers to walk or cycle to work for 3 months.

Supervised activity in the home

King et al. made a direct comparison of the efficacy of a structured versus a supervised home based programme in women and men aged 50–65 years.[113] Probably in part because of the lesser time demands of home based activities, programme adherence over a 1 year period was much better than for structured exercise. Perhaps for this same reason the women achieved larger gains of aerobic power with the home based than with the structured programme. Changes in body mass and blood lipids, however, were not significant for either type of exercise.

Issues age, sex, and ethnicity

How are conclusions regarding an appropriate dose of physical activity modified by issues of age, sex and ethnic group? The primary influence of such factors on the health response to physical activity comes from any peculiarities in the initial fitness of the target group. To the extent that elderly people, women, and minority groups enter trials with a low level of fitness, such individuals should gain more than average benefit from a programme of moderate physical activity, whether this be structured or unstructured. Thus rapid walking is much more likely to benefit an elderly immigrant woman than a young white man.

Against the potential advantage of a low initial level of fitness, there are obvious problems in recruitment and compliance for the groups identified. Moreover, the manner of participation in either structured or unstructured activities shows differences related to age, sex, and ethnic group. For example, a young person on average walks or cycles at a higher speed than an older adult. Data from the behavioural risk factor survey suggest that unstructured activities are on the increase in women and in elderly people but are decreasing in poorly educated and minority groups.[114,115]

Safety considerations

Children sustain a substantial proportion of their physical injuries during unstructured exercises.[116] In adults, however, one of the attractions of walking and similar activities is that the injury rate is extremely low relative to most other activities. Thus Pollock *et al.* noted that a deliberate 13 week exercise programme gave rise to only one injury in 57 healthy men and women aged 70–80 years.[117]

Conclusions

Current data suggest that structured exercise programmes may have a somewhat greater effect on health than unstructured leisure activity, particularly in young adults. It is easier to encourage unstructured activity, however, and thus there remains a need for a well designed and sustained prospective trial that compares the impact of the two approaches to physical activity in closely matched groups of participants. Further information is needed on how far the relative efficacy of structured and unstructured programmes differs between children, young men, women, and other adults. Present evidence suggests, however, that moderate lifestyle activity will enhance health in elderly, sedentary, and obese people, but not in young adults who are in good initial health.

1 Bouchard C, Shephard RJ, Stephens T, Sutton, J, McPherson B. *Exercise, fitness and health*. Champaign, Illinois: Human Kinetics Publishers, 1990.
2 Bouchard C, Shephard RJ, Stephens T. *Physical activity fitness and health*. Champaign, Illinois: Human Kinetics, 1994.
3 Blair SN, Kohl HW, Paffenbarger RS, *et al*. Phsyical fitness and all-cause mortality: a prospective study of healthy and unhealthy men. *JAMA* 1989;**262**:2395–401.
4 Blair SN, Kohl HW, Barlow CE, *et al*. Changes in physical fitness and all-cause mortality: a prospective study of healthy men and unhealthy men. *JAMA* 1995;**273**:1093–8.
5 Ekelund LG, Haskell WL, Johnson JL, *et al*. Physical fitness as a predictor of cardiovascular mortality in asymptomatic North American men: the lipid research clinics mortality follow-up study. *N Engl J Med* 1988;**319**:1379–84.
6 Leon AS, Connett J, Jacobs DR, *et al*. Leisure-time physical activity levels and risk of coronary heart disease and death: the multiple risk factor intervention trial. *JAMA* 1987;**258**:2388–95.
7 Lie H, Mundal R, Erikssen J. Coronary risk factors and incidence of coronary death in relation to physical fitness: seven-year follow-up of study of middle-aged and elderly men. *Eur Heart J* 1985;**6**:147–57.
8 Sandvik L, Eriksen J, Thaulow E, *et al*. Physical fitness as a predictor of mortality among healthy, middle-aged Norwegian men. *N Engl J Med* 1993;**328**:533–7.
9 Shaper AG, Wannamethee G. Physical activity and ischaemic heart disease in middle-aged British men. *Br Heart J* 1991;**66**:384–94.
10 American College of Sports Medicine. The recommended quantity and quality of exercise for developing and maintaining fitness in healthy adults. *Med Sci Sports Exerc* 1991;**22**:265–74.
11 American College of Sports Medicine. *Guidelines for graded exercise testing and exercise prescription*. 5th ed. Philadelphia: Lea and Febiger, 1995.
12 US Surgeon General. *Physical activity and health*. US Department of Health and Human Services, Washington, DC, 1996.
13 Haapanen N, Miilunpalo S, Vuori I, *et al*. Characteristics of leisure time physical activity associated with decreased risk of premature all-cause and cardiovascular disease mortality in middle-aged men. *Am J Epidemiol* 1996;**143**:870–80.
14 Morris JN, Clayton DG, Everitt MG, *et al*. Exercise in leisure time: coronary attack and death rates. *Br Heart J* 1990;**63**:325–34.
15 Lee I-M, Hsieh CC, Paffenbarger RS. Exercise intensity and longevity in men: the Harvard alumni health study. *JAMA* 1995;**273**:1179–84.

16 Lakka TA, Vanalainen JM, Rauamaa R, *et al.* Relation of leisure-time physical activity and cardiorespiratory fitness to the risk of acute myocardial infarction in men. *N Engl J Med* 1994;**330**:1549–54.

17 Slattery ML, Jacobs DR, Nichaman MZ. Leisure time physical activity and coronary heart disease death: the US railroad study. *Circulation* 1989;**79**:304–11.

18 Dishman R. *Exercise adherence.* Champaign, Illinois: Human Kinetics, 1995.

19 Dishman R, Buckworth J. Increasing physical activity: a quantitative synthesis. *Med Sci Sports Exerc* 1996;**28**:706–19.

20 Stephens T, Craig C. *The well-being of Canadians: the 1988 Campbell's survey.* Ottawa: Canadian Fitness and Lifestyle Research Institute, 1990.

21 Hillsdon M, Thorogood M, Anstiss T, Morris J. Randomized controlled trials of physical activity promotion in free-living populations: a review. *J Epidemiol Community Health* 1995;**49**:448–53.

22 Blamey A, Mutrie N, Aitchison T. Health promotion by encouraged use of stairs. *BMJ* 1995;**311**:289–90.

23 Brownell DK, Stunkard AJ, Albaum JM. Evaluation and modification of exercise patterns in a natural environment. *Am J Psychiatry* 1980;**137**:1540–5.

24 Vuori IM, Oja P, Paronen M. Physically active commuting to work: testing its potential for exercise promotion. *Med Sci Sports Exerc* 1994;**26**:844–50.

25 Young DR, Haskell WL, Taylor CB, Fortmann SP. Effect of community health education on physical activity knowledge, attitudes and behavior. *Am J Epidemiol* 1996;**144**:264–74.

26 Powell KE, Thompson PD, Caspersen CJ, Kendrick JS. Physical activity and the incidence of coronary heart disease. *Annu Rev Public Health* 1987;**8**:253–87.

27 Wyndham CH. An examination of the methods of physical classification of African labourers for manual work. *S Afr Med J* 1972;**46**:251–7.

28 Morris JN, Heady J, Raffle P. Physique of London busmen. *Lancet* 1956;**ii**:569–70.

29 Brunner D, Manelis G. Physical activity at work and ischemic heart disease. In: Larsen OA, Malmborg RO, eds. *Coronary heart disease and physical fitness.* Baltimore: University Park Press, 1971.

30 Berlin JA, Colditz GA. A meta-analysis of physical activity in the prevention of coronary heart disease. *Am J Epidemiol* 1990;**132**:612–18.

31 Rauramaa R, Tuomainen P, Väisänen S, Raukinen T. Physical activity and health-related fitness in middle-aged men. *Med Sci Sports Exerc* 1995;**27**:707–12.

32 Gardner AW, Poehlman ET. Leisure time physical activity is a significant predictor of body density in men. *J Clin Epidemiol* 1994;**47**:283–91.

33 Hickey N, Mulcahy R, Bourke GJ, *et al.* Study of coronary risk factors related to physical activity in 15,171 men. *BMJ* 1975;**iii**:507–9.

34 Cooper KH, Pollock ML, Martin RP, *et al.* Physical fitness levels vs selected coronary risk factors: a cross-sectional study. *JAMA* 1976;**236**:166–9.

35 Shephard RJ, Bouchard C. Population evaluations of health related fitness from perceptions of physical activity and fitness. *Can J Appl Physiol* 1994;**19**:151–73.

36 Davison RCR, Grant S, Mutrie N, *et al.* Walk for health? [abstract] *J Sports Sci* 1992;**10**:556.

37 Ohta T, Kawamura T, Hatano K, *et al.* Effects of exercise on coronary risk factors in obese, middle-aged subjects. *Jpn Circ J* 1990;**54**:1459–64.

38 Pollock ML, Miller HS, Janeway R, *et al.* Effects of walking on body composition and cardiovascular function of middle-aged men. *J Appl Physiol* 1971;**30**:126–30.

39 Whitehurst M, Menendez E. Endurance training in older women. Lipid and lipoprotein responses. *Physician and Sportsmedicine* 1991;**19**:95–103.

40 Duncan JJ, Gordon NF, Scott CB. Women walking for health and fitness. How much is enough? *JAMA* 1991;**266**:3295–9.

41 Ready EA, Naimark B, Ducas J, *et al*. Influence of walking volume on health benefits in women post-menopause. *Med Sci Sports Exerc* 1996;**28**:1097–105.

42 Hagberg JM, Montain SJ, Martin WH, *et al*. Effect of exercise training in 60 to 69-year-old persons with essential hypertension. *Am J Cardiol* 1989;**64**:348–53.

43 Seals DR, Reiling MJ. Effect of regular exercise on 24-hour arterial pressure in older hypertensive humans. *Hypertension* 1991;**18**:583–92.

44 Kingwell BA, Jennings GL. Effects of walking and other exercise programs upon blood pressure in normal subjects. *Med J Aust* 1993;**158**:234–8.

45 Cononie CC, Graves JE, Pollock ML, *et al*. Effect of exercise training on blood pressure in 70 to 79-year-old men and women. *Med Sci Sports Exerc* 1991;**23**:505–11.

46 Hamdorf PA, Withers RT, Penhall RK, *et al*. Physical training effects on the fitness and habitual activity patterns of elderly women. *Arch Phys Med Rehabil* 1992;**73**:603–8.

47 Hardman AE, Hudson A, Jones PMR, *et al*. Brisk walking and plasma high density lipoprotein cholesterol concentration in previously sedentary women. *BMJ* 1989;**290**:1204–5.

48 Leon AS, Conrad J, Humminghake DB, *et al*. Effects of a vigorous walking program on body composition, and carbohydrate and lipid metabolism of obese young men. *Am J Clin Nutr* 1979;**32**:1776–87.

49 Cook TC, Laporte RE, Washburn RA, *et al*. Chronic low level physical activity as a determinant of high density lipoprotein cholesterol and subfractions. *Med Sci Sports Exerc* 1986;**18**:653–7.

50 Tucker LA, Friedman GM. Walking and serum cholesterol in adults. *Am J Public Health* 1990;**80**:1111–13.

51 Wood PD, Haskell WL, Blair SN, *et al*. Increased exercise level and plasma lipoprotein alterations: a one-year randomized controlled study in sedentary middle-aged men. *Metabolism* 1983;**32**:31–9.

52 Santiago MC, Alexander JF, Stuff GA, *et al*. Physiological responses of sedentary women to a 20-week conditioning programme of walking or jogging. *Scand J Sports Sci* 1987;**9**:33–9.

53 Stensel DJ, Brooke-Wavell K, Hardman AE, *et al*. The influence of a one year programme of brisk walking on endurance fitness and body composition in previously sedentary men aged 42–59 years. *Eur J Appl Physiol* 1994;**68**:531–7.

54 White KM, Yeater RA, Martin RB, *et al*. Effects of aerobic dancing and walking on cardiovascular function and muscular strength in postmenopausal women. *J Sports Med* 1984;**12**:159–66.

55 Hardman AE, Jones PRM, Norgan NG, *et al*. Brisk walking improves endurance fitness without changing body fatness in previously sedentary men. *Eur J Appl Physiol* 1992;**65**:354–9.

56 Rowland TW, Varzeas MR, Walsh CA. Aerobic responses to walking training in sedentary adolescents. *J Adolesc Health* 1991;**12**:30–4.

57 Badenhop DT, Cleary PA, Schaal SF, *et al*. Physiological adjustments to higher or lower intensity exercise in elders. *Med Sci Sports Exerc* 1983;**15**:496–502.

58 Cramer SR, Nieman DC, Lee JW. The effects of moderate exercise training on psychological well-being and mood state in women. *Psychosom Res* 1991;**35**:437–49.

59 de Vries HA. Physiological effects of an exercise training regimen upon men aged 52 to 88. *J Gerontol* 1970;**25**:325–36.

60 Adams GM, de Vries HA. Physiological effects of an exercise training regimen upon women aged 52 to 79. *J Gerontol* 1973;**28**:50–5.

61 Gossard D, Haskell WL, Barr-Taylor C, *et al*. Effects of low and high intensity

home based exercise training on functional capacity in healthy middle aged men. *Am J Cardiol* 1986;**57**:446–9.

62 Hardman AE, Hudson A, Jones PMR, *et al*. Brisk walking influences the physiological responses to submaximal step test in women. *J Physiol (Lond)* 1989;**409**:22P.

63 Jetté M, Sidney KH, Campbell J. Effects of twelve-week walking programme on maximal and submaximal work output indices in sedentary middle-aged men and women. *J Sports Med Phys Fitness* 1988;**28**:59–66.

64 Durnin JVGA, Brockway JM, Whitcher HW. Effects of a short period of training of varying severity on some measurements of physical fitness. *J Appl Physiol* 1960;**15**:161–5.

65 Miyashita M, Haga S, Mizuta T. Training and detraining effects on aerobic power in middle aged and older men. *J Sports Med Phys Fitness* 1978;**18**:131–7.

66 Foster VL, Hume JGE, Byrnes WC, *et al*. Endurance training for elderly women. Moderate vs low intensity. *J Gerontol* 1989;**44M**:184–8.

67 Cavanaugh DJ, Cann CE. Brisk walking does not stop bone loss in postmenopausal women. *Bone* 1988;**9**:201–4.

68 Sandler RB, Cauley JA, Hom DL, *et al*. The effects of walking on the cross-sectional dimensions of the radius in postmenopausal women. *Calcif Tissue Int* 1987;**41**:65–9.

69 Nelson M, Fisher E, Dilmanian F, *et al*. A 1-year walking program and increased dietary calcium in postmenopausal women; effects on bone. *Am J Clin Nutr* 1991;**53**:1304–11.

70 Lau E, Donnan S, Bakrer DJP *et al*. Physical activity and calcium intake in fracture of the proximal femur in Hong Kong. *BMJ* 1988;**297**:441–3.

71 Krall EA, Dawson-Hughes B. Walking is related to bone density and rates of bone loss. *Am J Med* 1994;**96**:20–6.

72 Jones PRM, Hardman AE, Hudson A, *et al*. Influence of brisk walking on the broadband ultrasonic attenuation of the calcaneus in previously sedentary women aged 30–61 years. *Calcif Tissue Int* 1991;**49**:112–15.

73 Hatori M, Hasegawa A, Adachi H, *et al*. The effects of walking at the anaerobic threshold level on vertebral bone loss in post-menopausal women. *Calcif Tissue Int* 1993;**52**:411–14.

74 White MK, Martin RB, Yeater RA, *et al*. The effects of exercise on the bones of post-menopausal women. *Int Orthop* 1984;**7**:209–14.

75 Frändin K, Grimby G, Mellström D, *et al*. Walking habits and health-related factors in a 70-year-old population. *Gerontology* 1991;**37**:281–8.

76 Porcari J, Ward A, Morgan W, *et al*. Effects of walking on state anxiety and blood pressure [abstract]. *Med Sci Sports Exerc* 1988;**20**:S85.

77 Morgan WP, Roberts JA, Feinermann AD. Psychological effect of acute physical activity. *Phys Med Rehabil* 1971;**52**:422–5.

78 Porcari J, McCarron R, Kline G, *et al*. Is fast walking an adequate aerobic stimulus for 30 to 69-year-old men and women? *Physician and Sportsmedicine* 1987;**15**:119–29.

79 Fox SM, Skinner JS. Phsycial activity and cardiovascular health. *Am J Cardiol* 1964;**14**:731–46.

80 Morris JN, Raffle PAB. Coronary heart disease in transport workers: progress report. *Br J Ind Med* 1954;**11**:260–4.

81 Kahn H. The relationship of reported coronary heart disease mortality to physical activity of work. *Am J Public Health* 1963;**53**:1058–67.

82 Shephard RJ. The workload of the postal carrier. *J Hum Ergol (Tokyo)* 1983;**11**:151–64.

83 Shephard RJ. *Endurance fitness*. 1st ed. Toronto: University of Toronto Press, 1969.

84 Amerian College of Sports Medicine. The recommended quantity and quality

of exercise for developing and maintaining fitness in healthy adults. *Med Sci Sports Exerc* 1978;**10**:7–10.

85 Blair SN, Connelly JC. How much physical activity should we do? The case for moderate amounts and intensities of physical activity. *Res Q* 1996;**67**: 193–205.

86 Paffenbarger RS, Wing AL, Hyde RT, *et al*. Physical activity and incidence of hypertension in college alumni. *Am J Epidemiol* 1983;**117**:245–57.

87 Lochen ML, Rasmussen K. The Tromso study. Physical fitness, self-reported physical activity and their relationship to other coronary risk factors. *J Epidemiol Community Health* 1992;**46**:103–7.

88 Young DB, Steinhardt MA. The importance of physical fitness versus physical activity for coronary heart disease risk factors: a cross-sectional analysis. *Res Q* 1993;**64**:377–84.

89 American Heart Association. Statement on exercise: benefits and recommendations for physical activity programs for all Americans: a statement for health professionals by the Committee on Exercise and Cardiac Rehabilitation of the Council on Clinical Cardiology, American Heart Association. *Circulation:* 1992;**86**:340–4.

90 Pate RR, Pratt M, Blair SN, *et al*. Physical activity and public health: a recommendation from the Center for Disease Control and Prevention and the American College of Sports Medicine. *JAMA* 1995;**273**:402–7.

91 Health Canada/Canadian Society of Exercise Physiology. *Handbook for Canada's physical activity guide*. Ottawa: Health Canada, 1998.

92 Ballor DL, Keesey RA. A meta-analysis of the factors affecting exercise-induced changes in body mass, fat mass and fat-free mass in males and females. *Int J Obes* 1991;**15**:717–26.

93 Himann JE, Cunningham DA, Rechnitzer PA, *et al*. Age-related changes in speed of walking. *Med Sci Sports Exerc* 1988;**20**:161–6.

94 Danneskold-Samsoe B, Kofod V, Munter J, *et al*. Muscle strength and functional capacity in 78–81 year old men and women. *Eur J Appl Physiol* 1984;**52**:310–14.

95 Mahadeva K, Passmore R, Woolf B. Individual variations in the metabolic cost of standardized exercises: the effects of food, age, sex and race. *J Physiol (Lond)* 1953;**121**:225–31.

96 Goodman J, Goodman L. Exercise prescription for the sedentary adult. In: Welsh P, Shephard RJ, eds. *Current therapy in sports medicine 1985–1986*. Philadelphia: BC Decker, 1985:17–23.

97 Durnin JVGA, Passmore R. *Energy, work and leisure*. London: Heinemann, 1967.

98 Morris JN, Hardman AE. Walking to health. *Sports Med* 1997;**23**:306–32.

99 Hardman AD, Hudson A, Jones PRM, *et al*. Brisk walking improves endurance fitness without changing body fatness in previously sedentary women. *Eur J Appl Physiol* 1992;**65**:354–9.

100 Hardman AE, Morris JN. Walking to health. *Br J Sports Med* 1998;**32**:184 (letter).

101 Bassett DR, Vachon JA, Kirkland AO, *et al*. Energy cost of stair climbing and descending on the college alumnus questionnaire. *Med Sci Sports Exerc* 1997;**29**:1250–4.

102 Shephard RJ. How much physical activity is needed for good health. *Int J Sports Med* 1999;**20**:23–7.

103 Wynder EL. *The book of health. American Health Foundation*. New York: Franklin Watts, 1981.

104 Hopkins WG, Wilson NC, Russell DG. Validation of the physical activity instrument for the Life in New Zealand National Survey. *Am J Epidemiol* 1991;**133**:73–82.

105 DePietro L, Caspersen CJ, Otsfeld A, *et al*. A survey for assessing physical

activity among older adults. *Med Sci Sports Exerc* 1993;**25**:628–42.

106 Sallis JF, Haskell WL, Fortmann SP, *et al*. Moderate intensity physical activity and cardiovascular risk factors: the Stanford five-city project. *Prev Med* 1986;**15**:561–8.

107 Bhopal R, Unwin N. Cycling, physical exercise and the Millennium Fund. *BMJ* 1995;**311**:344.

108 Spelman CC, Pate RR, Macera CA, *et al*. Self-selected exercise intensity of habitual walkers. *Med Sci Sports Exerc* 1993;**25**:1174–9.

109 DiPietro L, Williamson DF, Caspersen CJ, *et al*. The descriptive epidemiology of selected physical activities and body weight among adults trying to lose weight: the behavioral risk factor surveillance system survey, 1989. *Int J Obes* 1993;**17**:69–76.

110 Shephard RJ. A critical analysis of work-site fitness programs and their postulated economic benefits. *Med Sci Sports Exerc* 1992;**24**:354–70.

111 Shephard RJ. Worksite fitness and exercise programs: a review of methodology and health impact. *Am J Health Promotion* 1996;**10**:116–32.

112 Blair SN, Piserchia PV, Wilbur CS, *et al*. A public health intervention model for work site health promotion: impact on exercise and physical fitness in a health promotion plan after 24 months. *JAMA* 1986;**255**:921–6.

113 King A, Haskell WL, Taylor B, *et al*. Group- vs home-based exercise training in healthy older men and women. A community-based clinical trial. *JAMA* 1991;**266**:1535–42.

114 Caspersen CJ, Merritt RK. Physical activity trends among 26 states, 1986–1990. *Med Sci Sports Exerc* 1995;**27**:713–20.

115 Heath GW, Smith JD. Physical activity patterns among adults in Georgia: results from the 1990 Behavioral Risk Factor Surveillance System. *South Med J* 1994;**87**:435–40.

116 Goldberg B, Witman PA, Gleim GW, Nicholas GA. Children's sports injuries: are they avoidable? *Physician and Sportsmedicine* 1979;**7**:93–101.

117 Pollock ML, Carroll JF, Graves JE, *et al*. Injuries and adherence to walk/jog and resistance training programs in the elderly. *Med Sci Sports Exerc* 1991;**23**:505–11.

Multiple choice questions

1 Which of the following statements are true?

(a) Health gains are minimal unless there is a large gain in aerobic fitness

(b) Health promotion experts currently advocate formal exercise classes rather than adoption of an active lifestyle

(c) It is easier to comply with exercise recommendations in the framework of a structured, supervised exercise class

(d) Lack of time is a commonly cited reason for non-compliance with exercise programmes

(e) Sports such as golf and tennis are the commonest forms of unstructured exercise

2 Which of the following statements are false?

(a) Cross sectional studies show a substantially lower risk of ischaemic heart disease in "heavy" work than in sedentary jobs

(b) Cross sectional studies show an inverse association between self reported leisure activity and ischaemic heart disease

(c) Longitudinal studies fail to confirm the inference from cross sectional data

(d) Inferences from randomised longitudinal studies are limited by recruitment bias and lack of adherence to the assigned programme

(e) The apparent benefit of exercise increases with the strength of study design

3 Which of the following statements are false?

(a) In occupational studies a reduction of cardiovascular or overall mortality is associated with a daily energy expenditure in the range 1.7–3.8 MJ (400–900 kcal)

(b) To enhance health the intensity of leisure activity must approach the anaerobic threshold, equivalent to 60–70% of maximum oxygen intake

(c) Current recommendations imply that a middle aged man should sustain a leisure activity of about 27 kJ/min (6.5 kcal/min) for at least 30 minutes on most days of the week

(d) In an elderly individual the requirement drops to 19 kJ/min (4.5 kcal/min), pursued for 30 minutes on most days of the week

(e) It would be acceptable to accumulate the 30 minutes through three bouts of 10 minutes duration

4 Which of the following statements are false?

(a) Exercising at a moderate walking pace (4.8 km/h or 3 mph) is as effective as much faster walking in decreasing body fat and serum cholesterol concentration

(b) Improvements in lipid profile are relatively independent of the distance covered by walkers

(c) Exercising at a moderate walking pace often does not enhance the individual's aerobic power

(d) Exercise at 60–70% of an individual's aerobic power will boost the maximal oxygen intake of young adults by 20%

(e) The self selected walking pace decreases with age

5 A large scale randomised trial of worksite fitness classes examined average responses for the entire worksite after a 2-year period of programme operation. Which of the following statements regarding benefits relative to a control worksite is false?

(a) Body fat content decreased by an average of 20%

(b) Aerobic power increased by an average of 6%

(c) Serum cholesterol concentration decreased by an average of 7%
(d) Systolic blood pressure decreased by an average of 4 mm Hg
(e) Diastolic pressure decreased by an average of 1 mm Hg

Answers are on p. 361.

2   A systematic review of strategies to promote physical activity

M Hillsdon, M Thorogood, C Foster

Introduction

Regular physical activity can play an important role in both the prevention and treatment of cardiovascular disease (CVD), hypertension, non-insulin-dependent diabetes mellitus, stroke, some cancers, osteoporosis and depression as well as improve the lipid profile.[1-8] A meta-analysis of the relationship between physical activity and coronary heart disease reported that the relative risk of coronary heart disease death in the least active compared with the most active was 1.9 fold.[9] The magnitude of this relative risk is similar to that of the other important CVD risk factors – cigarette smoking, hypertension and hyperlipidaemia.[10]

Despite this evidence, it is estimated that 70% of the English population takes inadequate physical activity[11] compared to 31% who smoke, 30% with a raised serum cholesterol concentration and 15% who are hypertensive.[12]

In 1995 the Centers for Disease Control and Prevention (USA) and the American College of Sports Medicine recognised the importance of physical activity and published a public health message recommending that "every adult should accumulate 30 minutes or more of moderate-intensity physical activity on most, preferably all days of the week."[13] In March of 1995 the Health Education Authority also recognised the public health potential of physical activity, by embarking on a three year national campaign (Active for Life) aimed at promoting the same message.

Although a large body of evidence exists about the health benefits of physical activity, far less is known about the effectiveness of strategies to achieve the increases in physical activity necessary to acquire these benefits.

In this chapter we report a revised and updated version of a previous systematic review of randomised controlled trials of physical activity promotion in apparently healthy, free-living adults.[14] We provide recent and reliable information on the effectiveness of physical activity promotion.

There are randomised, controlled trials using exercise as an intervention to study the physiological effects of exercise and in the management of health problems, notably hypertension, hyperlipidaemia and overweight. These show the effects of exercise on various physiological and biological outcomes and demonstrate the importance of exercise in the management of disease. However, because the main outcome of such trials is not physical activity, they do not help us understand the effectiveness of physical activity promotion strategies. For these reasons they were not considered.

Methods

Computerised searches were carried out using Medline, Embase, Amed, PsychLit, Sport and SCISearch from 1966–1999. The method described by Dickersin and colleagues[15] was used to search for randomised controlled trials on Medline. Key words for searching included "exercise", "physical activity", "Randomised-Controlled-Trial" and "Randomized-Controlled-Trial". The search was limited to English language journals. Additional searching was carried out using the references from both existing reviews[16–18] and the papers identified during the search. In addition to the studies described previously a further 5 were found. Those studies included in the previous review were re-read by two of us independently, as were the new studies identified during this search. Each paper was read and assessed using a shortened version of the EPI-Centre Review Guidelines.[19]

The criteria for inclusion of trials in the review were:

- A control group
- Subjects assigned to control or intervention by a process of randomisation
- Trials testing single factor interventions to increase activity
- Interventions tested on apparently healthy, free-living adults

- Minimum of 12 weeks duration
- Exercise behaviour was the dependent variable.

Results

Seventeen trials met the inclusion criteria and are described in table 2.1 (studies 5 and 6 are from the same paper and are reported separately for convenience). Most of the trials were from the USA with two from England (studies 16 and 17) and one from Australia (study 8). Subjects were mainly white, middle aged and well educated. Most subjects were volunteers, recruited via local advertisements. The trials include an even mix of men and women with an age range of 18–72 (mean of approximately 49).

Interventions

Table 2.1 summarises the main exercise components of the trials and table 2.2 the results. Both tables are sorted by location (home or facility) of exercise and then by outcome. Intervention periods ranged from 5 weeks to 2 years. Seven of the trials included follow up periods after intervention that ranged from 2 months to 12 years. Most outcomes were analysed on an intention to treat basis. In the trials, subjects were asked to exercise between three and five times a week for 20–60 minutes. Few studies described the exercise intensity, but when it was described there was a mixture of moderate and vigorous intensities.

Location of exercise

The location of the prescribed exercise was the home for 10 of the trials (table 2.1). By home location we refer to exercise that can take place in proximity to the subjects' homes rather than within their homes. Six out of the 10 home based trials (studies 1–5, 10) reported a positive outcome of the intervention. One of the trials not showing a significant difference between groups (study 6) was a comparison between subjects receiving telephone contact and those not receiving it. All of the subjects were sedentary at baseline and significantly increased their exercise level during the intervention. Those subjects receiving telephone support exercised more than those who did not but the difference did not reach significance.

Facility based trials normally required subjects to attend at least some specific sessions or groups at a local fitness centre or indoor track. Three of the seven facility based trials showed a significant

27

Table 2.1 Summary of interventions

Study	Authors, stated objectives	Length of intervention	Location of exercise (home or facility)	Authors' description of exercise	Prescribed frequency, intensity, and duration of exercise	Controls
home based						
1	Kriska[20] – To examine factors associated with exercise compliance in postmenopausal women	2 years	Home after initial 8 weeks	Walking	3 × wk 3 miles/session briskly	Assessment only
2	Lombard[21] – To determine the effect of frequency and structure of telephone prompts on frequency of walking	12 weeks	Home	Walking (group walking encouraged)	3 × wk at least 20 min/session	Initial instruction
3	King[22] – To determine the effectiveness of group v home based training of higher and lower intensities	1 year	2 groups home, 1 group facility	Walking and jogging	Two groups 3 × wk at 73–88% peak heart rate for 40 min/session, one group 5 × wk at 60–73% peak heart rate for 30 min each session	Assessment only
4	Noland[23] – To assess effects of behavioural techniques on adherence to unsupervised exercise	18 weeks	Home	Walking, jogging and swimming as preferred	3 × wk at 30–40% or 60–70% $\dot{V}O_2$ MAX for 30 min	Assessment and advice about exercise; no behavioural treatment
5	King[24] – To evaluate strategies for enhancing the maintenance of exercise training by healthy middle aged men and women (also see study 6)	6 months	Home	Walking and jogging	4 × wk at 65–77% peak heart rate for 30 min/session	Same as intervention group but reduced level of self monitoring

Table 2.1 Continued

Study	Authors, stated objectives	Length of intervention	Location of exercise (home or facility)	Authors' description of exercise	Prescribed frequency, intensity, and duration of exercise	Controls
6	King[24] – To evaluate strategies for enhancing the adoption of exercise training by healthy middle aged men and women (also see study 5)	6 months	Home	Walking and jogging	4 × wk at 65–77% peak heart rate for 30 min/session	Same as intervention group but less regular telephone contact
7	Godin[25] – To investigate the effectiveness of fitness testing and health appraisal on exercise intention and behaviour	3 months	Home	Physical activity lasting 20–30 min/session	None prescribed	Assessment only
8	Bull[26] – To test the effectiveness of verbal advice on exercise from a family physician, plus written materials, in a primary health care setting	2–3 min advice	Participants' choice	Not stated	Moderate intensity leisure time	Assessment only + written materials
9	Chen[27] – To evaluate a minimal behavioural intervention program designed to promote walking among initially sedentary ethnic minority women	8 weeks	Home	Walking	Individually determined	Brief phone call + educational materials
10	Marcus[28] – To compare the effectiveness of motivationally tailored and standard self help materials for physical activity adoption	6 months	Home	Moderate intensity	Not prescribed but focus on 5 × wk, 30 min	Standard self help materials via the post

Table 2.1 Continued

Study	Authors, stated objectives	Length of intervention	Location of exercise (home or facility)	Authors' description of exercise	Prescribed frequency, intensity, and duration of exercise	Controls
11	McAuley[29] – To determine the utility of an efficacy based intervention on exercise participation	20 weeks	Facility	Walking	3 × wk, 40 min	Initial instruction + exercise information classes
12	King[30] – To study the effect of two low cost methods of increasing the number of participant controlled jogging episodes	5 weeks	Facility	Jogging	4 × wk, individualised time and distance goals	Instructed to jog alone
13	MacKeen[31] – To study the effects of an 18 month exercise intervention on adherence	18 months	Facility and home	Jogging, swimming, games	3 × wk minimum, 35–75 min/ session	Assessment only
14	Reid[32] – To assess the effectiveness of a physician prescribed exercise programme with health education and self monitoring components	1 hour	Facility	Endurance activity	Advice about frequency, intensity, duration given but not described	Assessment and written exercise advice
15	Marcus[33] – To assess the effectiveness of a relapse prevention programme and reinforcement programme in increasing exercise adherence and short term maintenance	18 weeks	Facility	Exercise to music class	3 × wk, 35–50 min	Attendance at exercise group, no behavioural technique

Table 2.1 Continued

Study	Authors, stated objectives	Length of intervention	Location of exercise (home or facility)	Authors' description of exercise	Prescribed frequency, intensity, and duration of exercise	Controls
16	Stevens[34] – To assess the cost effectiveness of a primary care based intervention aimed at increasing physical activity in inactive people aged 45–74	10 weeks	Facility and home	Subjects' choice after discussion of options	Increase current activity	Educational materials
17	Taylor[35] – To examine the effects of a GP exercise referral scheme on modifying physical activity and other CHD risk factors	10 weeks	Facility	20 exercise sessions at facility up to 1 hour each time	2 sessions/week up to 60 min	Waiting list

Table 2.2 Summary of results

Study	Data analysed by "intention to treat"	No in study	Subjects	Follow up after intervention	Actual frequency, intensity, and duration of exercise intervention group	Main outcomes P<0.05	Outcome + or 0
1	Yes	229	Postmenopausal women aged 50–65	Annually	Mean miles walking/wk = 8.4	Self reported walking level significantly higher at years 1 and 2 compared to controls	+
2	Yes	135	University staff and faculty members, mean age 40, mainly female	12 weeks	46% of frequent prompt groups walking 3 × 20 min/week; 13% of low frequency prompts; 4% controls	Frequent telephone contact improved adherence to walking programme	+
3	Yes	357	160 women and 197 men aged 50–65; predominantly white and well educated	Ongoing	Mean frequency = HIG~1.2 × wk, HIH~2 × wk, LIH~3 × wk	Significant difference between intervention and control groups plus significant difference between home based and facility based groups	+
4	No	77	28 men (mean age 40) and 49 women (mean age 36)	Nil	Self monitoring group = mean of 2.4/wk for 26 min Reinforcement group = mean of 2.5/wk for 29 min	Behavioural interventions increased frequency of exercise compared to controls	+
5	Yes	51	Male and female middle aged subjects	Nil	11.4 sessions/month for daily self monitoring group; 7.5 sessions/month for weekly self monitoring group	Significant difference in number of exercise sessions/month between groups	+
6	Yes	52	Male and female middle aged subjects	Nil	12.4 sessions/month for 32 min in telephone group; 9.8 sessions/month for 28 min in comparison group	No significant difference in mean number of exercise sessions/month between groups; both groups increased exercise frequency over baseline	0

Table 2.2 Continued

Study	Data analysed by "intention to treat"	No in study	Subjects	Follow up after intervention	Actual frequency, intensity, and duration of exercise intervention group	Main outcomes P<0.05	Outcome + or 0
7	No	200	Average age 39 (±9)	None	~2–3 sessions/month	No difference between groups	0
8	Yes	763	Adults (aged 18–60+) attending health centre	12 months	33.1% "exercising" ≥5 hours in previous 2 wks	No significant difference between groups	0
9	Yes	125	Ethnic minority women aged 23–54	30 months	57 min walking/wk in behavioural group; 53 min walking/wk in education group	Both groups	0
10	No	194	Healthy sedentary men and women (76%) average age 44	Nil	151 min of physical activity/wk in motivation group; 98 min/wk standard group	Significant between group difference	+
11	Yes	125	Previously sedentary 45–64 year olds	None	Not stated	Intervention subjects exercised more frequently and for longer than controls	+
12	Yes	58	18–20 year old previously sedentary female psychology students	2 months	Mean frequency JAR and G = 2.4/wk; GR=1.4/wk	83% of jogging alone + relapse subjects still exercising at follow up compared to 36% of control subjects	+
13	No	171	Males aged 40–59 with CHD risk factors	12 years	Mean hours jogging/wk at year 13 = 0.3 hours	No difference between exercise and control conditions at follow up on jogging hours/wk	0
14	No	124	Male firefighters aged 24–56	6 months	Not stated	No significant difference between groups at follow up	0

Table 2.2 Continued

Study	Data analysed by "intention to treat"	No in study	Subjects	Follow up after intervention	Actual frequency, intensity, and duration of exercise intervention group	Main outcomes P<0.05	Outcome + or 0
15	Yes	120	Previously sedentary, female university employees with a mean age of 35 years	2 months	Percentage of classes attended during the 18 wks RP=51%, R=49%, controls=44%	No significant difference in attendance at 18 wks or 2 month follow up	0
16	Yes	714	45–74 year olds from 2 urban health centres	8 months	6 occasions of mod/vig exercise in previous 4 wks	10.6% reduction in number of intervention subjects classed as sedentary	+
17	No	142	40–70 year olds from 2 health centres	9 months	9.1 gym attendances/10 wks	No between group differences in energy expenditure at 37 wks	0

+ = positive significant difference; 0 = no significant difference.
HIG = high intensity group; HIH = high intensity home; LIH = low intensity home; JAR = jogging alone + relapse prevention; G = group jogging; GR = group jogging + relapse prevention; RP = relapse prevention; R = reinforcement

difference between intervention subjects and controls.

Study 3 compared home based and facility based exercise. After 1 year, subjects assigned to the two home based arms completed significantly more of the prescribed exercise sessions than subjects assigned to exercise at a facility (79%, 75%, and 53%, respectively), with no significant difference between the two home based arms. A significant contribution to this discussion has been made by Project Active – a large randomised (not controlled) trial that has shown that significant improvements in physical activity, fitness and other cardiovascular risk factors can be achieved without the need to attend supervised, structured physical activity.[36]

Components of prescribed exercise

Six of the eight trials that stated walking as the prescribed mode of exercise showed a significant increase in exercise when compared to controls. In one study (study 1), 80% of subjects were walking an average of at least 5 miles a week with 61% of subjects adhering to the prescribed level of 7 miles a week at 2 years. In a 10 year follow up of the same trial, intervention subjects were still walking significantly more than controls.[37] The trials in which walking was not specifically recommended included exercise to music classes, gym based "endurance activity", jogging and self determined activity. Three of the trials that did not specifically refer to walking showed an increase in exercise (studies 10,12,16). In one of the studies (study 12) subjects were women aged 18–20, who may have tolerated the prescribed jogging better than the older groups in the other trials. Study 16, which offered subjects the opportunity to attend a local facility at reduced cost, showed increases in physical activity not explained by attendances at the facility. Significant changes were only observed in moderate intensity activity suggesting that unstructured modes of activity were preferred.

Although the prescribed frequency of exercise averaged three to five times a week, most subjects were reporting lower frequency at follow up, with an average two to three times a week. Study 3 assigned subjects to three intervention arms of varying frequencies. One of the two home based arms prescribed three sessions a week for 40 minutes at a high intensity, while the other home based arm prescribed five sessions a week at a low intensity. The third arm, where subjects exercised at a local community hall prescribed three sessions a week. At one year there was no significant difference between the two home based arms on the percentage of prescribed sessions completed, with both completing significantly more than subjects in the facility based arm. Second year follow up data show that subjects in the three times a week home based arm were able to maintain significantly higher levels of adherence than those in the five times a week home based arm, who had reduced to a level similar to that of the facility based arm (68%, 49% and 36% of prescribed sessions, respectively).[38] Although the two home based arms were prescribed differing intensity levels, analysis of heart rate data showed that both arms actually exercised at an intensity normally described as moderate. Studies 10 and 16 were both able to make changes in the frequency of moderate intensity exercise. Study 16, which reported both moderate and vigorous, did not show any significant increases in the frequency of vigorous intensity exercise.

Strategies for improving compliance

A range of behavioural methods was used to improve compliance. It is difficult to measure the effect of some of these as they were often part of multi-faceted interventions taught to all groups. Methods included reinforcement (rewarding subjects for successful completion), self monitoring (keeping personal records of exercise performed) and relapse prevention training (learning to cope with situations that prompt inactivity and preventing a missed session leading to a return to pre-intervention exercise levels). Some trials investigated the impact of such strategies with varying results.

In study 4 subjects were randomly assigned to self monitoring, reinforcement and control arms. After 18 weeks subjects in the two behavioural treatment arms were exercising significantly more than those in the control arm. Study 14 found no difference in exercise levels between subjects instructed in self monitoring and control subjects. Study 5 took subjects from an earlier trial and randomised them to two "maintenance" groups with different frequencies of self monitoring. Subjects completing daily self monitoring forms performed 35% more exercise sessions than subjects completing forms weekly.

Relapse prevention training was compared with reinforcement strategies in a study of women attending exercise classes (study 15). Subjects in the relapse prevention arm attended weekly lessons on relapse prevention immediately following an exercise class, while subjects in the reinforcement group received T-shirts and other rewards for successful attendance at a number of classes.

Control subjects simply attended the exercise classes. At 18 weeks there was no difference between groups on number of exercise sessions attended with 72% of subjects attending less than the prescribed three classes a week.

In a trial of jogging alone or in a group, and of jogging with and without relapse prevention training (study 12), the impact of relapse prevention varied. Eighty-three per cent (10 of 12 subjects) of subjects with relapse prevention training who were jogging alone, were still exercising at 3 months compared with 36% (5 of 12 subjects) of those without such training. By contrast, in the two group jogging arms relapse prevention training did not increase jogging frequency at follow up.

Study 3 investigated the effect of subjects' perceptions of whether they had achieved expected physical or psychological benefits after 6 months on subsequent exercise adherence.[39] Those subjects who reported they had achieved expected benefits completed more exercise sessions in the next 6 months than those who did not achieve their expectations. It seems that to maintain adherence in the long term, subjects need to perceive a physical or psychological gain from exercise.

Studies 8 and 10 produced computer generated tailored reports based on data collected from baseline questionnaires. Study 10 showed significant differences in physical activity at 6 months in the tailored group compared to those receiving standard self help materials. Study 8 did not show any differences at 12 months follow up although there were differences at earlier stages.

Perhaps more important than any of these behavioural methods in achieving high rates of compliance is ongoing follow up.

Follow up

Telephone calling was a common method for following up participants in home based trials after an initial instruction session. All of the home based trials, apart from one (study 9), where researchers maintained contact by telephone, reported positive outcomes. Studies 2 and 6 investigated the effect of telephone prompting. Study 2 randomised subjects to four levels of telephone prompting or to a control arm. All subjects received 15 minutes of instruction on walking. At 6 months there was a significant difference in numbers of subjects still walking between the three prompted arms and the control arm, and between prompt frequency (once a week versus once every 3 weeks). Study 6 randomly assigned subjects who were waiting list controls from a previous trial[40] to two interventions, one of which received telephone contact (10 times during 6 months). All subjects received instructions in behavioural methods to improve compliance. Subjects in the telephone prompting arm exercised more frequently and for longer than those in the control arm (12.4 sessions/month for 32 minutes versus 9.8 sessions/month for 28 minutes). This difference did not achieve significance. Only subjects in the telephone arm significantly increased their fitness.

Discussion

We have not attempted a formal meta-analysis of the trials in this chapter as this would be inappropriate in view of the incompatible data and varying quality of the trials described. This is in accordance with the criteria for attempting a meta-analysis described by Eysenck.[41] The important public health question is whether evidence exists to guide policy makers considering strategies to increase the activity levels of a sedentary population. Trials that were able to demonstrate significant increases in activity involved exercise that was mainly home based, of moderate intensity, involved walking, and had regular follow up.

Walking from home was more successful than exercise that relied on attendance at structured exercise sessions. Only three facility based trials reported increases in exercise compared with six of the home based trials. All those trials prescribing walking reported increases in activity. Moderate intensity activity was also associated with higher compliance rates. Walking on level ground at a brisk pace would be a moderate intensity activity for most people.

In Britain, walking is the most popular leisure time physical activity.[42] Approximately half the subjects in a recent national survey[11] walked continuously for at least a mile (1·6 km) at least once in the past week. However, only 26% of men and 21% of women walked at a brisk or fast pace, and only 14% of men and 17% of women aged 55–74 walked at this pace. The 1993 Health Survey for England[12] confirmed these findings, reporting that 20% of women and 30% of men were classified as moderate walkers (fast or brisk pace), and 38% of women and 32% of men classified as light intensity walkers (slow or average pace). Brisk walking is recommended for improving population activity levels by the American College of Sports Medicine and the Centers for Disease Control and Prevention (USA).[13] In England, the Health Education Authority's Active for Life campaign emphasises the importance of brisk walking for improving one's health.

A United States survey has shown that people in lower income groups, older people, women, and black and hispanic people, participated in less exercise.[43] These differences were not seen in the numbers who were walking, which indicates that walking may be more universally accessible than other types of physical activity. In England, physical activity participation is lower in older people, women, those living in council properties, lower education groups[11] and lower socio-economic groups.[44]

Walking is also associated with a lower injury rate than other forms of physical activity.[45] Injuries are reported as a barrier to exercise particularly in older age groups.[11] Reviews of the determinants of physical activity report fewer barriers to walking than other types of physical activity.[46]

Some younger men and most other adults would improve their physical fitness if they took up regular brisk walking (figure 2.1).[47] Increases in cardiovascular fitness have been associated with reductions in cardiovascular and all-cause mortality.[48] A report on the health benefits of walking, which reviewed the impact of walking on various cardiovascular disease risk factors, concluded

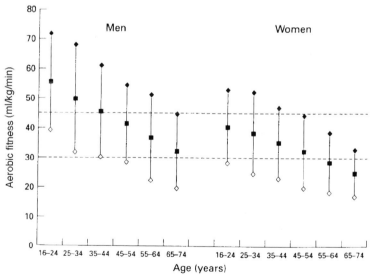

Fig 2.1 The dotted lines correspond to 45 ml/kg/min and 30/ml/kg/min. They define the range of values for aerobic fitness which would permit individuals to perform activities costing between 5 and 7.5 kcal/min (moderate intensity) at about 50% of their VO_2 max.

that "regular walking has the potential to lower blood pressure, improve the lipid profile, reduce body fat, enhance mental well-being and reduce the risk of coronary heart disease."[49]

This review has shown that when walking is recommended and attendance at a facility is not required, significant increases in activity can be achieved. When subjects are followed up regularly the increases can be maintained.

There has been a rapid growth in General Practitioner (GP) Prescription for Exercise Schemes. Estimates suggest that hundreds of such schemes exist in all parts of the country. A 1994 report[50] found that a large proportion of such schemes are leisure centre managed, and involve GPs referring patients at reduced or no cost for an average period of 10 weeks. The report estimated that less than 1% of a GP's patient list was referred into the schemes and also highlighted the fact that "no examples of good evaluation" were found, preventing any conclusions about effectiveness. A more recent review showed little improvement in levels of evaluation.[51] This review did not find any evidence of the effectiveness of these types of intervention. The emphasis placed on attending a leisure facility and the neglect of walking as a form of exercise is inconsistent with the findings of this review. Since the first review there has been an increase in the number of organised walking interventions and we await their results with interest.

Most of the studies used volunteers responding to advertisements to take part in a physical activity programme. One study (study 3) that used random digit dialling as a method of recruitment randomised only 27% of those actually contacted, suggesting a high degree of self selection.[52] These recruitment methods tell us little about how to increase the physical activity levels of the vast majority of people who are unlikely to respond to advertisements.

The findings of this review should be viewed with caution as they are based on only 17 trials most of which were carried out in the USA.

Future research

There is an urgent need for experimental research. In particular:

- There should be trials undertaken in the UK
- Trials should include groups other than the middle aged, middle class and white

- There is a need for trials specifically dealing with physical activity in the over 75s
- There is a need for evaluation of GP prescription schemes by randomised controlled trials
- There is a need to evaluate the effect of GPs advising their patients to exercise.

Conclusion

Levels of physical activity can be increased and the increase can be maintained for at least 2 years. Interventions that encourage walking and do not require attendance at a facility are most likely to lead to sustainable increases in overall physical activity. Regular follow up, which need not be time consuming and expensive, improves the proportion of people able to maintain initial increases.

Brisk walking has the greatest potential for increasing the overall activity levels of a sedentary population and meeting current public health recommendations. It is also the kind of exercise most likely to be adopted by a range of ages, socioeconomic and ethnic groups as well as both sexes.

In order to increase the attractiveness of walking for recreational purposes or as a mode of transport, attention will need to be paid to environmental factors that influence personal safety and convenience.

1 Powell KE, Thompson PD, Caspersen CJ, Kendrick JS. Physical activity and the incidence of coronary heart disease. *Ann Rev Public Health* 1987;**8**:253–87.
2 American College of Sports Medicine. Physical activity, physical fitness and hypertension. *Med Sci Sports Exerc* 1993;**25**:i–x.
3 Helmrich SP, Ragland DR, Leung RW, Paffenbarger RS. Physical activity and reduced occurrence of non-insulin dependent diabetes mellitus. *N Engl J Med* 1991;**325**:147–52.
4 Shinton R, Sagar G. Lifelong exercise and stroke. *BMJ* 1993;**307**:231–4.
5 Lee I, Paffenbarger RS, Hsieh C. Physical activity and risk of developing colorectal cancer among college alumni. *J Natl Cancer Inst* 1991;**83**:1324–9.
6 Drinkwater BL. Physical activity, fitness and osteoporosis. In: Bouchard C, Shephard RJ, Stephens T. *Physical activity, fitness and health: international proceedings and consensus statement 1992.* Champaign, Illinois: Human Kinetics, 1994:724–36.
7 North TC, McCullagh P, Vu Tran Z. Effect of exercise on depression. *Exerc Sports Sci Rev* 1990;**18**:379–416.
8 Wood PD, Stefanick ML, Williams PT, Haskell WL. The effects on plasma lipoproteins of prudent weight-reducing diet, with or without exercise, in overweight men and women. *N Engl J Med* 1991;**325**:461–6.
9 Berlin JA, Colditz GA. A meta-analysis of physical activity in the prevention of

coronary heart disease. *Am J Epidemiol* 1990;**132**:639–46.

10 Pooling Project Research Group. Relationship of blood pressure, serum cholesterol, smoking habit, relative weight and ECG abnormalities to incidence of major coronary events: final report of the pooling project. *J Chronic Dis* 1978;**31**:202–306.

11 Allied Dunbar National Fitness Survey. *Main findings*. London: Sports Council and Health Education Authority, 1992:46.

12 Office of Population Censuses and Surveys, *Health survey for England 1993*. London: HMSO, 1995.

13 Pate RR, Pratt M, Blair SN, Haskell WL, Macera CA, Bouchard C *et al.* Physical activity and public health: a recommendation from the Centers for Disease Control and Prevention and the American College of Sports Medicine. *JAMA* 1995;**273**:402–7.

14 Hillsdon M, Thorogood M. A systematic review of physical activity promotion strategies. *Br J Sports Med* 1996;**30**:84–9.

15 Dickersin K, Scherer R, Lefebvre C. Identifying relevant studies from systematic reviews. In: Chalmers I, Altman DG, eds. *Systematic Reviews*. London: BMJ Publishing, 1995:64–74.

16 Dishman RK. Determinants of participation in physical activity. In: Bouchard C, Shephard RJ, Stephens T, Sutton JR, McPherson BD, eds. *Exercise, fitness and health: a consensus of current knowledge 1988*. Champaign, Illinois: Human Kinetics, 1990:75–101.

17 King AC, Blair SN, Bild DE, Dishman RK, Dubbert PM, Marcus BH, Oldridge NB, Paffenbarger RS, Powell KE, Yeager KK. Determinants of physical activity and interventions in adults. *Med Sci Sports Exerc* 1992;**24**(suppl):221–36.

18 Dishman RK, Sallis JF. Determinants and interventions for physical activity and exercise. In: Bouchard C, Shephard RJ, Stephens T, eds. *Physical activity, fitness and health: International proceedings and consensus statement 1992*. Champaign, Illinois: Human Kinetics, 1994:214–38.

19 EPI-Centre. *EPI-Centre review guidelines*. Social Science Research Unit, London University of Education, London, 1996.

20 Kriska AM, Bayles C, Cauley JA, Laporte RE, Sandler RB, Pambiano G. A randomised exercise trial in older women: increased activity over two years and the factors associated with compliance. *Med Sci Sports Exerc* 1986;**18**:557–62.

21 Lombard DN, Lombard TN, Winett RA. Walking to meet health guidelines: the effect of prompting frequency and prompt structure. *Health Psychol* 1995;**14**:164–70.

22 King AC, Haskell WL, Barr Taylor C, Kraemer HC, DeBusk RF. Group vs home based exercise training in healthy older men and women. *JAMA* 1991;**266**:1535–42.

23 Noland MP. The effects of self monitoring and reinforcement on exercise adherence. *Res Q Exerc Sport* 1989;**60**:216–24.

24 King AC, Barr Taylor C, Haskell WL, DeBusk RF. Strategies for increasing early adherence to and long term maintenance of home based exercise training in healthy middle aged men and women. *Am J Cardiol* 1988;**61**:628–32.

25 Godin G, Deshamais R, Jobin J, Cook J. The impact of physical fitness and health age appraisal upon exercise intentions and behaviour. *J Behav Med* 1987;**10**:241–50.

26 Bull F, Jamrozik, K. Advice on exercise from a family physician can help sedentary patients to become active. *Am J Prev Med* 1998;**15**(2):85–94.

27 Chen A, Sallis J, Castro C, Lee R, Hickmann S, Williams C, Martin J. A home-based behavioral intervention to promote walking in sedentary ethnic minority women: project WALK. *Womens Health* 1998;**4**:19–39.

28 Marcus BH, Bock BC, Pinto BM, Forsyth LH, Roberts MB, Traficante RM. Efficacy of an individualised, motivationally-tailored physical activity inter-

vention. *Ann Behav Med* 1998;**20**:174–80.

29 McAuley E, Courneya KS, Rudolph DL, Lox CL. Enhancing exercise adherence in middle-aged males and females. *Prev Med* 1994;**23**:498–506.

30 King AC, Frederiksen LW. Low-cost strategies for increasing exercise behaviour. *Behav Modif* 1984;**8**:3–21.

31 MacKeen PC, Rosenberger JL, Slater JS, Channing NW, Buskirk ER. A 13 year follow up of a coronary heart disease risk factor screening and exercise programme for 40–59 year old men: exercise habit maintenance and physiologic status. *J Cardiopulm Rehab* 1985;**5**:510–23.

32 Reid EL, Morgan RW. Exercise prescription: a clinical trial. *Am J Public Health* 1979;**69**:591–5.

33 Marcus BH, Stanton AL. Evaluation of relapse prevention and reinforcement interventions to promote exercise adherence in sedentary females. *Res Q Exerc Sport* 1993;**64**:447–52.

34 Stevens W, Hillsdon M, Thorogood M, McArdle D. Cost-effectiveness of a primary care based physical activity intervention in 45–74 year old men and women: a randomised controlled trial. *Br J Sports Med.* 1998;**32**:236–41.

35 Taylor A, Doust J, Webborn N. Randomised controlled trial to examine the effects of a GP exercise referral programme in Hailsham, East Sussex, on modifiable coronary heart disease risk factors. *J Epidemiol Community Health* 1998;**52**:595–601.

36 Dunn A, Marcus B, Kampert J, Garcia M, Kohl H, Blair S. Comparison of lifestyle and structured interventions to promote physical activity and cardio-respiratory fitness: a randomised trial. *JAMA* 1999;**281**:327–34.

37 Perieira M, Kriska A, Day R, Cauley J, LaPorte R, Kuller LH. A randomised walking trial in postmenopausal women: effects on physical activity and health 10 years later. *Arch Internal Med* 1998;**158**:1695–701.

38 King AC, Haskell WL, Young DR, Oka RK, Stefanick ML. Long term effects of varying intensities and formats of physical activity on participation rates, fitness and lipoproteins in men and women aged 50–65 years. *Circulation* 1995;**91**:2596–604.

39 Neff KL, King AC. Exercise programme adherence in older adults: the importance of achieving one's expected benefits. *Med Exerc Nutr Health* 1995;**4**:355–62.

40 Juneau M, Rogers F, de Santos V *et al.* Effectiveness of self monitored, home based moderate intensity exercise training in middle aged men and women. *Am J Cardiol* 1987;**60**:60–70.

41 Eysenck HJ. Problems with meta-analysis. In: Chalmers I, Altman DG, eds. *Systematic reviews.* London: BMJ Publishing 1995:64–74.

42 Office of Population Censuses and Surveys. *General household survey 1990.* London: HMSO, 1992.

43 Siegel PZ, Brackbill RM, Heath GW. The epidemiology of walking for exercise: implications for promoting activity among sedentary groups. *Am J Public Health* 1995;**85**:706–9

44 Cox BD, Huppert FA, Whichelow MJ. *The health and lifestyle survey: seven years on.* Aldershot: Dartmouth, 1993.

45 Pollock M, Carroll JF, Graves JE, Leggett SH, Braith RW, Limacher M, Hagberg JM. Injuries and adherence to walk/jog and resistance training programs in the elderly. *Med Sci Sports Exerc* 1991;**23**:1194–200.

46 Hovell MF, Hofstetter CR, Sallis JF, Rauh MJD, Barrington E. Correlates of change in walking for exercise: an exploratory analysis. *Res Q Exerc Sport* 1992;**63**:425–34.

47 Killoran AJ, Fentem P, Caspersen C. *Moving on: international perspectives on promoting physical activity.* London: Health Education Authority, 1994.

48 Blair SN, Kohl HW, Barlow CE, Paffenbarger RS, Gibbons LW, Macera CA. Changes in physical fitness and all-cause mortality. *JAMA* 1995;**273**:1093–8.

49 Davidson RRC, Grant S. Is walking sufficient for health? *Sports Med* 1993;**16**:369–73.
50 Biddle S, Fox K, Edmunds L. *Physical activity promotion in primary health care in England*. London: Health Education Authority, 1994.
51 Riddoch C, Puig-Ribera M, Cooper A. *Effectiveness of physical activity promotion schemes in primary care: a review*. London: Health Education Authority, 1998.
52 King AC, Harris RB, Haskell WL. Effect of recruitment strategy on types of subjects entered into a primary prevention clinical trial. *Ann Epidemiol* 1994;**4**:312–20.

Multiple choice questions

1 Which of the following exercise frequencies are typical post intervention?
(a) Once per week
(b) 2–3 times per week
(c) 4–5 times per week
(d) 6–7 times per week
(e) No change is usually observed

2 Which of the following are behavioural strategies used in exercise trials?
(a) Self monitoring
(b) Relapse prevention
(c) Punishment
(d) Reinforcement
(e) (a), (b), (d)

3 According to the Allied Dunbar National Fitness Survey, which of the following statements are true?
(a) Approximately 40% of adults aged 55–74 years walk regularly at a brisk to fast pace
(b) Approximately 25% of adults aged 16–74 years walk a mile at least once a week
(c) Approximately 70% of adults aged 16–74 years take an inadequate amount of exercise
(d) Cycling is the most popular leisure time physical activity
(e) 3 out of 10 adults aged 16–74 play a sport at least once a week

4 Which of the following can be said about exercise interventions?
(a) Regular follow up does not have an effect on exercise adherence
(b) Increases in physical activity are more likely if the activity can be performed from the home

(c) Supervised, gym based exercise interventions lead to greater increases in physical activity than walking interventions

(d) Subjects find it easier to adhere to vigorous intensity exercise rather than moderate intensity

(e) No evidence exists that regular physical activity can be maintained after 12 months

5 Based on current evidence, which of the following has the greatest potential for increasing the level of physical activity in the population?

(a) Build more fitness centres

(b) Increase the number of cycling lanes in the country

(c) Focus on environmental changes that make walking safe and enjoyable

(d) Encourage more GPs to refer patients to leisure centres

(e) Develop more opportunities for sport

Answers are on p. 361.

3   A systematic review of promotion of physical activity in primary care

C B Eaton, L M Menard

Introduction

The risks of sedentary lifestyles[1-3] and the apparent health benefits of physical activity[4-7] in the prevention and treatment of coronary heart disease, hypertension, non-insulin dependent diabetes mellitus, depression, osteoporosis and some cancers are well documented. Estimates of the relative risk of sedentary lifestyle on coronary heart disease range from 1.3 to 1.9 and suggest that physical inactivity is of the same order of magnitude as cigarette smoking, hypertension, and hyperlipidaemia as a risk factor for cardiovascular disease.[1,4] Public health officials in the United States and Great Britain have recognised the importance of physical activity and have recently published a health message that, "every adult should accumulate 30 minutes or more of moderate-intensity physical activity on most days of the week."[1,8] Despite this message, most of the British (70%) and American population (60%) remain sedentary.[1,9]

One potential way of increasing physical activity in the population is for primary care doctors or general practitioners to provide counselling in their offices with regard to physical activity. Most of the population of the United States and Great Britain visit a general practitioner or primary care doctor at least once every 2 years.[10] Thus office based counselling on physical activity has the potential to be an important preventive strategy if performed effectively.

The purpose of this systematic review is to answer the following questions:

- What is the quality of the evidence that physical activity counselling in primary care is efficacious?
- If efficacious, how generalisable are these results to normal primary care?

Methods

Search methods

Computerised searches were carried out with Medline, Dialog(R) of Dissertation Abstracts, and Sci Li Reference from 1961 to 1998. Keywords for searching included "exercise", "physical fitness", "trials", "meta-analysis", and "outcome assessment". The search was limited to the English language. Additional searches were carried out by using papers identified in the search and from previous reviews. In addition, experts in the specialty were asked to provide additional published or unpublished studies.

Data extraction

Papers were reviewed if they met the following criteria:

- A control group had to exist
- Subjects had to be assigned to a control group or intervention status
- Interventions had to be performed in the doctor's office practice and not at homes, worksites, churches or community organisations
- Exercise behaviour had to be assessed a minimum of 4 weeks

Box 3.1 Why should primary care physicians prescribe exercise?

- Over 100 scientific studies have consistently shown that the health benefits of regular exercise far outweigh the small risks
- Public health officials in the United States and Great Britain have recognised this fact and have promoted a health message "Every adult should accumulate 30 minutes or more of moderate-intensity physical activity on most days of the week (5 days)"
- Despite this message most of the British (70%) and American (60%) population remain sedentary
- One potential approach is to have a patient's general practitioner or primary care doctor counsel patients regarding physical activity as most patients see their personal doctor at least once every 2 years

---

after the intervention and had to be interpretable as a dichotomous variable so that odds ratios (ORs) could be calculated

The following factors were evaluated in each study by two independent reviewers: study design, practice location, number of study subjects, recruitment rate, number of practices, practice intervention, patient intervention, duration of the study, year of the study, physical activity at baseline and after the intervention, selection bias, measurement error of outcome variable, confounding bias, competing interventions, and generalisability of results.

Statistical methods

Two by two tables were generated by comparing physically active with sedentary subjects for intervention and control groups in each study. Odds ratio and 95% confidence intervals were calculated by comparing the odds of the intervention group increasing physical activity or being active at follow up with those of a control group. The 95% confidence intervals were calculated by using the formula, antilog $(\log_e OR + 1.96SE)$, where the standard error $SE = (1/A + 1/B + 1/C + 1/D)^{1/2}$ for a standard two by two table.[11] A summary odds ratio with meta-analytic techniques was not determined because of the small number of studies and the large degree of heterogeneity between studies, making summary estimates of effect misleading.

Results

Over 20 potentially relevant articles were reviewed. Ten clinical trials met the inclusion criteria and the results are tabulated in table 3.1A&B. Most studies used different methods in terms of recruitment of patients and practices, interventions, outcome measures and methods of analyses and are discussed below.

The INSURE (Industry-wide Network for Social, Urban and Rural Efforts) study performed in 1984, was a prospective study of 2218 adults (1409 study subjects and 809 controls) and used a quasi-experimental design to determine if patients' health risk behaviours changed 1 year after a preventive intervention by primary care doctors.[12] Three of 6 multispecialty practices and 2 of 5 control practices agreed to participate in the study and 74–100% of the primary care doctors from each practice agreed to participate. About 28% of the random sample of patients were

Table 3.1A Clinical trials of physical activity promotion in primary care offices

Article	Study design	Randomised trial	Practice	Study
INSURE 1984 Wisconsin, Pennsylvania, Florida	Quasi-experimental; multiple behaviours; 1 year follow up	No; volunteer practices	5 multispecialty group practices, (72 physicians)	Exp = 203, control = 83; age >18; men and women
Kelly 1987 Cleveland, Ohio	Quasi-experimental; multiple behaviours; 6 week follow up	No; control group a random sample of non-participants due to office scheduling with non-physician provider	Single model FP residency, (18 physicians)	Exp = 134, control = 58; age 18-60; men and women
PACE 1996 San Diego County	Quasi-experimental; stage of change approach to physical activity; 4-6 week follow up	No; volunteer practices	17 volunteer primary care physician offices	Exp = 98, control = 114; age >18; men and women free of coronary heart disease
Johns Hopkins Medicare Preventive Services Demonstration Project 1989 Eastern Baltimore	Randomised clinical trial; 1 year follow up	Yes, patients randomised to preventive health exams	3 hospital clinics, 13 community group practices, 103 solo/partnership practices	1573 intervention; 1524 controls. Medicare beneficiaries age 65 and older; 32.6% sedentary with good health and 72.9% with poor health
Physician Advice 1991 Colorado	Quasi-experimental; 1 month follow up	No, both groups with high frequency of advice	24 residents, academic family practice	82 advice; 111 no advice group; age >18; scheduled patients
Oxcheck 1989-92 Bedfordshire, England	Randomised clinical trial; 3 year follow up	Yes, patients randomised	5 urban general practices	2205 study patients;1916 controls;age 35-64, men and women

Table 3.1A Continued

Article	Study design	Randomised trial	Practice	Study
Green Prescription Auckland and Dunedin, New Zealand	Randomised clinical trial; 6 week follow up	Yes; but convenience sample of sedentary patients assessed to most likely benefit and succeed over next 6 weeks in increasing physical activity	37 general practices	218 intervention group of written prescription; 238 verbal advice only for subjects with <1 hr of vigorous activity or <3 hrs of moderate activity per week
Leeds Yorkshire, and SW Thames 1992	Quasi-experimental; 1 and 2 year follow up	No; 12% sample was chosen for health check	18 general practices	1687 intervention group; 3937 control group
PAL 1997 Southeastern Mass, USA	Randomised clinical trial; 6 week and 8 month follow up	Yes; 13% of orginal patient list enrolled	22 community-based primary care practices, 34 physicians	Exp= 181, control= 174; age > 50; not disabled
Advice on Exercise 1998 Perth, Australia	Controlled trial	No; balanced assignment each day	10 general practices	Exp=416, control= 347 sedentary patients

Table 3.1B Clinical trials of physical activity promotion in primary care offices

Article	Practice intervention	Patient intervention	Outcome	Odds ratio 95% CI	Comments
INSURE 1984 Wisconsin, Pennsylvania, Florida	CME seminars; review protocols, discuss problems	15 minutes' patient education and risk factor counselling	Self reported started vigorous exercise at least once per week with unvalidated telephone or mail questionnaire	1.39 (0.99 to 1.96); total study; 1.65 (1.12 to 2.43) post hoc treated only	External validity questionable as only 28% of sample responded; unit of intervention practice, unit of analysis patient
Kelly 1987 Cleveland, Ohio	Physician education on lifestyle prescription form, and education materials	Lifestyle assessment, educational materials, booster phone calls	Self reported making some or significant change in exercising with unvalidated question on telephone follow up 4 wks after intervention	2.84 (1.49 to 5.42)	Potential selection bias with use of non-participants as control group. Benefits of "some change" in exercise not clear
PACE 1996 San Diego County	Physician manual, physician role playing with trainer for two visits	Stages of change assessment; 3-5 minutes counselling, physician recommendations, 10 minute booster phone call	Self reported stage of change and physical activity with validated walking question and overall activity; subsample with Caltrac accelerometer; telephone interview 4-6 wks after intervention	6.56 (4.61 to 9.33) moving from contemplation to active stage; intervention increased walking 37 minutes/week compared to 7 minutes/week for controls	Volunteer physicians; 52% of eligible patients evaluated. Intervention group while increasing only average 11 minutes/day of exercise compared to 30 minutes/day recommended

Table 3.1B Continued

Article	Practice intervention	Patient intervention	Outcome	Odds ratio 95% CI	Comments
Johns Hopkins Medicare Preventive Services Demonstration Project 1989 Eastern Baltimore	Orientation sessions with CME credits on preventive exams and counselling visits	Two preventive exams a year apart reviewing lifestyle risk assessment and reimbursed follow up counselling within 6 months; controls received usual care	Self reported performance of physical activities such as walking, gardening, or heavy housework > 3 times/ week	1.04* (0.78 to 1.39) good health; 1.17* (0.69 to 1.97) poor health; *adjusted for age, sex, race, marital status, health status	Well designed, large sample size, multiple interventions, PA discussed in 89% of preventive visits; 70% of intervention patients had preventive visits
Physician Advice 1991 Colorado	15 minutes' physician training on protocol	2-3 minutes of exercise advice, educational handout, 1 month follow up	Self reported activity levels, frequency and duration at baseline and 1 month telephone follow up	1.91 (1.25 to 2.94); increase of 109 minutes/ week in advice group compared with decrease of 24 minutes/week in no advice group	Randomised control trial abandoned due to high percentage of advice in control physicians; biased sample with 80% of patients at baseline exercising
Oxcheck 1989-92 Bedfordshire, England	Nurse trained in patient centred communication model during 2 day course, annual study day, monthly evening training sessions	1 hour nurse health check including lifestyle evaluation and 10-20 minute follow up appointments	Self reported vigorous exercise < 1 month at baseline and 3 years later	1.19 (1.11 to 1.27); attenders only 1.25 (1.16 to 1.34)	Mutiple risk factor intervention; health benefits of increased vigorous exercise to > 1 /month unclear; significant time spent on recruiting patients limit practicality

Table 3.1B   Continued

Article	Practice intervention	Patient intervention	Outcome	Odds ratio 95% CI	Comments
Green Prescription Auckland & Dunedin, New Zealand	Training session of GPs to assess and prescribe physical activity	Assessment and advice of approximately 5 minutes with written prescription of exercise	Self reported time spent over preceding 2 weeks in walking, sport, or leisure time activities measured at baseline by personal interview and at 6 weeks by telephone interview	1.81 (1.42 to 2.32); increase of 156 min/2 week period in Green experimental group	Patients and GPs selected for high compliance; the majority of intervention and control groups did not reach goal of 30 minutes of walking 5 days/week
Leeds Yorkshire & SW Thames, UK 1992	None	Health check up by GP	Self reported vigorous activity in previous 2 weeks at baseline and 2 years later with mailed questionnaires	0.91 (0.83 to 0.99) health check in past 2 years; 1.0 (0.95 to 1.05) health check in past 12 months	Multiple risk factor intervention; 75% compliance with health check up; 75% of respondents had no vigorous exercise in past two weeks at survey 2
PAL 1997 Southeastern Mass, USA	Staff orientation, 2 training sessions, physician manual, office poster, desktop reminder, reimbursement for patients with follow up interview	Stage of readiness for exercise adoption, physician advice, written exercise prescription, patient manual	PASE scale of self reported activity, SF-36 QOL scale, stage of exercise adoption, % moderate exercise for 30 minutes 5 days/week	1.41 (1.03 to 1.74) moderate exercise for 30 minutes 5 days/week at 6 weeks	More patients in intervention group adopted preparation or action stage of readiness than control group. PASE score, minutes walking and % moderately active not affected.
Advice on Exercise 1998 Perth, Australia	One hour of individual training to FP	2-3 minutes verbal advice followed by standard or tailored pamphlet sent to patient's home address	Self report of "now active", total number of sessions of physical activity	1.43 (1.22 to 1.68) at 6 months assuming non-responders are sedentary	Significant bias due to non-random selection for intervention and large drop out rate

53

evaluated with a response rate of 61% to the initial postal survey, 57% for the initial health examination and 80% response for the follow up appointments. Thus the experimental group consisted of 203 subjects and the control group 83 subjects. The intervention group received about 15 minutes of education and counselling on risk reduction. At baseline, 55.4% of the intervention group and 55.3% of the controls were sedentary. Of these sedentary patients, 31.5% of those randomised to the intervention group started exercising compared with 24.1% of the control group. This 39% increase in vigorous activity in a previously sedentary population fell just short of significance (P = 0.06). In a post hoc analysis of participants who actually received the preventive intervention, 33.8% increased self reported vigorous exercise at least once a week compared with 24.1% in the control group, and this 65% increase was found to be significant (P = 0.02). Concerns exist about the external validity of this study due to the use of volunteer practices and the low response rate (28%). Measurement error inherent in the use of unvalidated, self reported measures of physical activity in this trial would tend to bias the results towards no effect. It is unclear from this trial if the degree of exercise change of 33.8% of sedentary patients in the intervention group from less than once a week of vigorous exercise to more than once a week has any clinically relevant health benefits.

The "controlled trial of a time-efficient method" by Kelly[13] was a randomised trial in one family practice residency consisting of 3 doctors and 15 residents. Several risk behaviours were assessed in 412 adults aged 18-60 who were eligible for health promotion. Sedentary patients defined as exercising less than twice a week (n = 192) who received any lifestyle education were compared to those who were non-participants because of office scheduling problems. Those participants who made some change or significant change defined as exercising two or more times a week were compared with those that made no change over a 4 week interval, as assessed from a structured phone interview. Those in the intervention group were significantly more likely (odds ratio 2.84; 95% confidence interval 1.49-5.42) than non-participants to increase physical activity. Although these results were significant, concerns exist about the clinical relevance of some or "significant" change in self reported exercise of more than twice a week after only 1 month of follow up. In addition, the selection bias inherent in the selection of the control group leads to questions of internal validity of this study.

The controlled trial of physician counselling to promote the adoption of physical activity by Calfas *et al.*, evaluated a physician based assessment of counselling for exercise protocol by using a stage of change model in 17 volunteer primary care doctors' offices in San Diego County.[14] Sedentary patients defined as engaging in vigorous physical activity less than 3 times a week or moderate activity less than 2 hours a week who were aged over 18 and free of coronary heart disease or other conditions that could limit mobility were recruited for the study. A 52% response rate (n = 212) was obtained after 4 to 6 weeks of follow up. The intervention focused on increasing moderate levels of physical activity such as walking by using a patient centred stage of change approach. Of those patients in the intervention group, 52% moved from contemplation to the active stage compared with 12% of the control group, odds ratio of 6.56; confidence interval 4.61 to 9.33. The intervention group increased activity by 37 minutes a week compared with 7 minutes a week in the control group (P < 0.05). However at follow up assessment, patients reported walking an average of 11 minutes a day which has questionable clinical relevant health benefits particularly in light of short term follow up noted in this study. In addition, the selection bias of using volunteer practices suggests a best case scenario that may not be applicable to most primary care office practices.

The "Johns Hopkins Medicare preventive services demonstration project" evaluated the effects of preventive examinations on smoking, excessive alcohol drinking, and sedentary lifestyle at baseline and 1 year later in Medicare beneficiaries in Eastern Baltimore in 1989.[15] This randomised controlled trial involved 1573 intervention and 1524 control patients from 3 hospital clinics, 13 community group practices and 103 solo/partnership practices. Definition of sedentary lifestyle was based upon self reported performance of physical activity such as walking, gardening and heavy housework less than three times a week. During preventive examinations, doctors discussed physical activity in 89% of the encounters. Compliance with the preventive examinations was good, with 70% of those randomised to intervention receiving an examination. No statistically or clinically significant increases in physical activity occurred as a result of the intervention with an odds ratio of 1.04 (0.78 to 1.39) for patients with good health and 1.17 (0.69 to 1.97) for patients in poor health after adjustment for age, sex, race, marital status, and health status. This study reflects a generalisable, well designed clinical trial with a large sample size of elderly patients, with little bias or confounding.

The "effect of physician advice on exercise behavior" study by Lewis and Lynch was designed as a randomised clinical trial to evaluate the efficacy of a physician advice protocol to increase the frequency and duration of self reported activity levels after 1 month of follow up.[16] The study location was one family practice residency in Colorado with 24 residents in 1991. Of the 396 patients admitted to the study, 35% refused to cooperate, and 12% were lost to follow up, resulting in a 53% response rate. Baseline assessment showed that 70% of the patients were exercising before the intervention and that a sizeable percentage (30–40%) of the control group doctors were giving unprompted physical activity promotion advice. For this reason the investigators adopted a quasi-experimental design and assessed the effect of physician advice (intervention group) versus no advice (control group) on increasing physical activity levels. A significant difference, odds ratio of 1.91; confidence interval 1.25–2.94, was found when those reporting exercising at the end of 1 month in the physician advice group were compared with the no advice group. This increase appeared to be related to an increase in duration but not frequency of exercise. There are concerns about the internal validity of this study's conclusions because of uncontrolled confounding bias resulting from the abandonment of the intention to treat analysis of this study. Also the high rate of exercise, over 70% at baseline, limits the generalisability of these findings.

Oxcheck (Oxford and collaborators health check) was a randomised controlled trial focused on the effect of a general health check on several cardiovascular disease and cancer risk behaviours including vigorous exercise; it was performed in Bedfordshire, between 1989 and 1992.[17] Nurses trained in patient centred communication performed health checks, including lifestyle assessment, and provided counselling and follow up appointments in 5 urban general practices. Assessment of 2205 intervention patients and 1916 control patients after 3 years of follow up showed that 70.9% of the control group and 67.6% of the intervention group reported undertaking vigorous exercise less than once a month. These results from this well designed clinical trial with high internal validity and generalisability were significant with an odds ratio of 1.19, confidence interval 1.11–1.27. However, the clinical relevance of a 4.5% absolute difference when the intervention group was compared with the control group in performing vigorous exercise more than once per month is probably limited.

The Green prescription by Swinburn *et al.*, was a randomised clinical trial that was performed to determine if written advice increased physical activity among selected sedentary patients more than verbal advice alone after 6 weeks of follow up.[18] This study, performed in 37 general practices in Auckland and Dunedin, New Zealand, trained general practitioners to assess and prescribe physical activity, focusing on walking as the main intervention. From a convenience sample of sedentary patients defined as undertaking less than 1 hour of vigorous activity or 3 hours of moderate activity a week during work or recreation time, who were deemed by their general practitioner to be likely to benefit from enhanced physical activity and who were able to do so over the ensuing 6 weeks, 218 intervention patients were randomised to written prescription and patient education materials and 238 control patients were given only verbal advice. Physician assessment and advice averaged 5 minutes. After 6 weeks of follow up, a significant increase in physical activity (odds ratio 1.81; confidence interval 1.42–2.32) was found in the intervention group (85% active) compared with the verbal advice alone group (76%). This increase in physical activity averaged 156 minutes per 2 week period. Long term benefits in the intervention group were assessed by telephone interview at 11 months only in those who successfully increased activity and maintained increased physical activity. Bias inherent in selecting patients during practice consultations convenient to the practitioner rather than a random sample of patients places considerable restraints on the generalisability of these findings. While the intervention group significantly increased their level of walking, the absolute levels of walking were greater in the verbal advice group (249 minutes/2 weeks) at 6 weeks than in the intervention group (217 minutes/2 weeks). The health benefits of the average level of physical activity for both groups (17 minutes a day of walking) are unclear as it is far below the recommended 30 minutes per day of moderate level activity. Ascertainment bias of the investigators by failing to follow up on the control group and those who initially had not increased physical activity may invalidate the results of the 11 month follow up data in this study.

The "prevention in practice" study by Dowell *et al.* in Leeds used a quasi-experimental design to compare self reported vigorous exercise in the 2 weeks before and 2 years after a health check aimed at changing multiple risk factors for the prevention of stroke and heart disease.[19] A 12% stratified sample of patients was chosen from 18 general practices in the Yorkshire and Southwest Thames regions, and these patients were invited for a health check, yielding 1687 patients in the intervention group and 3937 patients in the control group without a health check. The investigators found a significant decrease in exercise (odds ratio 0.91; confidence interval 0.83 to 0.99) after 2 years of follow up in the health check group and a non-significant null effect after 1 year of follow up (odds ratio 1.0; confidence interval 0.95 to 1.05). The population was largely sedentary with 75% of the respondents reporting no vigorous exercise in the preceding 2 weeks. Significant concerns about the potential role of confounding bias exist in this study because of its quasi-experimental design.

The "physician active for life project" (PAL)[20] by Goldstein M *et al.* was a randomised clinical trial in relatively healthy older patients that used a practice based intervention with a stage of change model (transtheoretical model of behaviour change). In total 2674 patients scheduled for non-acute appointments were contacted by phone from 12 single handed and 12 group primary care practices in southeastern Massachusetts. Of those screened, 13% were enrolled in the study; 181 in the intervention group and 174 in the control group. Physician groups randomised to the intervention received two sessions of training focusing on the five As of counselling (address the agenda, assess, advise, assist, and arrange follow up), a physician manual, a desk reminder, an office poster regarding exercise, and monetary incentives for each follow up patient seen according to protocol.

Patients in the intervention practices were more likely to report entering a stage of preparation or action for adopting a more physically active lifestyle than control patients. The physicians in the intervention practices did not report more exercise counselling nor did patients in the intervention practices report increased physical activity with a PASE score or minutes walked a day at 6 weeks or 8 months of follow up. The percentage of patients participating in moderate exercise for 30 minutes 5 days a week was significantly greater at 6 weeks in the intervention group compared with the control (odds ratio 1.41; confidence interval 1.03–1.74).

"Advice on exercise from a family physician" by Bull and Jamrozik in Perth, Western Australia, was a non-randomised clinical trial in which 10 general practices were assigned on alternate days to give verbal advice plus a mailed pamphlet versus no advice or follow up pamphlet to sedentary patients.[21] Of 6351 adult patients, 763 sedentary adults were recruited for the project

(12%). A postal survey response at 1, 6, and 12 months after intervention was analysed. Treating non-responders as sedentary, 40% of the intervention group was "now active" at 1 month compared with 31% of the control group (P < 0.05). This difference persisted at the 6 month follow up (38% v 30%) but diminished at 1 year (36% v 31%). The lack of randomisation, and the frequent decision by the family physician not to prescribe physical activity because of the patient's underlying disease, time constraints, etc. as well as the modest follow up at 6 months (57%) and 1 year (50%) are problematic in this study.

Synthesis

In table 3.2 each study's results are evaluated as either positive, negative or equivocal based upon its odds ratio and its 95% confidence interval. Factors that might explain these differences such as study design, length of follow up, single versus multiple risk factor intervention, type of physical activity measured, and methodological flaws are also tabulated to determine if they associated with positive results.

Six of 10 trials were positive with significant odds ratios > 1.0. The odds ratios ranged from 0.91 to 6.56 but significant biases or limited clinical relevance of the outcomes were found in all trials. Two of 10 trials were positive with odds ratios > 1.0, but the results were not significant at P < 0.05 and therefore are judged to be equivocal. Short term trials of less than 1 year (five of six positive, one of six equivocal), single risk factor trials (five of six positive, one of six equivocal) and randomised clinical trials (two of four positive, one of four equivocal) were most likely to find benefit in

---

Box 3.2   Does physician exercise counselling work?

- Ten clinical trials have assessed whether physical activity counselling performed by primary care physicians is effective
- Eight out of 10 clinical trials showed that advice from a doctor or nurse increased physical activity if only for short periods of follow up
- Clinical trials that focused on only one physical activity (5/6 positive) and that promoted moderate intensity physical activity (4/6 positive) were the most likely to be successful
- No well-designed randomised trials have shown long term clinically and statistically significant results to date

---

Table 3.2 Comparison of physical activity promotion trials by selected factors

Article	Randomised clinical trial	Intervention physical activity only	Duration of follow up	Outcome measure	Methodological flaws	Interpretation
INSURE	No	No	1 year	Vigorous activity	Significant	+/- (post hoc analysis +)
Kelly	No	No	4 weeks	Exercise	Significant	++ (OR>2.0)
PACE	No	Yes	4-6 weeks	Walking; validated	Significant	+++ (OR>5.0)
Johns Hopkins	Yes	No	1 year	Walking, Gardening, household	None	- (OR=1.0)
COLORADO	No	Yes	4 weeks	Walking	Significant	+ (OR>1.0)
OXCHECK	Yes	No	3 years	Vigorous activity	None	+ (OR>1.0)
Green Rx	Yes	Yes	6 weeks	Walking; validated	Significant	+ (OR>1.0)
Leeds	No	No	1 and 2 years	Vigorous	Significant	-- (OR<1.0)
PAL	Yes	Yes	6 weeks and 8 months	Walking; total validated	Few	+/- (OR>1.0)
Perth	No	Yes	6 months, 1 year	Now active	Significant	+ (OR>1.0) at 6 months but not 1 year

office based physical activity promotion. Only one of five large trials from primary care practices that lasted a year or more were positive.

Discussion

There is a large body of evidence from cardiac rehabilitation programmes, worksites and facility based programmes that highly motivated participants can increase their physical activity and adhere to exercise programmes that improve exercise tolerance, cardiac risk factors, and body composition.[22-26] However, the percentage of the population that participate in such programmes is small[1] and it is unlikely that a sizeable percentage of the population will participate in such supervised exercise programmes in the near future. The concept that primary care doctors, who provide the majority of health promotion services to most of the population, can by their personal relationship with their patients motivate them to change their sedentary lifestyles remains appealing as an approach to physical activity health promotion. This analysis shows that to date the scientific evidence for the efficacy of such an approach is modest but increasing. From the reviewed studies it does appear that well designed, unifactorial intervention studies aimed at increasing moderate activity in a currently sedentary population by using an intention to treat analysis with the practice as the unit of analysis as well as intervention are most likely to show a short term increase in physical activity that would be scientifically valid. The failure of long term studies to be effective suggests that long term changes in physical activity may require more active follow up programmes such as a reminder phone call system, increased social support – that is, a buddy system – and other incentives, perhaps financial, to be successful.

Given the paucity of valid scientific evidence that promotion of physical activity is worthwhile in primary care settings, what is a busy primary care doctor to do? It seems that by selecting sedentary patients with medical conditions in which physical activity improves prognosis or control and who are motivated to change, that 3–5 minutes of verbal advice regarding physical activity, associated with a written prescription and some follow up mechanism – such as a mailed leaflet and an exercise diary – can be helpful and can increase activity by 30% to 50% compared with no intervention. Further research – such as the ACT trial[27] – should

61

help us to reach the necessary intensity and resources effective for counselling in primary care.

1 US Department of Health and Human Services. *Physical activity and health: a report of the surgeon general.* Atlanta, Georgia: US Department of Health and Human Services, Centers for Disease Control and Prevention, National Center for Chronic Disease Prevention and Health Promotion, 1996.

2 Paffenbarger RS, Hyde RT, Wing AL, Hsieh CC. Physical activity, all-cause mortality, and longevity of college alumni. *N Engl J Med* 1986;**314**:605–13.

3 Eaton CB, Medalie JH, Flocke SA, *et al.* Self-reported physical activity predicts long-term coronary heart disease and all-cause mortalities: twenty-one-year follow-up of the Israeli ischemic heart disease study. *Arch Fam Med* 1995;**4**:323–9.

4 Eaton CB. Relation of physical activity and cardiovascular fitness to coronary heart disease. Part I. A meta-analysis of the independent relation of physical activity and coronary heart disease. *J Am Board Fam Pract* 1992;**5**:31–42.

5 Albanes D, Blair A, Taylor PR. Physical activity and risk of cancer in NHANES I population. *Am J Public Health* 1989;**79**:744–50.

6 Taylor CB, Sallis JF, Needle R. The relation of physical activity and exercise to mental health. *Public Health Rep* 1985;**100**:195–201.

7 Helmrich SP, Ragland DR, Leung RW, Paffenbarger RS. Physical activity and reduced occurrence of non-insulin dependent diabetes mellitus. *N Engl J Med* 1991;**325**:147–52.

8 Secretary of State for Health. *The health of the nation: a strategy for health in England.* London, HMSO, 1992; (Cmnd 1986).

9 Activity and Health Research. *Allied Dunbar national fitness survey: a report on the activity patterns and fitness levels. Main findings.* London: Sports Council and Health Education Authority, 1992.

10 Marcus BH, Goldstein MG, Jette A, *et al.* Training physicians to conduct physical activity counseling. *Prev Med* 1997;**26**:382–8.

11 Rothman K, ed. *Modern epidemiology.* Boston/Toronto: Little, Brown, 1986:217–21.

12 Lodgsdon DN, Lazaro CM, Meier RV. The feasibility of behavioral risk reduction in primary medical care. *Am J Prev Med* 1989;**5**:249–56.

13 Kelly RB. Controlled trial of a time-efficient method of health promotion. *Am J Prev Med* 1988;**4**:200–7.

14 Calfas KJ, Long BJ, Dallis JF, *et al.* A controlled trial of physician counseling to promote the adoption of physical activity. *Prev Med* 1966;**25**:225–33.

15 Burton LC, Paglia MJ, German PS, *et al.* The effect among older persons of a general preventive visit on three health behaviors: smoking, excessive alcohol drinking, and sedentary lifestyle. *Prev Med* 1995;**24**:492–7.

16 Lewis BL, Lynch WD. The effect of physician advice on exercise behavior. *Prev Med* 1993;**22**:110–21.

17 Imperial Cancer Research fund OXCHECK study group. Effectiveness of health checks conducted by nurses in primary care: final results of the OXCHECK study. *BMJ* 1995;**310**:1099–104.

18 Swinburn B, Walter L, Arroll B, *et al.* The Green prescription study: A randomized controlled trial of exercise prescription in general practice. *Am J Public Health* 1998;**88**:288–91.

19 Dowell AC, Ochera JJ, Hilton SR, *et al.* Prevention in practice: results of a 2-year follow-up of routine health promotion interventions in general practice. *Fam Pract* 1996;**13**:357–62.

20 Goldstein MG, Pinto BM, Marcus BH, Eaton CB, Menard LM, Milan F. Office based physical activity counseling in healthy adults. In: *Textbook of medicine, exercise, nutrition and health.* Oxford: Blackwell, 1999, (in press).

21 Bull FC, Jamrozik K. Advice on exercise from a family physician can help sedentary patients to become active. *Am J Prev Med* 1998;**15**:85–94.

22 O'Connor GT, Buring JE, Yusuf S, *et al.* An overview of randomized trials of rehabilitation with exercise after myocardial infarction. *Circulation* 1989;**80**:234–44.

23 DeBusk RF, Miller NH, Superko HR, *et al.* A case-management system for coronary risk factor modification after acute myocardial infarction. *Ann Intern Med* 1994;**120**:721–9.

24 Leon AS, Certo C, Comoss P, *et al.* Scientific evidence of the value of cardiac rehabilitation services with emphasis on patients following myocardial infarction: section I: exercise, conditioning component (position paper). *J Cardiopulm Rehab* 1990;**10**:79–87.

25 Blair SN, Piserchia PV, Wilbur CS, Crowder JH. A public health intervention model for worksite health promotion: impact on exercise and physical fitness in a health promotion plan after 24 months. *JAMA* 1986;**255**:921–6.

26 Heirich MA, Foote A, Erfurt JC, Konopka B. Work-site physical fitness programs: comparing the impact of different program designs on cardiovascular risks. *J Occup Med* 1993;**35**:510–17.

27 King AC, Sallis JF, Dunn AL, *et al.* Overview of the activity counselling trial (ACT) intervention for promoting physical activity in primary health care settings. *Med Sci Sports Exerc* 1998;**30**:1086–96.

Multiple choice questions

1 Physical activity has been shown in valid scientific studies to prevent or prolong survival for the following diseases:

(a) Coronary heart disease

(b) Osteoporosis

(c) Obsessive compulsive disorder

(d) Hypertension

(e) Type 2 diabetes mellitus

2 Exercise science has shown the following:

(a) Only vigorous exercise done for more than 20 minutes at least 3 times a week has significant health benefits

(b) Walking or moderate activity for 10 minutes 3 times a day is better than regular vigorous exercise

(c) All the benefits from exercise come from changes in body composition (for instance, weight loss) therefore if you don't lose weight you get no benefit from exercise

(d) Regular vigorous physical activity increases the chance of injury and death during the exercise period

(e) The benefits of regular physical activity outweigh the risks for most individuals

3 Office based counselling of sedentary patients in primary care settings:

(a) Has been shown to be effective at increasing physical activity to a level that has documented health benefits in well designed clinical trials

(b) Has been shown to be effective in increasing physical activity in most well designed clinical trials

(c) Has been shown to be effective increasing physical activity for short periods of time in selected patients in several clinical trials

(d) Has shown that exercise counselling is better done by exercise specialists than primary care providers

4 Sedentary lifestyle or no regular physical activity is:

(a) Common in both Great Britain and the United States

(b) Associated with higher risk of obesity, hypertension, diabetes mellitus, and low HDL cholesterol

(c) An independent risk factor for coronary heart disease regardless of body mass, and diabetes and HDL cholesterol concentration

(d) Unlikely to be changed by simple advice and therefore not worth the time and effort for busy general practitioners

5 Scientific studies in general practice have shown:

(a) That interventions focusing on increasing physical activity alone are more likely to be successful than preventive health visits dealing with multiple behaviours such as smoking, diet, and screening test compliance

(b) That a written exercise prescription plus verbal advice is better than verbal advice alone

(c) That exercise counselling to motivated patients is more likely to be successful than randomly selected patients from a practice list

(d) That exercise counselling by a doctor during a visit for illness leads to better compliance than during a prevention health checkup

(e) That exercise counselling by a doctor is better than that done by a nurse or exercise specialist

(f) That referring patients to an exercise specialist is better than office based counselling by general practitioners

Answers are on p. 361.

4 Getting started—a review of physical activity adoption studies

A L Dunn

Introduction

The naming of physical inactivity as a major risk factor for cardiovascular disease[1] combined with the high prevalence of physical inactivity in industrialised nations is spurring development of research efforts that examine how to increase physical activity. Experts have conceptualised becoming physically active as a process consisting of four phases: adoption, maintenance, relapse, and resumption.[2] The first phase, adoption, or getting people started, is the focus of this chapter.

Systematic research of why people begin a programme of exercise or regular physical activity is becoming increasingly important as we learn of the increased risks of inactivity and as we shift our thinking from treatment of disease to disease prevention. Since Dishman's early review of exercise adherence,[3] there is an increasing appreciation that exercise and physical activity behaviours are complex, with multiple determinants.[2] Many excellent reviews are available that summarise and criticise existing exercise adherence research,[2,4,5] clinical and community interventions to increase physical activity,[5] and most recently environmental and policy approaches to intervention. These reviews document important multilevel research efforts and indicate that we are beginning to develop the tools and strategies necessary to intervene in the high risk behaviour of physical inactivity. They provide the conceptual scheme of this review because they delineate the phases of exercise behaviour, provide a framework for examining multiple approaches, and illustrate how we have broadened our programmes and research efforts from more rigidly defined exercise behaviours in supervised gym based programmes to include many types of moderate intensity physical activities in more naturalistic settings.

In 1989, Winett *et al.* proposed a multilevel, multidisciplinary approach emphasising the need to combine behavioural science, exercise science, and public health expertise to develop effective intervention strategies aimed at individuals and small groups, organisations and environments, and even social policy.[7] This approach provides a coherent framework for identifying the focus of past research, the strategies found to be effective and goals for future research. I shall adopt that framework for this present review on how to get sedentary adults to be physically active. I shall summarise representative observation, quasi-experimental, and experimental studies that have contributed to our understanding of how to get sedentary adults to adopt a physically active way of life.

The selection of observational studies is based on the following criteria: (1) being specifically focused on getting sedentary adults to adopt a programme of exercise or physical activity; and (2) using reliable and valid measures to assess exercise adoption—that is, valid measures of physical activity. Selection of quasi-experimental and experimental studies is based on criterion 1 above, being representative of important trends in getting sedentary adults to adopt an exercise or physical activity programme, having a complete description of methods and strategies used, and demonstrated effectiveness. Effectiveness is broadly defined as a statistically significant increase in physical activity or physical fitness over a period of one to six months.

Methods

Several computerised searches were conducted on Medline for studies published between 1966 and 1999. Combinations of the following key words were used to develop a comprehensive list. These included exercise, physical activity, primary prevention, intervention, adherence, compliance, leisure activity, evaluation, effectiveness, behaviour, psychology, public health, health promotion, and epidemiology. The search was limited to studies in adults. The rationale for limiting the review to adults is based on evidence that determinants of physical activity differ between children and adults[2] and on my belief that adoption of physical activity by children should be a topic for a separate review.

Other studies were identified from these references and from existing reviews on determinants of exercise or physical activity. Studies were classified as being either observational studies of populations, examining the question of adoption of physical activity or exercise, or quasi-experimental or experimental studies. Quasi-experimental and experimental studies were subdivided into the multilevel framework of Winnett *et al.*[7] The majority of these were categorised as personal level interventions. The personal level intervention studies were further divided into studies that examined some aspect of physical activity or exercise or some aspect of behaviour – for example, theories of exercise adoption, comparison of behavioural techniques. Representative studies were then selected for inclusion based on the criteria listed earlier.

Results

Observational studies

Over 200 studies have examined barriers to physical activity adoption or have studied dropping out of exercise. These have been summarised by Dishman *et al.*[8] and by King *et al.*[9] A major criticism is that these studies may not be applicable to most people because they have mostly studied self selected physically active volunteers in specific exercise programmes.[10] In other words, we have accumulated data for what keeps people from starting a programme and what makes them stop; however, we know very little about what makes them start. Only two prospective studies were found that examined the factors that were important to adopting vigorous physical activity in adults.[10,11] In their earliest studies Sallis *et al.*[11] found that there were different predictors for adoption and maintenance of vigorous physical activity. Further, there were some shared similarities between men and women in predictors for adopting exercise but there also were some significant differences. Their second study[10] extended these findings and was more complete because of an expanded multivariate approach.

This study of 1719 mostly non-Hispanic white residents in San Diego, California, used a multivariate approach to predict adoption of physical activity, based on Bandura's social cognitive theory[12] and principles of operant learning.[13] Social cognitive theory takes into account that behaviour has multiple determinants that include biological variables (for example, sex, obesity, age), psychological variables (for example, intentions, beliefs), and external social and environmental variables (for example, weather, access to facilities and programmes). At baseline and follow up 2 years later, 25 indices of physiological, psychological, social, and environmental variables were assessed in addition to demographic, historical, and contemporary policy variables and self report measures of physical activity. Change measures were calculated for two groups of women and men: those between the ages of 18 and 49 and those of 50 years or older. This study confirmed the previous findings that predictors of change in vigorous physical activity are different for adoption and maintenance and that there are differences between men and women. More predictors were found for adoption than for maintenance. Specifically, self efficacy or exercise confidence and physical activity history were significant predictors for both men and women. For men, exercise adoption was predicted by age and neighbourhood environment. For women, adoption of vigorous exercise was predicted by years of education and by support from family and friends.

These findings have important implications for physical activity interventions. First, it is possible that interventions may need to be different for men and women, particularly for older men and less educated women. Second, interventions that emphasise social support may be more successful for women, and interventions that target the physical environment may lead to greater success for men.

These findings also are important because of similarities and differences with cross sectional studies.[14] In both cross sectional and prospective analyses, associations were found between self efficacy, age, education, social variables, and some environmental variables. However, relations were not found in the prospective analysis between physical activity and body mass index (BMI), exercise knowledge, smoking behaviour, alcohol use, dietary behaviour, and perceived barriers.

These results suggest several recommendations. First, more intervention studies are needed to test the sex differences and more prospective observational research could help clarify the discrepancies between prospective and cross sectional studies. Further, the paucity of data of this type underscores the need to conduct similar studies in populations that are associated with a higher rate of physical inactivity such as those who have less education, older adults, and non-white populations. Another recommendation concerns the type of physical activity. These studies examined vigorous physical activity. Cross sectional studies that have examined correlates of moderate intensity activity indicate that predictors for adopting moderate intensity activity may differ from those for adopting vigorous activity.[15] Longitudinal studies that identify predictors for adopting moderate intensity activity are also needed.

Personal level interventions—aspects of physical activity

Personal level interventions also show how various aspects of physical activity influence whether individuals begin a programme. Exercise guidelines developed by the American College of Sports Medicine prescribe large muscle aerobic exercise based on frequency, intensity, and duration.[16] Although understudied, there is some evidence that there may be different determinants of each of these components. Courneya and McAuley[17] examined this question in undergraduate volunteers at three time points by assessing self efficacy, attitude, intention, and effect based on modifications of the theory of planned behaviour.[18] Hierarchical regression analyses showed that self efficacy was the most important determinant for each of the three components and that it was a unique contributor to frequency and intensity but not duration. Intention was a stronger predictor of duration than of frequency and intensity. Attitude was a unique contributor to frequency and duration and positive effect was a unique contributor to intensity. These different predictors are likely to be important in moving individuals along the path of starting a programme of regular exercise. However, they may be important only to individuals who are already intending to start an exercise programme. Other aspects of activity might also be important and might have wider applicability to those not intending to start a programme of regular exercise. These include the types of activity and the format of those activities.

For example, King et al. compared higher intensity group based training, higher intensity home based training, and lower intensity home based training with controls.[19] For all intensities of activity, improvements in physical fitness were equivalent. However, participants in both of the home based conditions had significantly higher adherence rates for every month of the 12 month programme than participants in the higher intensity, group based programme. The advantages of home based programmes include greater convenience and flexibility compared to group based programmes. A more convenient format could enable a large number of individuals to begin a programme of regular physical activity.

Recently, the Centers for Disease Control and Prevention and the American College of Sports Medicine issued public health recommendations for physical activity, stating that individuals need to accumulate 30 minutes or more of moderate intensity activity on most, preferably all, days of the week.[20] The scientific foundation for this recommendation is based on consistent epidemiological findings that the greatest decrease in mortality risk comes by moving from the no activity category into the moderate activity category and observations that the prevalence of those engaging in vigorous activity has not increased since the fitness boom of the 1980s. One idea that has emerged from these recommendations is that individuals can engage in moderate intensity activities like brisk walking in several shorter bouts – for example, 10 minutes – several times over the course of the day. The hope is that by increasing the convenience and flexibility that more sedentary individuals will participate in activity.[21,22] While the impact of these recommendations has not been evaluated, the concept of using short bouts to increase participation has been tested in a recent study in overweight women.[23] In this study, participants were randomised to either a long bout or a short bout exercise group. The long bout group was instructed to progress from 20 to 40 minutes a day 5 days a week, and the short bout group were instructed to perform multiple 10 minute bouts to accumulate 20 to 40 minutes a day, 5 days a week. The length of the intervention was 20 weeks. The short bout group had significantly greater physical activity participation (35 minutes more a week), equivalent increases in physical fitness, and slightly greater weight loss than the long bout group.

These studies provide evidence that there are different determinants of the components of exercise prescription and that the types and formats of physical activity programmes do influence participation. The convenience and flexibility of home based programmes and use of shorter bouts are likely to play an important part in adoption of physical activity, but no published studies have specifically examined this question in relation to exercise adoption. More studies need to be conducted on how different aspects of physical activity might influence adoption in sedentary populations.

Personal level interventions—cognitive and behavioural aspects

The discussion on the types and formats of activities shows there has been an evolution in thinking about what kinds of activity are necessary to produce health benefits. Similarly there has been an evolution in our thinking about what is necessary to get people to adopt a physically active way of life. Few exercise scientists now believe that education alone will increase the proportion of individuals who engage in a programme of either moderate or vigorous physical activity. Since the 1980s, the proportion of individuals who engage in regular physical activity of a sufficient intensity has plateaued.[24] This has spurred the development of behavioural interventions to increase physical activity that is directed at the personal level. These interventions have evolved from theoretical, supervised, gym based interventions to theoretically driven, home and lifestyle interventions delivered through a variety of channels. In this section, I shall trace examples of this evolution and pinpoint important trends that have led to improvements in our understanding of how to get individuals to adopt a programme of regular physical activity.

One can see in table 4.1 that personal level interventions have moved from comparison of behavioural skill building techniques to theoretically driven interventions that use operationally defined valid behavioural measures, derived from theoretical constructs. For example, various paper and pencil assessments of self efficacy have been developed for physical activity.[25–27] Furthermore, as the table shows, several interventions use the concept of self efficacy to develop intervention strategies – for example, McAuley's use of social modelling,[28] and mastery accomplishments. The use of more sophisticated behavioural theories and models is one important trend.

In addition to the trend of moving from comparison of behavioural skills to theory driven interventions, another important trend has been comparison of various theories and use of regression analyses and path analysis techniques to determine what constructs predict adoption of physical activity. For example, Godin[29] examined the role of intention to exercise or participate in regular physical activity and showed that attitude-behaviour theories[30] predict 25–59% of the variance for participating in physical activity.[31] This work on theoretical models will enable us to develop better models of physical activity behaviour. This in turn

71

will help us develop more effective interventions.

This concept of intention has become more fully developed in the work of Marcus and colleagues,[27] who have adapted the transtheoretical model[32] to physical activity behaviour. This model includes many of the concepts from Bandura's social learning theory but also categorises individuals in terms of their motivational readiness to change. In the case of physical activity, individuals are classified as being in: *precontemplation*—not intending to change; *contemplation*—intending to change; *preparation*—doing some physical activity but not on a regular basis; *action*—accumulating 30 minutes of moderate intensity activity on most days of the week; or *maintenance*—having been in action for at least 6 months. This categorisation is an innovation for those who are interested in getting sedentary adults to be physically active because it changes our idea of exercise adoption from being an all or none phenomenon to being a continuous process. Knowing a person's stage of change allows those who are developing interventions to target sedentary populations more effectively and perhaps establish more realistic expectations of themselves and the population they are targeting. Marcus *et al.* have demonstrated the efficacy of this model in both worksite[33] and community interventions,[34] and it is my belief that this is a third important trend.

Use of the transtheoretical model is rapidly expanding. It was the basis for a mail mediated intervention conducted by Cardinal and Sachs[35] and the PAGE intervention.[36] We are currently conducting a randomised clinical trial, Project Active, that is comparing a 2 year traditional structured exercise intervention with a lifestyle intervention. Our 6 month results indicate that both types of intervention were able to move nearly 80% of the sedentary adults originally in contemplation into action. Furthermore, both of these groups had significant increases in fitness and physical activity at 6 months and similar significant decreases in cardiovascular risk factors.[37,38]

The intervention described by Cardinal and Sachs[35] and by Calfas and colleagues[36] is also indicative of a fourth important trend in personal level intervention – that is, the use of different channels for intervention – for example, mail mediated interventions and interventions by primary care physicians. Use of these different channels has not been well studied in the past, but new technologies, combined with theoretically driven interventions, will allow us to expand interventions in ways that have not been used in the past.

Table 4.1 Studies representing important trends in personal level behavioural interventions

Study	Representation	Intervention
Wysocki et al., 1979[39]	One of the earliest studies to use a behaviour change strategy	Contracts based on expectation. Attendance earned back deposited items
Epstein et al., 1980[40]	Example of comparison of behaviour change strategies	Compared contracting and lottery procedures with no treatment control. Higher attendance with both behaviour change strategies
King and Frederickson, 1984[41]	Example of comparison of behaviour and cognitive strategies	Compared social support and relapse prevention in a 2 x 2 design. Found either social support alone or relapse prevention alone predicted significant increases in jogging
Noland, 1989[42]	Example of behaviour change strategies	Compared self monitoring and reinforcement with unsupervised exercise. Both groups who received behavioural interventions increased fitness compared with the control group
King et al., 1988[43]	Example of one of the first home based interventions to determine the influence of social support strategies that were necessary for adoption of physical activity and increases in fitness	Compared two groups who both received relapse prevention strategies, daily self monitoring, adherence tips. One group received staff contact by telephone. Both groups increased the number of sessions and duration; however, only the group which received staff support by telephone increased fitness by 12 months
McAuley, 1992[44]	What is the role of self efficacy? Test of different types of self efficacy in adoption and maintenance of physical activity	General self efficacy and exercise self efficacy were found to have different roles in adoption and maintenance phase. Exercise self efficacy was most important in the adoption phase
McAuley et al., 1994[28]	What is the role of self efficacy? Examined effects of self efficacy based treatment on exercise adherence and self efficacy	Treatment was based on providing efficacy information from mastery accomplishments, social modelling, social persuasion, and interpretation of physiological states. These were compared with attention control. Found intervention had a direct effect on exercise adherence. The treatment was not found to have a direct effect on efficacy as a mediator

Table 4.1 Continued

Study	Representation	Intervention
Courneya and McAuley, 1993[45]	What is the role of self efficacy? Examined the role of exercise intentions on physical activity participation	Compared short range and longer range intentions to predict participation in physical activity. Shorter range intention is a better predictor than longer range intention
Valois et al., 1988[46]	Comparison of psychological theories	Compared theory of reasoned action[47] with Triandis model on exercise intention and behaviour. Support was found for both theories. Concluded exercise never becomes "automatic"; intention is associated with attitude, therefore it is important that any type of programme be positive and enjoyable
Marcus et al., 1992[27]	Use of concept of motivational readiness to adopt physical activity, "stages of change"	Examined the relation between stage of readiness to exercise and self reported physical activity and the relation between stage of readiness and self efficacy. Those in higher stages had higher self reported physical activity and higher self efficacy
Calfas et al., 1996[36]	One of the first physician counselling interventions to promote adoption of physical activity	This was an efficacy study to test the effects of the physician based assessment and counselling for exercise (PACE) protocol. PACE patients reported significantly more walking than control patients. Physician counselling can produce increases in physical activity in sedentary patients
Cardinal and Sachs, 1995[35]	Example of mail mediated intervention using stages of change	Examined three types of mail mediated exercise packets: lifestyle, structured, and fitness feedback. Regardless of group, participants in earlier stages improved their stage

To summarise, this section has identified four important trends in behavioural approaches to personal level interventions. These are: (1) increasing use of theories to develop interventions; (2) use of regression analyses and path analysis techniques to predict important factors for adoption of physical activity; (3) use of stages of motivational readiness to target interventions; and (4) use of different channels for personal level interventions. Clearly more work needs to be done in relation to the efficacy of these interventions, but we also need to begin to develop interventions to test their effectiveness – for example, how well will worksite and community interventions using stages of change materials generalise to other worksites and communities? We also need to continue to develop theories with more explanatory power to develop more effective interventions.

Interpersonal level approaches

Interpersonal approaches have not been widely used in physical activity interventions to get sedentary adults to be more physically active. These approaches focus on group – for example, families or class formats – and include involvement of peers in the format. For example, one study conducted by Nader and colleagues[48] targeted Mexican-American and Anglo-American families and randomly assigned half to a year long dietary education and physical activity intervention. Although physical activity was not significantly increased by this intervention, knowledge of exercise was increased. It is possible that family interventions such as these need to use less traditional approaches to increasing physical activity such as discussed above and should also incorporate stages of motivational readiness measures as part of outcome measures. More interventions targeting families need to be done.

In addition to intervening in families, use of peer counsellors may be another way to increase adoption of physical activity in the community. My search reveals there are no studies that have specifically examined physical activity adoption by using this type of approach. However, the approach has been used with other risk factor interventions such as the Zuni Indian diabetes project in New Mexico[49] and the heart, body, and soul project in East Baltimore.[50] Results from these programmes have been encouraging and they have been shown to increase physical activity. However, more work needs to be done with peer counsellor approaches to determine their effectiveness in getting individuals to adopt physical activity.

Organisational and community approaches

Interventions that are designed for the organisational and environmental level could include a change in rules – such as limiting car traffic in parks, expanding hours, and making facilities or programmes available to either enhance the behaviour or remove barriers.[5] Programmes offered in worksites and health maintenance organisations (HMO) are examples of these types of programme. In the United States, the government has established a physical activity objective for worksites for the year 2000.[51] This is one of the few physical activity goals that will be met by the year 2000 and this is probably due to the increase in employee wellness programmes, which include health risk appraisals (HRA), fitness facilities, and exercise programmes as part of sophisticated multifactorial interventions. (See Pelletier[52] for a review and analysis of health and cost effective outcomes studies on worksite health promotion programmes.)

Several studies have shown that it is possible to increase physical activity levels in the worksite.[53,54] However, a recent study that compared four different multifactor cardiovascular disease risk factor interventions at a worksite deserves mention. This study compared health risk assessment, risk factor education, behavioural counselling, and behavioural counselling plus incentives.[55] It was hypothesised that the behavioural counselling interventions would be superior to the health risk assessment and the risk factor education. In the case of increasing fitness, all groups significantly increased their aerobic fitness by 3 months and there were no differences between any of these groups. However, by the end of 12 months, fitness levels for all groups had returned to baseline. Use of health risk assessments was studied recently by Mayer and colleagues[56] in an HMO. In this study, a health risk appraisal combined with one face to face session and two follow up phone calls offered to elderly Medicare beneficiaries showed that individuals who received these sessions increased their level of physical activity significantly over 12 months compared with controls.

Both of these studies indicate that it is possible to increase the adoption of physical activity with these broad based approaches in targeted populations. However, the study by Gomel and colleagues[55] showed the importance of evaluating their effectiveness, particularly over time, since these same strategies may not be effective in helping to maintain the behaviour. More evaluations of these programmes need to be conducted to identify the important factors for physical activity adoption within these types of programme.

Multiple risk factor interventions aimed at reducing cardiovascular disease have also included a physical activity component. These have also been done in a number of community settings including the Pawtucket heart health programme,[57] the Stanford five cities project,[58] the Minnesota heart health programme,[59] the County health improvement project in Pennsylvania,[60] and the North Karelia project.[61] Most of these programmes have used a variety of the approaches described above and have shown modest increases in physical activity. The reader is referred to King[62] for a comprehensive review of these studies.

As part of these community based studies, some workers have used large scale mass media campaigns. To my knowledge only one study has evaluated the effects of such campaigns on increasing physical activity participation in the community.[63] This study evaluated the effects of two national campaigns conducted in 1990 and 1991. The goals of these campaigns were (1) to increase awareness of the message; (2) to increase physical activity participation in modern intensity activity; and (3) to increase the intention to become more physically active. The results from the 1990 campaign show that these goals were achieved, though not for all age groups for actual increases in physical activity participation. Only age groups 40 and over showed significant increases in physical activity participation after the 1990 campaign. Results from the 1991 campaign, however, only showed increases in awareness of the message, though this increase was a much smaller magnitude than the 1990 campaign. For example, the 1990 campaign showed message awareness before the campaign was 46% compared with 71% after. In 1991 message awareness was 63% before compared with 74% after. These results seem to indicate that it is possible to increase physical activity participation with large scale mass media campaigns; however, it is possible that these types of campaign might have limited effectiveness – that is, ceiling effects might have occurred as a result of the 1990 campaign. It is possible that more targeted approaches with different messages aimed at different stages of motivational readiness could be more effective. At this time, these approaches remain untried.

Environmental/policy approaches

Policy approaches refer to either explicit or implicit statements or rules that have been established at all levels of government. These approaches are more fully discussed by King and colleagues[6] and my search found that only one study evaluated changes in policy community wide. This evaluation compared building bicycle paths, extending hours at recreation facilities, installing new exercise equipment at gyms, scheduling broadly based athletic events, marking running courses throughout the community, and organising running and cycling clubs.[64] Release time and rewards for fitness improvements were authorised by commanding officers. There were significant improvements in fitness in the community that changed these policies compared with a similar community that did not incorporate any of these changes.

Many communities may be instituting these changes but few are evaluating the effects of these programmes on increasing physical activity participation. Evaluations of these policy changes need to be conducted to determine their effects on increasing the adoption of physical activity in sedentary populations.

Conclusions

In this chapter I have described important predictors of exercise adoption from observational studies. I have also described important factors that have been found to increase physical activity adoption at multiple levels including personal, interpersonal, organisational/community, and environmental/policy levels. Most interventions have been conducted at the personal level. For those wishing to begin programmes to increase physical activity for sedentary adults, it is important to determine the target population and the level of intervention; select a theory to guide intervention development; include components that will increase self efficacy and realistic outcome expectations; take into account motivational readiness of the target population; take into account important demographic factors such as education, socioeconomic status, and sex; and perform evaluations of methods and results.

1 Fletcher GF, Blair SN, Blumenthal J, *et al.* Position statement. Statement on exercise – benefits and recommendations for physical activity programs for all Americans. A statement for health professionals by the committee on Exercise and Cardiac Rehabilitation of the Council on Clinical Cardiology, American Heart Association. *Circulation* 1992;**86**:340–4.

2 Sallis JF, Hovell MF. Determinants of exercise behavior. *Exerc Sports Sci Rev* 1990;**18**:307–30.
3 Dishman RK. Compliance/adherence in health-related exercise. *Health Psychol* 1982;**1**:237–67.
4 Dishman RK, Sallis JF. Determinants and interventions for physical activity and exercise. In: Bouchard C, Shephard RJ, Stephens T, eds. *Physical activity, fitness, and health*. Champaign, Illinois: Human Kinetics, 1994:214–38.
5 King AC. Clinical and community interventions to promote and support physical activity participation. In: Dishman RK, ed. *Advances in exercise adherence*. Champaign, Illinois: Human Kinetics, 1994:183–212.
6 King AC, Fridinger F, Dusenbury L, *et al.* Environmental and policy approaches to cardiovascular disease prevention through physical activity: issues and opportunities. *Health Educ Q* 1995;**22**:499–511.
7 Winett RA, King AC, Altman DG. *Health psychology and public health: an integrative approach.* Elmsford, New York: Pergamon Press, 1989.
8 Dishman RK, Sallis JF, Orenstein DR. The determinants of physical activity and exercise. *Public Health Rep* 1985;**100**:158–72.
9 King AC, Blair SN, Bild DE, *et al.* Determinants of physical activity and interventions in adults. *Med Sci Sports Exerc* 1992;**24**(suppl):221–36.
10 Sallis JF, Hovell MF, Hofstetter CR. Predictors of adoption and maintenance of vigorous physical activity in men and women. *Prev Med* 1992;**21**:237–51.
11 Sallis JF, Haskell WL, Fortmann SP, *et al.* Predictors of adoption and maintenance of physical activity in a community sample. *Prev Med* 1986;**15**:331–41.
12 Bandura A. Self-efficacy: toward a unifying theory of behavior change. *Psychol Rev* 1977;**84**:192–215.
13 Skinner BF. *Science and human behavior.* New York: MacMillan, 1953.
14 Sallis JF, Hovwell MF, Hofstetter CR, *et al.* A multivariate study of determinants of vigorous exercise in a community sample. *Prev Med* 1989;**18**:20–34.
15 Hovell MF, Sallis JF, Hofstetter CR, *et al.* Identifying correlates of walking for exercise: an epidemiologic prerequisite for physical activity promotion. *Prev Med* 1989;**18**:856–66.
16 American College of Sports Medicine. The recommended quantity and quality of exercise for developing and maintaining cardiorespiratory and muscular fitness in healthy adults. *Med Sci Sports Exerc* 1990;**22**:265–74.
17 Courneya KS, McAuley E. Are there different determinants of the frequency, intensity, and duration of physical activity? *Behav Med* 1994;**20**:84–90.
18 Ajzen I. The theory of planned behavior. *Org Behav Human Dec Proc* 1991;**50**:179–211.
19 King AC, Haskell WL, Taylor CB, *et al.* Group vs home-based exercise training in healthy older men and women: a community-based clinical trial. *JAMA* 1991;**266**:1535–42.
20 Pate RR, Pratt M, Blair SN, *et al.* Physical activity and public health: a recommendation from the Centers for Disease Control and Prevention and the American College of Sports Medicine. *JAMA* 1995;**273**:402–7.
21 Blair SN, Kohl HW, Gordon NF. Physical activity and health: a lifestyle approach. *Med Exerc Nutr Health* 1992;**1**:54–7.
22 Blair SN, Kohl HW, Gordon NF, *et al.* How much physical activity is good for health? *Annu Rev Public Health* 1992;**13**:99–126.
23 Jakicic JM, Wing RR, Butler BA, *et al.* Prescribing exercise in multiple short bouts versus one continuous bout: effects on adherence, cardiorespiratory fitness, and weight loss in overweight women. *Int J Obes* 1995;**19**:893–901.
24 Stephens T. Physical activity and mental health in the United States and Canada: evidence from four population surveys. *Prev Med* 1988;**17**:35–47.
25 Garcia AW, King AC. Predicting long-term adherence to aerobic exercise: a

comparison of two models. *J Sport Exerc Psychol* 1991;**13**:394–410.

26 Sallis JF, Pinski RB, Grossman RM, *et al.* The development of self-efficacy scales for health related diet and exercise behaviors. *Health Educ Res* 1988;**3**:283–92.

27 Marcus BH, Selby VC, Niura RS, *et al.* Self-efficacy and the stages of exercise behavior change. *Res Q Exerc Sport* 1992;**63**:60–6.

28 McAuley E, Courneya KS, Rudolph DL, *et al.* Enhancing exercise adherence in middle-aged males and females. *Prev Med* 1994;**23**:498–506.

29 Godin G. Theories of reasoned action and planned behavior: usefulness for exercise promotion. *Med Sci Sports Exerc* 1994;**26**:1391–4.

30 Ajzen I, Fishbein M. *Understanding attitudes and predicting social behavior.* Englewood Cliffs, New Jersey: Prentice-Hall, 1980.

31 Godin G, Shephard RJ. Use of attitude-behaviour models in exercise promotion. *Sports Med* 1990;**10**:103–21.

32 Prochaska JO, DiClemente CC. The stages and processes of self-change in smoking: towards an integrative model of change. *J Consult Clin Psychol* 1983;**51**:390–5.

33 Marcus BH, Rossi JS, Selby VC, *et al.* The stages and processes of exercise adoption and maintenance in a worksite sample. *Health Psychol* 1992;**11**:386–95.

34 Marcus BH, Banspach SW, Lefebvre RC, *et al.* Using the stages of change model to increase the adoption of physical activity among community participants. *Am J Health Promotion* 1992;**6**:424–9.

35 Cardinal BJ, Sachs ML. Prospective analysis of stage-of-exercise movement following mail delivered, self-instructional exercise packets. *Am J Health Promotion* 1995;**9**:430–2.

36 Calfas KJ, Long BJ, Sallis JF, *et al.* A controlled trial of physician counseling to promote the adoption of physical activity. *Prev Med* 1996;**25**:225–33.

37 Garcia ME, Dunn AL, Kampert JB, Kohl HW, Blair SB. Changes in cardiovascular disease risk factors in a lifestyle versus a structured exercise intervention. *Med Sci Sports Exerc* 1996;**28**:S144.

38 Dunn AL, Kampert JB, Garcia ME, *et al.* Structures vs life-style approaches: 6 month physical activity and fitness changes. *Med Sci Sports Exerc* 1996;**28**:S145.

39 Wysocki T, Hall G, Iwata B, *et al.* Behavioral management of exercise: contracting for aerobic points. *J Appl Behav Anal* 1979;**12**:55–64.

40 Epstein LH, Wing RR, Thompson JK, *et al.* Attendance and fitness in aerobics exercise: the effects of contract and lottery procedures. *Behav Modif* 1980;**4**:465–79.

41 King AC, Frederiksen LW. Low-cost strategies for increasing exercise behavior: relapse preparation training and social support. *Behav Modif* 1984;**8**:3–21.

42 Noland MP. The effects of self-monitoring and reinforcement on exercise adherence. *Res Q Exerc Sport* 1989;**60**:216–24.

43 King AC, Taylor CB, Haskell WL, *et al.* Strategies for increasing early adherence to and longterm maintenance of home-based exercise training in healthy, middle-aged men and women. *Am J Cardiol* 1988;**61**:628–32.

44 McAuley E. The role of efficacy cognitions in the prediction of exercise behavior in middle aged adults. *J Behav Med* 1992;**15**:65–88.

45 Courneya KS, McAuley E. Can short-range intentions predict physical activity participation? *Percept Motor Skills* 1993;**77**:115–22.

46 Valois P, Desharnais R, Godin G. A comparison of the Fishbein and Ajzen and the Triandis attitudinal models for the prediction of exercise intention and behavior. *J Behav Med* 1988;**11**:459–72.

47 Fishbein M, Ajzen I. *Belief, attitude, intention and behavior: an introduction to theory and research.* Reading, Massachusetts: Addison-Wesley, 1975.

48 Nader PR, Sallis JF, Patterson TL, *et al.* A family approach to cardiovascular risk

reduction: results from the San Diego family health project. *Health Educ Q* 1989;**16**:229–44.

49 Heath GW, Leonard BE, Wilson RH, *et al.* Community-based exercise intervention: Zuni diabetes project. *Diabetes Care* 1987;**20**:579–83.

50 Levine DM, Becker DM, Bone LR, *et al.* Community-academic health center partnerships for underserved minority populations: one solution to a national crisis. *JAMA* 1994;**272**:309–14.

51 Public Health Service, Centers for Disease Control and Prevention, National Center for Health Statistics. *Healthy people 2000 review 1993.* Hyattsville, Maryland: National Center for Health Statistics, 1994.

52 Pelletier KR. A review and analysis of the health and cost-effective outcome studies of comprehensive health promotion and disease prevention programs at the worksite: 1993–1995 update. *Am J Health Promotion* 1996;**10**:380–8.

53 Blair SN, Piserchia PV, Wilbur CS, *et al.* A public health intervention model for work-site health promotion: impact on exercise and physical fitness in a health promotion plan after 24 months. *JAMA* 1986;**255**:921–6.

54 Altman DG, Evans AJ, Flora JA, *et al.* A worksite exercise content. In: *Proceedings of the Society of Behavioral Medicine's Seventh Annual Scientific Sessions.* Washington, DC: Society of Behavioral Medicine, 1994:38.

55 Gomel M, Oldenburg B, Simpson JM, *et al.* Work-site cardiovascular risk reduction: a randomized trial of health risk assessment, education, counseling, and incentives. *Am J Public Health* 1993;**83**:1231–8.

56 Mayer JA, Jermanovich A, Wright BL, *et al.* Changes in health behaviors of older adults: the San Diego Medicare preventive health project. *Prev Med* 1994;**23**:127–33.

57 Lefebvre RC, Lasater TM, Carleton RA. Theory and delivery of health programming in the community: the Pawtucket health program. *Prev Med* 1987;**16**:80–95.

58 Farquhar JW, Fortmann SP, Maccoby N. The Stanford five-city project: design and methods. *Am J Epidemiol* 1985;**122**:323–34.

59 Blackburn H, Luepker RV, Kline FG. The Minnesota health program: a research and demonstration project in cardiovascular disease prevention. In: Matarazzo JD, Weiss SM, Herd JA, eds. *Behavioral health: a handbook for health enhancement and disease prevention.* New York: John Wiley, 1984:1171–8.

60 Stunkard AJ, Felix MRJ, Cohen RY. Mobilizing a community to promote health: the Pennsylvania County health improvement program (CHIP). In: Rosen JC, Solomon LF, eds. *Prevention in health psychology.* Hanover, New Hampshire: University Press of New England, 1985:143–90.

61 Puska P, Nissinen A, Salonen JT. Ten years of the North Karelia project: results with community-based prevention of coronary heart disease. *Scand J Soc Med* 1983;**11**:65–8.

62 King AC. Community intervention for promotion of physical activity and fitness. *Exerc Sports Sci Rev* 1991;**19**:211–59.

63 Owen N, Bauman A, Booth M, *et al.* Serial mass-media campaigns to promote physical activity: reinforcing or redundant? *Am J Public Health* 1995;**85**:244–8.

64 Linenger JM, Chesson CV, Nice SN. Physical fitness gains following simple environmental change. *Am J Prev Med* 1991;7:298–310.

Multiple choice questions

Which of the following is true/false?

1 Becoming more active is simply a matter of deciding to exercise

2 Exercising in the gym is the only sensible method of getting started

3 The stages of change model is a useful theoretical construct but has yet to be validated

4 The four phases in becoming physically active are adoption, maintenance, improvement, and excellence

5 There are many studies exploring the barriers to physical activity

6 The factors encouraging people to be active are similar for men and women

7 People who exercise at home are more likely to continue than those who go to an organised class

8 Educating people about the benefits of physical activity is the key to increasing physical activity

9 Those who are sedentary and become active have relatively greater health gains than active people who become more active

10 There are many more people who are vigorously active now than there were in the 1980s

11 Mass media campaigns have rarely been shown to be effective

12 Interventions should be targeted differently at men and women

Answers are on p. 361.

5 Sudden death from cardiovascular disease in young athletes

S Sharma, G Whyte, W J McKenna

Introduction

The cardiovascular benefits of exercise are well established and epidemiological studies suggest that long term exercise programmes reduce the development of atheroma and the risk of sudden cardiac death (SCD).[1-5] It is well recognised that a small but significant proportion of athletes may die suddenly. The precise incidence of SCD in young athletes is unknown but estimates from the United States suggest that it is very low. Such tragedies are highly publicised, particularly when high profile athletes are involved, causing major concern in the general community who perceive athletes as the most healthy segment of society.[6] The sudden and unexpected death of athletes has evoked considerable interest among doctors and pathologists and led to the detection of a wide number of cardiovascular disorders causing sudden death in this population.[7-17]

Most non-traumatic sudden deaths in young athletes are due to inherited structural and functional cardiovascular abnormalities. Hypertrophic cardiomyopathy (HCM) accounts for 40–50% of all such deaths. Other well recognised causes include arrhythmogenic right ventricular cardiomyopathy, congenital anomalous coronary arteries, premature coronary artery disease, Wolff-Parkinson-White syndrome, long QT syndrome, myocarditis, and Marfan's syndrome (table 5.1). With the exception of mitral valve prolapse the prevalence of these inherited disorders in the general population is relatively low (table 5.2). The exact prevalence in athletes is unknown. Early identification of affected individuals should prevent sudden death. There is controversy about the extent of the problem, the significance of cardiovascular abnormalities detected at postmortem examination in athletes, and whether or not exercise related sudden death in apparently healthy individuals should be a cause for alarm in the sporting community.[18]

Definitions

Before proceeding further, it is prudent to define the terms "young", "competitive athlete", and "sudden cardiac death". Sporting individuals aged below 25 years will be classified as young. Although a substantial proportion of the population consider themselves to be athletes, we consider a competitive athlete as an individual who participates in an organised team or individual sport in which regular competition is a component.[19] SCD is defined as an event that is non-traumatic, non-violent, unexpected, and resulting from sudden cardiac arrest within 6 hours of previously witnessed normal health.

SCD in young athletes is thought to be uncommon, but precise data on its exact incidence are lacking. Estimates from the United States suggest an incidence of 1 in 200 000.[20–22] This is unlikely to represent the true incidence for several reasons. When faced with SCD in a young athlete, the coroner's mandate is to exclude foul play rather than provide the cause of death. An expert pathologist with experience of conditions causing SCD is rarely responsible for carrying out postmortem examination, thus subtle conditions may not be detected. The cause of death is difficult to ascertain in conditions predisposing to fatal cardiac arrhythmias, and SCD in the absence of structural cardiac abnormalities—for example, the long QT syndrome. Furthermore, the evident lack of a systematic national registry for SCD in athletes means that the compilation of statistics on SCD relies heavily on reports from the media, which usually concentrate on the most elite athletes rather than the general young athletic population, and on voluntary referrals from hospital based pathology registries. Such crude methods of data collection undoubtedly lead to a significant underestimation of exercise related SCDs.

Some 80% of non-traumatic sudden deaths in young competitive athletes are due to inherited or congenital structural or functional cardiovascular abnormalities, most of which provide a pathological substrate for fatal cardiac arrhythmias predisposing to sudden death. A proportion of affected athletes are capable of

Table 5.1   Causes of sudden cardiac death in young competitive athletes

Common	Uncommon
Hypertrophic cardiomyopathy	Myocarditis
Idiopathic concentric left ventricular hypertrophy	Premature coronary artery disease
	Long QT syndrome
Coronary artery anomalies	Marfan's syndrome (aortic rupture)
Arrhythmogenic right ventricular cardiomyopathy*	Mitral valve prolapse

*Commonest cause of death in northern Italy.

incredibly high levels of performance, and reports on the sudden deaths of athletes have shown that many had competed at intercollegiate, professional, and national level (table 5.1).

The majority of deaths occur during or immediately after strenuous physical activity, suggesting that exercise is a strong trigger factor for cardiac arrhythmias in athletes harbouring potential lethal cardiac conditions. Most deaths occur in men. This may be due to a higher participation rate and competition in more rigorous sports compared with women. Most athletes are allegedly asymptomatic before death. In a recent review of SCD in 157 young athletes (mean age 17) in the United States between 1985 and 1995, 90% died during or immediately after a training session and only 18% had prodromal symptoms thought to be cardiovascular in origin in the preceding 36 months.[23] The lack of prodromal symptoms may be due to underreporting on the part of the victim through fear of being perceived as "unfit" by sporting bodies, or, more importantly, to false reassurance as the result of the triviality attached to potentially serious symptoms by medical practitioners who perceive athletes to be extremely healthy. An apparently healthy young athlete presenting with chest pain or syncope during exertion is often inappropriately reassured rather than investigated.

The commonest cause of SCD in young athletes is hypertrophic cardiomyopathy, which accounts for between 40% and 50% of deaths.[1,7,23] Other important causes include arrhythmogenic right ventricular cardiomyopathy, coronary artery anomalies, Wolff-Parkinson-White syndrome, long QT syndrome, Marfan's syndrome, mitral valve prolapse, myocarditis, and premature coronary artery disease. Premature coronary artery disease is the most predominant cause of death in older athletes.[24,25]

Table 5.2   Prevalence of inherited or congenital cardiovascular disorders associated with sudden death

Condition	Estimated prevalence	Estimate no affected in United Kingdom
HCM	1/500	100 000
ARVC	1/10 000	5000
Wolff-Parkinson-White syndrome	1.5/1000	75 000
Long QT syndrome	?*	?
CAA	?	?
Mitral valve prolapse	2/100	1 000 000
Marfan's syndrome	1/5000	10 000

*Incidence of long QT syndrome is between 1/10 000 and 1/15 000 but the prevalence is unknown.

Hypertrophic cardiomyopathy

Hypertrophic cardiomyopathy (HCM) is defined as ventricular hypertrophy in the absence of a cardiac or systemic cause.[26] It is inherited as an autosomal dominant trait with a high degree of penetrance. Missense mutations within genes encoding six different cardiac sarcomeric contractile proteins are responsible for the disease. These include β myosin heavy chain, cardiac troponin T, cardiac troponin I, troponin light chain, α tropomyosin, and myosin binding protein C.[27] The most common pattern of hypertrophy is asymmetric septal but almost any pattern is possible.[28,29] Left ventricular outflow tract obstruction secondary to systolic anterior motion of the mitral valve apparatus is present in 20%. The histological hallmark of the disease is myocyte and myofibrillar disarray, which contributes to a variety of pathophysiological disturbances and electrical instability.[30,31] The prevalence of the disease in young adults is 0.2%, which means there are about 100 000 affected individuals in the United Kingdom.[32]

Box 5.1   SCD in athletes

- SCD in athletes is uncommon
- 80% of non-traumatic sudden deaths are attributed to inherited or congenital cardiovascular disorders
- 40–50% of all deaths are from hypertrophic cardiomyopathy
- Most deaths occur during or immediately after physical activity
- Prodromal symptoms of cardiovascular disease may be absent

Box 5.2 Symptoms of cardiovascular disease

- Chest pain on exertion
- Disproportionate breathlessness in relation to the exercise being performed
- Dizziness on exertion
- Syncopal episodes during or after exertion
- Palpitations

Chest pain and dyspnoea are the commonest symptoms of HCM. Other symptoms include palpitation, dizziness on exertion, and syncope. The majority of young patients are asymptomatic or have minor symptoms.[33,34] Physical examination is helpful in those individuals with left ventricular outflow tract obstruction for which palpation of the carotid artery may show up a jerky pulse, and palpation and auscultation of the pericardium may detect a double apical impulse and a harsh ejection systolic murmur, respectively.

Sudden death is often the first presentation. Data from referral institutions show a death rate of about 2.5% a year, reaching a maximum of 6% during childhood and adolescence. The exact death rate among young athletes is not known but is probably significantly higher than in the non-exercising population. In a study comparing sports related and non-sports related SCD in young athletes, HCM was a much more common cause of death in sports related deaths than in non-sports related deaths: eight of 34 deaths compared with 20 of 656 (P=0.00019).[36] The highly significant increase in exercise related sudden death from HCM in young athletes suggests that the propensity to life threatening supraventricular and ventricular arrhythmias resulting from myocardial disarray may be triggered by the stress of exercise.

The antagonist for HCM being an important cause of SCD may argue that left ventricular hypertrophy is common in athletes participating in regular endurance sport, and there is a possibility that postmortem demonstration of ventricular hypertrophy is often falsely attributed to HCM rather than physiological adaptation to exercise.[18] However, physiological hypertrophy is usually mild, and left ventricular hypertrophy exceeding 13 mm is rare even in the most elite athletes.[37-39] Major publications documenting HCM as the cause of death have based their findings on the demonstration of gross left ventricular hypertrophy with a heart weight usually

87

exceeding 500 g or a maximum left ventricular wall thickness of 20 mm in the absence of a dilated ventricular cavity, together with histological evidence of extensive myocardial disarray and scarring.[7-9,11,23] To date there is a conspicuous lack of reputable reports on athletes with a ventricular wall thickness exceeding 16 mm or left ventricular mass exceeding 400 g.

Patients with HCM have extensive disarray with about 20% of the myocardium affected. There are reports on SCD in athletes where postmortem examination has shown concentric left ventricular hypertrophy with a wall thickness range of 15–19 mm, a non-dilated left ventricular cavity, and a modest increase in left ventricular mass with heart weights between 400 g and 490 g. Histological examination of the myocardium has failed to detect myocardial disarray, and the cause of SCD in this group has been classified under a separate entity termed "idiopathic concentric ventricular hypertrophy" even though the macroscopic findings are compatible with the diagnosis of HCM.[7-9] Most affected athletes have been black, and it is possible that these changes may be an exaggerated race related response to undetected hypertension during life.[40] Alternatively, the protagonists for HCM causing SCD in athletes may argue that these cases represent mild or atypical forms of HCM.[41-43] The latter is in keeping with the fact that HCM is a significantly more common cause of SCD in young black athletes.[23]

The genetic heterogeneity of HCM currently makes it impractical to perform genetic testing on all individuals suspected of having HCM. Two dimensional echocardiography and Doppler studies continue to serve as the gold standard test for the diagnosis of HCM. The demonstration of left ventricular hypertrophy with a wall thickness exceeding 15 mm and a small left ventricular cavity is usually diagnostic. Additional features such as systolic anterior motion of the mitral valve, redundant mitral valve leaflets, a gradient across the left ventricular outflow tract, and Doppler evidence of abnormal ventricular filling may also be present.

The autosomal dominant inheritance of HCM makes it prudent that all first degree relatives of patients with HCM are screened for the condition with echocardiography. Thus athletes with affected first degree relatives should be offered screening. The early diagnosis of HCM in competitive athletes should reduce the death rate by preventing affected individuals from participating in vigorous training and further competition[44] and, where appropriate, undergoing treatment to prevent sudden death.[45]

Differentiation of the normal athlete's heart from the condition of HCM with non-invasive cardiac tests

Regular physical training induces structural and functional cardiac changes as part of a normal adaptive physiological process which may simulate cardiac pathology.[46–49] The structural features of an athlete's heart include a 10% increase in left ventricular cavity, 10–20% increase in left ventricular wall thickness, and a 45% increase in left ventricular mass.[39] Although cavity dilatation and hypertrophy are common, absolute cardiac dimensions are usually within normal limits irrespective of body surface area. In a few cases, left ventricular hypertrophy is quite pronounced and may raise the differential diagnosis of HCM. This is highlighted by a recent echocardiographic study involving 947 elite Italian athletes in which about 2% had left ventricular hypertrophy of between 13 mm and 15 mm.[37–39] The distinction between the athlete's heart and HCM in this rare situation has important implications because identification of HCM in an athlete may be the basis of disqualification from competition to minimise the risk of sudden death. An erroneous diagnosis of HCM in an athlete may lead to unnecessary withdrawal from sport with profound consequences in terms of physical, financial, and psychological wellbeing.

A large number of studies on elite athletes have led to proposed echocardiographic criteria for the differentiation of physiological hypertrophy from HCM (table 5.3). However, there are cases where echocardiography cannot reliably differentiate physiological from pathological hypertrophy, and, if undue reliance is placed on this investigation alone, then there is a risk of generating false positives and false negatives. Additional information from family history and the 12 lead electrocardiograph may be helpful in these circumstances. The demonstration of HCM in a first degree relative of an athlete with left ventricular hypertrophy will increase the possibility of the diagnosis of HCM. Voltage criteria of left ventricular hypertrophy and ST segment repolarisation changes on the electrocardiogram (ECG) are common in both conditions; however, the presence of prominent Q waves, left bundle branch block, and deep T wave inversion favours the diagnosis of HCM.

Despite the ECG criteria, there are cases where differentiation of the normal athlete's heart from HCM remains difficult. A definitive method of resolving the diagnosis is demonstration of regression of ventricular hypertrophy after a 3 month period of detraining, a feature characteristic of physiological but not

Table 5.3 Differentiation of the normal athlete's heart from hypertrophic cardiomyopathy (HCM) by using non-invasive cardiac testing

Measure	Athlete's heart	HCM
Left atrial dimension	Common	Unusual
LVH (mm)	<16	>16
Patterns of LVH	Concentric	Heterogeneous distribution
LV cavity size in diastole (mm)	>55	<45
Indices of diastolic function	Enhanced	Reduced
ECG patterns	Large complexes. Voltage LVH (Sokolow) in absence of deep T wave inversion in left precordial leads	Large complexes. Voltage criteria LVH and deep T wave inversion in left precordial leads
	Elevation of J point	ST depression or ST elevation. Q waves
	Right axis deviation	Leftward axis
	RV conduction delay	Partial LBBB

LV = left ventricular; LVH = left ventricular hypertrophy; LBBB = left bundle branch block.
Sokolow criterion for LVH is present when sum of RVI + SV6 > 35 mV.

pathological hypertrophy.[50] This is usually unacceptable to the athlete striving to achieve honours in competitive sport because it hinders fitness and team selection, but it may be feasible during injury or during the off season. Future developments in molecular genetics should allow DNA testing in all individuals with suspected HCM. In the meantime, the development of more specific and sensitive cardiac tests for differentiation between physiological and pathological hypertrophy may obviate the need to detrain.

Arrhythmogenic right ventricular cardiomyopathy

Arrhythmogenic right ventricular cardiomyopathy (ARVC) is a heart muscle disorder characterised by patchy fibrofatty replacement of right ventricular myocardium. The replacement of myocardium by fatty tissue predisposes to inhomogeneous and fatal re-entrant ventricular arrhythmias.[51] It is the commonest cause of exercise related SCD in young athletes in the Veneto region of northern Italy.[52-54] The strong association with strenuous physical activity incriminates exercise as a trigger factor for arrhythmias. The exact incidence and prevalence are unknown, but the prevalence is estimated to be 1 in 10 000, which means there are potentially 5000 affected individuals in the United Kingdom. In about 30–50% of cases the condition is familial, the commonest pattern of inheritance being autosomal dominant,[55-57] although an autosomal recessive pattern has also been described.[58] The main clinical features are palpitation, dyspnoea, presyncope, syncope, and sudden death.[59,60] The results of physical examination are usually normal. The definitive diagnosis of ARVC relies on histological demonstration of transmural fibrofatty replacement of ventricular myocardium. This is difficult in most living patients and not without risk of perforation. Diagnosis based on endomyocardial biopsy may generate false negatives because of the segmental nature of the disease. In addition, the potential errors in histological interpretation means that an expert pathologist with ample experience in ARVC histology is generally necessary. The limitations of histological diagnosis means that diagnosis before death usually relies on the combination of cardiovascular symptoms, family history of ARVC, electrocardiographic evidence of T wave inversion in the right precordial leads, multiple ventricular ectopics or ventricular tachycardia of left bundle branch block morphology,[61,62] delayed potentials on the signal averaged ECG,[63] and demonstration of abnormalities of the right ventricle with cardiac imaging techniques.[64–68]

The diagnosis of ARVC in a competitive athlete is an indication for disqualification from competitive sport to prevent sudden death. Individuals with persistent life threatening ventricular arrhythmias are managed with anti-arrhythmic medication or by implantation of an automatic cardioverter defibrillator.[69]

Differentiation of the normal athlete's heart from the condition of ARVC with non-invasive cardiac tests

Some highly trained athletes may show right ventricular enlargement[70] and a variety of repolarisation ECG changes in the right precordial leads, raising the differential diagnosis of ARVC. In this situation the demonstration of right ventricular aneurysms, hypokinetic segments, or gross dilatation would support the diagnosis of ARVC, whereas the presence of mild global enlargement together with a slightly dilated hypertrophied left ventricle with good systolic function would be more in keeping with the athlete's heart.

Congenital coronary artery anomalies (CAAs)

Sudden death can complicate anomalous insertion of the coronary arteries, particularly when the left coronary artery originates from the anterior sinus of Valsalva.[7–9] In a review of 51 cases of CAAs there were nine sudden deaths. All deaths occurred either during or just after physical activity. In all nine cases the left coronary artery arose from the anterior sinus of Valsalva.[71] The acute leftward passage of the coronary artery along the aortic wall is thought to cause the entrance into the left coronary system to be slit-like. During exercise there is stretching of the left coronary artery and a flap-like closure of the orifice of the left coronary artery causing myocardial ischaemia. There were no deaths when both coronaries arose from the left coronary sinus of Valsalva in this study, but there have been reports of SCD in this type of CAA.[72] Before these reports, CAAs were thought to be minor and associated with a normal life expectancy. CAA is now recognised as the second most common cause of SCD in young athletes in the United States. Most affected patients are asymptomatic, but some may present with exercise induced chest pain, fatigue, and collapse. Exercise testing rarely shows up inducible myocardial ischaemia.[73] The visualisation of the left main stem and right coronary artery is important in the evaluation of all symptoms of athletes suggestive of a cardiovascular abnormality. This is achieved by non-invasive means on the short axis views of the aortic root on two dimensional echocardiography. Magnetic resonance imaging is useful in demonstrating CAA in cases where echocardiography fails to do so. Detection and correction of this anomaly can prevent SCD.

Premature coronary artery disease

Coronary atherosclerosis is a rare cause of SCD in young athletes.[74] Almost all individuals have a family history of premature coronary artery disease from hypercholesterolaemia. SCD is almost always the first presentation. Prodromal symptoms of myocardial ischaemia are rare, and most individuals are free from established risk factors for coronary artery disease. This is in contrast with older athletes in whom prodromal symptoms are common, and risk factors are identified in about 50%.[11] ECG and exercise testing performed before death on young athletes with premature coronary artery disease have often failed to show evidence of myocardial ischaemia.

Death is usually from single vessel disease, predominantly affecting the left anterior descending artery. The macroscopic findings show obstructive atheromatous lesions with acute thrombosis superimposed on a ruptured atheromatous plaque.

Wolff-Parkinson-White syndrome

Wolff-Parkinson-White syndrome is characterised by an accessory conduction pathway with a predilection to re-entrant supraventricular tachyarrhythmias which may precipitate ventricular fibrillation.[75,76] It is reported as a rare cause of sudden death in athletes. This may be due to failure to identify or appreciate abnormalities of cardiac conduction tissue disease at postmortem examination. Affected patients may present with rapid palpitation, presyncope, or syncope. Wolff-Parkinson-White syndrome can be identified by the presence of δ waves and a short PR interval on the ECG. Exercise testing is useful for predicting the risk of fatal arrhythmias. High risk pathways should be investigated further by electrophysiological studies. Radiofrequency ablation of the accessory is the therapeutic technique most widely used and is particularly attractive for athletes in whom antiarrhythmic agents prove ineffective because of the high sympathetic drive.

Long QT syndrome

The long QT syndrome is a rare familial disorder characterised by prolongation of the QT interval (>440 msec; corrected) on the ECG, and the propensity to syncope and fatal ventricular arrhythmias.[77,80] The prevalence of the disorder is between 1/10 000 and 1/15 000. Both autosomal dominant and autosomal recessive modes of inheritance are recognised. In 10% of cases it is a result of de novo genetic mutations. Mutations on at least four gene loci located on chromosomes 3, 4, 7, and 11 have been identified. The mutations result in defective sodium or potassium channels within cardiac myocytes and are the basis of fatal cardiac rhythm disturbances. The clinical course is variable, ranging from malignant ventricular arrhythmias with recurrent syncope and sudden death in some patients to an asymptomatic course throughout life. Syncope is usually due to polymorphic ventricular tachycardia, which, in most patients, is initiated by acute auto-somic change precipitated by fear, sudden auditory stimuli, intense emotion, and physical exertion. Patients at high risk are those with a history of syncope and a strong family history of syncope and premature sudden death. Cardiac morphology is normal, and therefore postmortem identification is not usually possible in the absence of ECG information before death or a family history of the condition.

Affected individuals can be identified by ECG. Twenty four hour ambulatory ECG recordings and exercise testing may be helpful in evaluating the seriousness of the disorder. Recent advances in the molecular genetics of the long QT syndrome should prove helpful in the preclinical diagnosis of young patients at risk and in the diagnosis of equivocal or sporadic cases. Avoidance of vigorous physical activity and treatment with β blockers may prevent sudden death in athletes who are identified early.

Myocarditis

Myocarditis is a rare cause of exercise related SCD in young athletes. Viruses and occasionally drugs have been implicated as the cause.[81] Most deaths are related to strenuous physical activity. Myocardial inflammation with lymphocytic infiltration and focal necrosis shown at postmortem examination may be the substrate for exercise induced arrhythmias. Symptoms are non-specific, with coryzal symptoms or a mild febrile illness predominating the clinical picture. Specific signs include tachycardia, evidence of cardiomegaly, and rarely cardiac failure. The ECG information is non-specific but may show cardiac arrhythmias. In severe cases, there may be evidence of ventricular dilatation and impairment at echocardiography, but there are cases where the ECG is entirely normal,[82] and therefore a high index of suspicion is required if deaths caused by myocarditis are to be prevented. All athletes with coryzal symptoms or a febrile illness should be rested until completely asymptomatic.

Marfan's syndrome

Marfan's syndrome is an inherited connective tissue disorder characterised by skeletal, ocular, and cardiac abnormalities. The gene is located in the long arm of chromosome 15 and encodes the glycoprotein fibrillin. The prevalence based on clinical criteria is 1 in 5000. Affected patients are excessively tall, have chest wall abnormalities, kyphoscoliosis, arachnodactyly, and high arched palates. Lens dislocation is common. Cardiac involvement is almost always characterised by mitral valve prolapse with or without mitral regurgitation. Aortic root dilatation is a potentially serious cardiac manifestation, and sudden death is usually from aortic dissection or rupture. There may be a family history of premature sudden death. Physical examination should raise suspicion of Marfan's syndrome. Patients should be referred for assessment of the aortic root by echocardiography. Prophylactic surgery is indicated once the aortic root diameter exceeds 6 cm. Abstinence from competitive sport and treatment with β blockers may retard aortic dilatation and prevent death from aortic rupture.

Mitral valve prolapse

Mitral valve prolapse is extremely common in the general population. It is thought to affect up to 5% of the population. The condition is generally benign, but there are 60 cases of SCD in the medical literature thought to be associated with mitral valve prolapse. Only four deaths occurred in young individuals, and in only three of the 60 cases was death related to exercise.[83] Symptoms include atypical sharp inframammary chest pain, fatigue, dizziness, and occasionally syncope. Mitral valve prolapse can be clinically detected by auscultation and confirmed by echocardiography. Controversy remains about its association with

SCD. The detection of mitral valve prolapse after sudden death may be coincidental rather than causal, or it may be due to its association with Wolff-Parkinson-White syndrome or long QT syndrome. The approach to mitral valve prolapse in relation to participation in competitive sport should be pragmatic. In the absence of symptoms and signs and a family history of sudden death, full participation is allowed. It would be reasonable to disqualify athletes with a history of syncope, disabling chest pain, complex ventricular arrhythmias, significant mitral regurgitation, prolonged QT interval, Marfan's syndrome, and a family history of sudden death.

Screening and prevention of sudden death

The incidence of cardiovascular conditions predisposing to SCD is low. The ultimate question remains whether all cases of SCD could be prevented if every competitive athlete was screened for cardiovascular disease. The Italian experience is of interest in this

---

Box 5.3 Cardiovascular assessment of an athlete

- Screening for cardiovascular disease is warranted in athletes with symptoms of cardiovascular origin and a family history of premature (<40 years) non-traumatic sudden death
- Initial screening should involve thorough cardiovascular examination with particular reference to blood pressure and cardiac murmurs, 12 lead ECG, and two dimensional echocardiography
- Physical examination will detect forms of HCM with obstruction (20–25%) valvular disorders, and Marfan's syndrome with or without cardiovascular involvement
- The ECG is abnormal but not diagnostic in almost all patients with HCM and 90% of patients with ARVC
- The presence of a long QT interval or accessory pathway on the 12 lead ECG should raise the suspicion of the long QT syndrome and Wolff-Parkinson-White syndrome, respectively, and should prompt referral to a specialist cardiology unit for further evaluation with exercise testing and electrophysiological studies
- Echocardiography with particular reference to left ventricular thickness, right ventricular architecture and function, aortic root dimension, and demonstration of the origins of the coronary arteries will detect all HCM, Marfan's syndrome, mitral valve prolapse, and a large proportion of ARVC and CAA
- Further invasive diagnostic investigations may be warranted in some individuals

---

respect because all young athletes require an annual certificate of fitness based on a normal physical examination, normal ECG, and a limited exercise test. The systematic evaluation shows that HCM is a very rare cause of SCD in young athletes. This contrasts with published reports from other countries showing that HCM is by far the commonest cause of SCD. One interpretation is that individuals with HCM are identified early and excluded from sporting activities by the requirements of the Italian fitness certificate.[84] Similarly the potential of detecting Wolff-Parkinson-White syndrome and long QT syndrome on ECG during such fitness screens may reduce the incidence of sudden death from these conditions.

The financial constraints of public health services mean that large scale screening programmes are not cost effective; a substantial number of athletes would need to be screened to detect a small proportion at risk of SCD.[85-87] This should not deter major independent financially endowed sporting bodies from protecting their athletes by providing funds for cardiovascular screening because a significant proportion of deaths occur in the absence of symptoms. Where cost is a major issue, raising public awareness of the risk of SCD in athletes with emphasis on the warning features may be more practical. Athletes with a family history of premature sudden death or symptoms of palpitation, chest pain disproportionate breathlessness in relation to the intensity of the exercise being performed, dizziness, or syncope should undergo evaluation in a specialist cardiology centre to exclude underlying cardiovascular disease. Initial investigation with ECG will detect Wolff-Parkinson-White syndrome and long QT syndrome.

Echocardiography with particular reference to left ventricular wall thickness, right ventricular architecture and function, aortic root dimension, and demonstration of the origins of the coronary arteries will detect all HCM, Marfan's syndrome, mitral valve prolapse, and a large proportion of ARVC and CAA. Further invasive diagnostic investigations may be warranted in some individuals. Many athletes at risk may not present with warning features, but many will, and greater sensitivity and awareness within the athletic community should improve identification of those athletes who are at risk of sudden death.

Conclusion

SCD in athletes is rare, but the true incidence of the problem is not known. Most deaths are due to HCM. SCD from HCM is more common in athletic than in sedentary individuals. Exercise is a recognised trigger of fatal arrhythmias culminating in sudden death. There have been claims that ventricular hypertrophy from physiological adaptation to exercise may be misinterpreted as HCM when detected at postmortem examination; however, the diagnosis of HCM in athletes who die suddenly has been based on the demonstration of gross ventricular hypertrophy, massive left ventricular mass, and histological evidence of widespread myocardial disarray, fibrosis, and scarring, none of which are characteristic of physiological hypertrophy. In addition to HCM, there are several other recognised cardiovascular abnormalities that predispose to sudden death in athletes. Early identification of all causes of SCD in young athletes should help to prevent death by allowing the recommendation of abstinence from vigorous exercise and, if appropriate, initiation of medical treatment. Individuals with symptoms suggestive of cardiovascular disease or those with a family history of premature sudden death should undergo thorough cardiovascular evaluation at a specialist centre.

1 Paffenbarger RS, Hyde RT, Wing AL, Hsieh CC. Physical activity, all cause mortality and longevity of college alumni. *N Engl J Med* 1986;**314**:605–13.
2 Slattery ML, Jacobs DR, Nichmann MZ. Leisure time physical activity and coronary artery disease. The US railroad study. *Circulation* 1989;**79**:304–11.
3 Morris JN, Clayton DG, Everitt MG, Semmence AM, Burgess EH. Exercise in leisure time: coronary attack and death rates. *Br Heart J* 1990;**63**:325–34.
4 Siskovick DS, Weiss NS, Fletcher RH. The incidence of primary cardiac arrest during vigorous exercise. *N Engl J Med* 1994;**311**:874–7.
5 Powell KE, Thompson PD, Caspersen CJ, Kendrick JS. Physical activity and the incidence of coronary artery disease. *Annu Rev Public Health* 1987;**8**:253–87.
6 Maron BJ. Sudden death in athletes: lessons from the Hank Gathers affair. *N Engl J Med* 1993;**329**:55–7.
7 Maron BJ, Roberts WC, McAllister HA, Rosing DR, Epstein SE. Sudden death in young athletes. *Circulation* 1980;**62**:218–29.
8 Maron BJ, Epstein SE, Roberts WC. Causes of death in competitive athletes. *J Am Coll Cardiol* 1986;**7**:204–14.
9 Tsung SH, Huang TY, Chang MH. Sudden death in young athletes. *Arch Pathol Lab Med* 1982;**106**:168–70.
10 Corrado D, Thiene G, Nava A, Rossi L, Pennelli N. Sudden death in young competitive athletes: clinicopathologic correlations in 22 cases. *Am J Med* 1990;**89**:588–96.
11 Burke AP, Farb A, Virmani R. Causes of sudden death in athletes. *Cardiol Clin* 1992;**10**:303–17.
12 Hillis W, McIntyre PD, Maclean J, Goodwin JF, McKenna WJ. ABC of sports medicine. Sudden death in sport. *BMJ* 1994;**309**:657–60.
13 Opic LH. Sudden death and sport. *Lancet* 1975;**i**:263–6.
14 Northcote RJ, Ballantyne D. Sudden cardiac death in sport. *BMJ* 1983;**287**:1357–9.
15 Van Camp SP, Bloor CM, Mueller FO, Cantu RC, Olson HG. Non traumatic

sports death in high school and college athletes. *Med Sci Sports Exerc* 1995;**27**:641–7.

16 James TN, Froggat P, Marshall TK. Sudden death. *Ann Intern Med* 1982;**106**:168–70.

17 Furlanello F, Bettini R, Cozzi F, Del Favero A, Disertori M, Vergara G, *et al.* Ventricular arrhythmias and sudden death in athletes. *Ann N Y Acad Sci* 1984;**427**:253–79.

18 Shephard RJ. The athlete's heart: is big beautiful? *Br J Sports Med* 1996;**30**:5–10.

19 Maron BJ, Epstein SE, Mitchell JH. The competitive athlete with cardiovascular disease: definitions, guidelines, and considerations. Introduction to Bethesda Conference No 16. *J Am Coll Cardiol* 1986;**6**:1189–90.

20 Epstein SE, Maron BJ. Sudden death and the competitive athlete: perspectives on preparticipation screening studies. *J Am Coll Cardiol* 1986;**7**:220–30.

21 Braden DS, Strong WB. Preparticipation screening for sudden cardiac death in high school and college athletes. *Physician and Sportsmedicine* 1988;**16**:128–40.

22 Ades PA. Preventing sudden death. *Physician and Sportsmedicine* 1992;**20**:75–9.

23 Maron BJ, Shirani J, Poliac LC, Mathenge R, Roberts WC, Mueller FO. Sudden death in young competitive athletes. Clinical, demographic, and pathological profiles. *JAMA* 1996;**276**:199–204.

24 Waller BF, Roberts WC. Sudden death whilst running in conditioned runners aged 40 years or over. *Am J Cardiol* 1980;**45**:1292–300.

25 Noakes TD, Opie HL, Rose AG. Autopsy proved coronary atherosclerosis in marathon runners. *N Engl J Med* 1979;**310**:86–95.

26 Report of the WHO/ESFC task force on the definition and classification of cardiomyopathies. *Circulation* 1996;**93**:841–2.

27 McKenna WJ, Watkins HC. In: Scriver CR, Beaudet AL, Sly WS, Valle E, eds. *The metabolic and molecular bases of inherited disease.* 7th ed. Volume III. New York: McGraw-Hill Inc, 1995:4523–72.

28 Shapiro LM, McKenna WJ. Distribution of left ventricular hypertrophy in hypertrophic cardiomyopathy: a two-dimensional echocardiographic study. *J Am Coll Cardiol* 1983;**2**:437–44.

29 Maron BJ, Gottdiener JS, Epstein SE. Patterns and significance of distribution of left ventricular hypertrophy in hypertrophic cardiomyopathy. A wide angle, 2-dimensional echocardiographic study of 125 patients. *Am J Cardiol* 1981;**48**:418–28.

30 Davies MJ. The current status of myocardial disarray in hypertrophic cardiomyopathy. *Br Heart J* 1984;**51**:361–3.

31 McKenna WJ, England D, Doi YL, Deanfield JE, Oakley C, Goodwin JF. Arrhythmia in hypertrophic cardiomyopathy. Influence on prognosis. *Br Heart J* 1981;**46**:168–72.

32 Maron BJ, Gardin JM, Flack JM. Prevalence of hypertrophic cardiomyopathy in a general population of young adults: echocardiographic analysis of 4111 subjects in the CARDIA study. *Circulation* 1995;**92**:785–9.

33 McKenna WJ, Camm AJ. Sudden death in hypertrophic cardiomyopathy: assessment of patients at high risk. *Circulation* 1989;**80**:1489–92.

34 Maron BJ, Bonow RO, Cannon RO, Leon MB, Epstein SE. Hypertrophic cardiomyopathy. Interrelations of clinical manifestations, pathophysiology, and therapy. *N Engl J Med* 1987;**26**:780–89, 844–52.

35 McKenna WJ, Deanfield J, Faruqui A. Prognosis of hypertrophic cardiomyopathy: role of age and clinical, electrocardiographic and haemodynamic features. *Am J Cardiol* 1978;**41**:1133–40.

36 Burke AP, Farb A, Virmani R. Sports-related and non-sports related sudden cardiac death in young adults. *Am Heart J* 1991;**121**:568–75.

37 Pellicia A, Maron BJ, Spataro A, Proschan MA, Spirito P. The upper limit of physiological hypertrophy in highly trained elite athletes. *N Engl J Med*

1991;**324**:295–301.

38 Maron BJ, Pellicia S, Spirito P. Cardiac disease in young trained athletes. Insights into methods for distinguishing athletes heart from structural heart disease, with particular emphasis on hypertrophic cardiomyopathy. *Circulation* 1995;**91**:1596–601.

39 Maron BJ. Structural features of the heart as defined by echocardiography. *J Am Coll Cardiol* 1986;**7**:190–203.

40 Lewis J. Considerations for racial differences in the athlete's heart. *Cardiol Clin* 1992;**10**:329–33.

41 McKenna WJ, Stewart JT, Nihoyannopoulos P, McCinty F, Davies MJ. Hypertrophic cardiomyopathy without hypertrophy. *Br Heart J* 1990;**63**: 287–90.

42 Maron BJ, Kragel AH, Roberts WC. Sudden death in hypertrophic cardiomyopathy with normal left ventricular mass. *Br Heart J* 1990;**65**:308–10.

43 Thierfelder L, Watkins H, MacRae C, *et al*. Alpha tropomyosin and cardiac troponin T mutations causing familial hypertrophic cardiomyopathy, a disease of the sarcomere. *Cell* 1994;**77**:701–12.

44 Mitchell JH, Maron BJ, Epstein SE. 16th Bethesda conference: cardiovascular abnormalities in the athlete: recommendations regarding eligibility for competition. *J Am Coll Cardiol* 1985;**6**:1186–232.

45 McKenna WJ, Oakley CM, Krikler DM, Goodwin JF. Improved survival with amiodarone in patients with hypertrophic cardiomyopathy and ventricular tachycardia. *Am J Cardiol* 1981;**48**:252–7.

46 Oakley DG, Oakley CM. Significance of abnormal ECGs in highly trained athletes. *Am J Cardiol* 1982;**50**:985–9.

47 Shapiro LM. Physiological left ventricular hypertropy. *Br Heart J* 1984;**52**:130–5.

48 Roeske WR, O'Rourke RA, Klein A, Leopold G, Karliner JS. Non invasive evaluation of ventricular hypertrophy in professional athletes. *Circulation* 1976;**53**:286–92.

49 Huston TP, Puffer JC, McMillan R. The athletic heart syndrome. *N Engl J Med* 1985;**313**:24–32.

50 Ehsani AA, Hagberg JM, Hickson RC. Rapid changes in left ventricular dimensions and mass in response to physical conditioning and deconditioning. *Am J Cardiol* 1978;**42**:52–6.

51 McKenna WJ, Thiene G, Nava A, *et al*. Diagnosis of arrhythmogenic right ventricular dysplasia cardiomyopathy. Task force of the Working Group Myocardial and Pericardial Disease of the European Society of Cardiology and the Scientific Council on Cardiomyopathies of the International Society and Federation of Cardiology. *Br Heart J* 1994;**71**:215–8.

52 Thiene G, Nava A, Corrado D, Rossi L, Pennelli L. Right ventricular cardiomyopathy and sudden death in young people. *N Engl J Med* 1988;**318**:129–33.

53 Maron BJ. Right ventricular cardiomyopathy: another cause of sudden death in the young. *N Engl J Med* 1988;**318**:178–80.

54 Nava A, Thiene G, Canicani B, *et al*. Clinical profile of concealed form of arrhythmogenic right ventricular cardiomyopathy presenting with apparently idiopathic ventricular arrhythmias. *Int J Cardiol* 1992;**35**:195–206.

55 Laurent M, Descaves C, Biron Y, Deplace C, Almange C, Daubert JC. Familial form of arrhythmogenic right ventricular dysplasia. *Am Heart J* 1987; **113**:827–9.

56 Nava A, Thiene G, Canicani B, *et al*. Familial occurrence of right ventricular dysplasia. A study involving nine families. *J Am Coll Cardiol* 1988;**12**:1222–8.

57 Ruder MA, Winston SA, Davis JC, Abbot JA, Eldar M, Scheinmann L. Arrhythmogenic right ventricular dysplasia in a family. *Am J Cardiol* 1985;**56**:799–800.

58 Coonar AS, Protonotarios N, Tsatsopolou A, Mattu RK, Needham EWA, McKenna WJ. Linkage analysis in a recessive form of arrhythmogenic right ventricular cardiomyopathy. *Eur Heart J* 1996;**17**(abstract suppl):165, P932.

59 Marcus FI, Fontaine GH, Guiraudon G, *et al*. Right ventricular dysplasia: A report of 24 adult cases. *Circulation* 1982;**65**:384–98.

60 Rossi P, Massumi A, Gillette P, Hall RJ. Arrhythmogenic right ventricular dysplasia: clinical features, diagnostic techniques, and current management. *Am Heart J* 1982;**3**:415–20.

61 Lemery R, Brugada P, Janssen J, Cheriex E, Dugernier T, Wellens HJ. Nonischaemic sustained ventricular tachycardia: clinical outcome in 12 patients with arrhythmogenic right ventricular dysplasia. *J Am Coll Cardiol* 1989;**14**:96–105.

62 Buxton AE, Waxman HL, Marchlinski FE, Simson MB, Cassidy D, Josephson ME. Right ventricular tachycardia: clinical and electrophysiologic characteristics. *Circulation* 1983;**68**:917–27.

63 Fontaine G, Frank R, Gallais-Hamonno F, Allali I, Phan-Thuc H, Grosgogeat Y. Electrocardiographie des potentiels tardifs du syndrome de post-excitation. *Arch Mal Coeur Vaiss* 1978;**71**:854–64.

64 Kisslo J. Two dimensional echocardiography in arrhythmogenic right ventricular dysplasia. *Eur Heart J* 1989; **10**(suppl D):22–6.

65 Chiddo A, Locuratolo N, Gaglione A, *et al*. Right ventricular dysplasia: angiographic study. *Eur Heart J* 1989;**10**(suppl D):42–5.

66 Robertson JH, Brady GH, German LD. Comparison of two dimensional echocardiographic and angiographic findings in arrhythmogenic right ventricular cardiomyopathy. *Am J Cardiol* 1985;**55**:1506–8.

67 Casolo GC, Poggesi I, Boddi M, *et al*. ECG-gated magnetic resonance imaging in right ventricular dysplasia. *Am Heart J* 1987;**113**:1245–8.

68 Ricci C, Longo R, Pagnan L, *et al*. Magnetic resonance imaging in right ventricular dysplasia. *Am J Cardiol* 1992;**70**:1589–95.

69 Breihardt G, Wichter T, Haverkamp W, *et al*. Implantable cardioverter defibrillator therapy in patients with arrhythmic right ventricular cardiomyopathy, long QT syndrome, or no structural heart disease. *Am Heart J* 1994;**4**:1151–8.

70 Hauser AM, Dressendorfer RH, Vos M, Hashimoto T, Gordon S, Timmis GC. Symmetric cardiac enlargement in highly trained endurance athletes: a two dimensional echocardiographic study. *Am Heart J* 1985;**109**:1038–44.

71 Cheitlin MD, de Castro CM, McAllister HA. Sudden death as a complication of anomalous left coronary origin from the anterior sinus of Valsalva: a not so minor congenital abnormality. *Circulation* 1994;**50**:780–7.

72 Roberts WC, Siegal RJ, Zipes DP. Origin of the right coronary artery from the left sinus of Valsalva and its functional consequences. Analysis of 10 necroscopy patients. *Am J Cardiol* 1982;**49**:863–8.

73 Corrado D, Thiene G, Cocco P, Fresura C. Non-atherosclerotic coronary artery disease and sudden death in the young. *Br Heart J* 1992;**68**:601–7.

74 Corrado D, Thiene G, Pennelli N. Sudden death as the first manifestation of coronary artery disease in young people (< 35 years). *Eur Heart J* 1988;**9**:39–44.

75 Dreifus LS, Haiat R, Watanabe Y, Arriaga J, Reitman N. Ventricular fibrillation: a possible cause mechanism of sudden death in patients with Wolff-Parkinson-White syndrome. *Circulation* 1971;**43**:520–7.

76 Gallagher JJ, Pritchett EL, Sealy WC, Kassell J, Wallace AG. The pre-excitation syndromes. *Prog Cardiovasc Dis* 1978;**20**:285–327.

77 Schwartz PJ, Periti M, Malliani A. The long QT syndrome. *Am Heart J* 1975;**89**:378–90.

78 Moss AJ, Robinson I. Clinical features of the idiopathic long QT syndrome. *Circulation* 1992;**85**:140–4.

79 Moss AJ. Prolonged QT syndromes. *JAMA* 1986;**256**:2985–7.
80 Towbin JA. New revelations about the long QT syndrome. *N Engl J Med* 1995;**333**:380–1.
81 Virmani R, Robinowitz M, Smialek JE, Smyth DF. Cardiovascular effects of cocaine: an autopsy study of 40 patients. *Am Heart J* 1988;**115**:1068–76.
82 Corrado D, Basso C, Angelini A, Thiene G. Sudden arrhythmic death in young people with apparently normal heart. *J Am Coll Cardiol* 1995;**22**:19–22.
83 Jeresaty RM. Mitral valve prolapse: definition and implications in athletes. *J Am Coll Cardiol* 1986;**7**:231.
84 Corrado D, Basso C, Schiavon M, Thiene G. Screening for hypertrophic cardiomyopathy in young athletes. *N Engl J Med* 1998;**339**:364–9.
85 Maron BJ, Bodison SA, Wesley YE, Tucker E, Green KJ. Results of screening a large group of intercollegiate competitive athletes for cardiovascular disease. *J Am Coll Cardiol* 1987;**10**:1214–21.
86 La Corte MA, Boxer RA, Gottersflied B, *et al.* ECG screening program for school athletes. *Clin Cardiol* 1989;**12**:42–4.
87 Lewis JF, Maron BJ, Diggs JA, Spencer JE, Mehrotra PP, Curry CL. Pre participation echocardiographic screening for cardiovascular disease in a large, predominantly black population of college athletes. *Am J Cardiol* 1989;**64**:1029–33.

Multiple choice questions

1 Which of the following statements are correct?
   (a) Sudden cardiac death in elite athletes is common
   (b) Premature coronary artery disease is the most common cause of death in young (< 25 years) athletes
   (c) Most deaths occur during or just after exercise
   (d) 40–50% of all sudden cardiac deaths in athletes in the United States are due to hypertrophic cardiomyopathy
   (e) Sudden death may occur in the absence of prodromal symptoms

2 Which of the following symptoms may be suggestive of underlying cardiovascular disease in an athletic individual?
   (a) Chest pain during exertion
   (b) Blackouts
   (c) Breathlessness disproportionate to the amount of exercise being performed
   (d) Palpitation
   (e) Dizziness during or after exertion

3 Recognised causes of sudden cardiac death in athletes include:
   (a) Aortic rupture
   (b) Myocarditis
   (c) Cocaine abuse
   (d) Arrhythmogenic right ventricular cardiomyopathy
   (e) Coronary artery anomalies

4 In an athlete with left ventricular hypertrophy of 13–16 mm, which of the following would be suggestive of hypertrophic cardiomyopathy?

(a) A left ventricular cavity size of 44 mm

(b) A history of premature sudden death in a first degree relative

(c) ECG showing isolated Sokolow voltage criteria for left ventricular hypertrophy

(d) Regression of hypertrophy after a 6 month period of detraining

(e) Pathological Q waves on the ECG

5 Which of the following statements concerning cardiovascular evaluation of athletes is false?

(a) Screening for cardiovascular disease is warranted in a young athlete with symptoms suggestive of cardiac disease

(b) Screening for cardiovascular disease is warranted in athletes with a family history of premature sudden death in first degree relatives

(c) Physical examination will identify most individuals with underlying cardiac disease

(d) The 12 lead ECG is useful in identifying accessory conduction pathways and long QT syndrome

(e) Echocardiography may be useful in identifying coronary artery anomalies

Answers are on p. 362.

6   Exercise for older women

J E Taunton, A D Martin, E C Rhodes, L A Wolski,
M Donelly, J Elliot, R E Rhodes

Introduction

Many industrially developed countries are confronted with the
practical problems of a rapidly expanding geriatric population.
Ageing and a subsequent loss of strength will have a pronounced
effect on the capacity of this population to lead viable and
independent lives. Approximately 10% of non-disabled community
dwelling adults aged 75 or older lose independence in basic
activities of daily living each year.[1] This functional dependence is
associated with increased mortality[2] and leads to additional adverse
outcomes, such as hospital, nursing home placement, and greater
use of formal and informal home services.[3-5] Strategies for reducing
the frequency of this common cause of morbidity and mortality are
needed.

The increased rate of healthcare expenditure due to loss of
physical function is a major economic issue in industrially
developed countries. For example, in Canada, 40% of current
healthcare expenditures is devoted to treatment of the older adult
population.[6] However, the most important focus of any geriatric
programme is not to reduce healthcare costs, but rather to
maintain physical independence as this has been shown to increase
the wellbeing and quality of life of elderly people.[7,8]

There is a parallel between inactivity and ageing; inactivity is, to
a great degree, responsible for the physiological decline attributed
to the ageing process,[9-11] a decline that is more apparent in women
than men.[12] Increasing evidence shows that some of the age related
declines in physiological and cognitive function may be attenuated,
or even reversed, by regular physical activity, thus preserving
functional independence.[13]

> **Box 6.1 The population**
>
> - Most elderly women in our society are not physically active enough to maintain physical independence
> - Much of the current research on exercise does not include very old women (>80 years)
> - Osteoporosis affects a quarter of women aged >50 years and over a half of those aged >75 in our population

Women outlive men by approximately 7 or 8 years, which means that after the age of 80, 88% of women live on their own and make up most of our elderly population. A recent study by Van Den Hambergh *et al.* found that elderly widowed or unmarried women tend to be less active than married women of the same age and that most elderly women in our society are not physically active enough to maintain physical independence.[14] Disability is also disproportionately more common in women.[3,15] Therefore, women should be the initial target for intervention to help maintain the ability to perform everyday tasks and activities.[16] It is essential that exercise scientists and other healthcare professionals understand the interplay between decreased physical activity and increased age, particularly in women.

Unfortunately, much of the current data on the impact of exercise on strength and function in the elderly includes a minimal number of women in the upper age ranges.[17] This group typically exhibits a lack of familiarity with exercise and low functional capacity and may possibly experience an acceleration of the age related declines in functional capacity.[18] It is imperative that the barriers to exercise that inhibit elderly women from participating be identified and strategies for promoting physical activity in these same women be developed. Current research in this area has suggested that maintenance of strength and of bone mineral density can help to maintain physical function. The purpose of this chapter is to highlight the research focusing on the impact of exercise on elderly women. In particular, the effects of strength-training exercise on their ability to function, strength, bone mineral density and psycho-social health of elderly women will be discussed.

Exercise and strength

Although ageing is a universal biological phenomenon, its various morphological and physiological manifestations make it impossible to provide a single process or theory which adequately describes it. As time progresses, the cumulative biological changes that occur in all species ultimately result in decreased ability to function in the environment.[19] True age related declines include intrinsic impairments in cross bridges, changes in the concentrations of substances in the cytosol,[11] loss of entire motor units [20] and a loss of muscle membrane excitability.[21] Motor unit impairments from a decrease in the number of motor units, a decrease in the innervation ratio or the cross-sectional area of individual fibres, whole muscle atrophy, weakness, fatigue, and injury are evidenced by impaired mobility in the activities of daily living as well as an increased incidence of soft tissue injuries and falls. These age related deteriorations may be, in part, biologically inherited, but they may also be modified by environmental conditions such as nutrition, stress, and physical inactivity.[22]

The decline of muscle strength with age has been quantified as approximately 15% per decade after the age of about 60.[23] Additionally, lower limb muscles appear to be more affected by ageing than upper limb muscles.[24] Increased sedentary activity and the lack of fast and forceful movements during standing and walking severely compromise the large muscles of the legs. However, the age related loss of muscle strength, which reduces the capacity for physical activity performance, can be slowed down or even reversed by resistance training thereby possibly improving the quality of life for elderly people.

Females are weaker than males in overall body strength at all ages.[25] A survey in the United States showed that after the age of 74, 66% of women cannot lift objects weighing more than 4.5 kg.[10] Young found that the typical healthy 80 year old woman is at, or very near, the threshold value of quadriceps strength required to rise from a chair.[26] Thus, any reduction in strength for elderly women may lead to loss of physical independence in activities of daily living and is also a risk factor for both falls and hip fractures.

Most studies concerning the adaptation of skeletal muscle to strength training in elderly people have been conducted on men. From the research that has been done on elderly women, there seems to be a positive relationship between activity level and strength.[27-30] Knee extension strength and walking speed were higher in a group of elderly (66–85 year old) physically trained women than in a group of age matched controls[27] and elderly female athletes (endurance and strength) were found to have better muscle performance than age matched controls.[28] However, training mode may have an impact on maintenance of strength in elderly people. Klitgaard *et al.* reported superior muscle performance among elderly strength trained athletes when compared with endurance athletes or age matched untrained controls.[31]

Although the differences between untrained and trained elderly women provides solid evidence that training can positively influence muscle performance and strength, of more interest to us is the impact of an exercise programme on the strength of previously inactive women, as most elderly women in our society are not involved in physical activity. Recent research showed that general land based and water based training programmes improved maximum aerobic power in elderly women (aged 65–75 years) but did not increase muscular strength or change body composition.[32] It was suggested that specific strength training programmes may be required to improve strength and balance in elderly women. Subsequent research showed that a 1 year progressive resistance exercise programme in women, aged 65–75, resulted in significant changes in strength.[33]

Other strength training studies in elderly women have had mixed success in improving strength. Generally, programmes of longer duration have resulted in improvements in strength whereas those of shorter duration have produced equivocal results. For example, Morganti *et al.* trained 16 women twice a week at 80% of 1 repetition maximum for 12 months and found that 1 repetition maximum strength test scores improved 82%, 41% and 84% for the knee extensor, double leg press and lateral pull down exercises, respectively.[34] They concluded that high intensity progressive resistance training resulted in substantial, continual increases in strength in postmenopausal women. Pyka *et al.* studied 25 men and women who exercised three times a week for 12 months on a 12 exercise circuit at 75% of 1 repetition maximum.[35] They found that average strength increased by 30% (hip extensors) to 97% (hip flexors) and found hypertrophy of both type 1 and type 2 fibres.

In strength training programmes of shorter duration, some researchers have shown improvements in strength after 8 to 16 weeks of strength training,[36,37] whereas others found that strength training programmes of 18 weeks were not effective in inducing fibre transformation or hypertrophy in muscle fibres of healthy elderly women.[38]

The results of these studies suggest that training programmes for elderly women need to focus on longer durations than programmes designed for young adults. Because ageing muscle adapts more slowly to stress, it is essential that elderly women are encouraged to begin a lifetime change in exercise patterns to maintain or increase strength. Training benefits such as increases in strength are lost with cessation of training. For most of the population, this means a decrease in physical fitness and limitations in physical activity. However, for elderly women, the loss of strength can mean the loss of physical function, independence and mobility. Recently, Gill *et al.* established a battery of simple functional tests that assess physical performance and identify subgroups of older people who are at increased risk for functional dependence.[1] This group found that in a community sample of adults aged 72 years and older, who were independent in activities of daily living, nearly 10% became dependent in one or more of these activities by 1 year. Thus, the relationship between increasing activity and maintenance of function becomes increasingly important as women age.

Exercise and function

Although it is inevitable that ageing produces physiological change, some of the declines in physical and mental dexterity can be slowed down through exercise. It is well documented that physical activity in old age can help to sustain muscle mass[39,40] and bone density.[41] It also helps to maintain other aspects of physical fitness such as maximal aerobic power,[18] motor performance,[42] grip strength,[43] reaction time[44-46] and flexibility.[47] However, the applicability of the improvements in the various components of fitness with functional ability remains unclear. Buchner and Wagner showed that impaired balance and decreased lower limb strength are important risk factors for the loss of physical function.[48] Few researchers have attempted to correlate the benefits of exercise with improvements in the ability to carry out daily functional tasks. The risk factors that are generally assessed – such as smoking, hypertension, body mass index and heart disease – are not strong predictors of functional decline.

Simonsick *et al.* examined the association between recreational physical activity among physically capable older adults and functional status, incidence of selected chronic conditions and mortality over 3 and 6 years.[30] They found that a moderate to high activity level (activity being vigorous exercise performed at least weekly or frequent walking) reduced the likelihood of developing limitations in physical functioning over 3 years, particularly in the areas of walking and doing heavy housework. Fitness level was not measured; however, it can reasonably be assumed that the fitness of the more active subjects was higher than that of the sedentary subjects. Thus increased fitness seems to decrease the risk of loss of function of daily living.

In the past few years, researchers have been using training studies with elderly women in an effort to show a direct link between functional ability and fitness. The results have been positive in that many have found that strength training improves functional ability in elderly people. For example, Fiatarone et al.[49] and Sauvage et al.[50] found that walking speed and stair-climbing ability were positively related to muscle strength and were improved after strength conditioning in frail elderly people. Additionally, Hunter et al. found that women aged 60–77 and living independently, significantly improved their ability to rise from a chair and carry a box of groceries after 16 weeks of strength conditioning.[36] They also showed significant increases in walking speed even though walking was not part of the exercise pro- gramme. Furthermore, Connelly and Vandervoort found that strength as well as scores on functional tests such as self paced walking and timed up and go results improved significantly in 10 women, mean age 81.6 years, who completed an 8 week strengthening programme.[37]

The above studies certainly indicate that strength training programmes can help to maintain or even improve activities of daily living. However, Skelton et al. found that a general strength training programme in women aged 75 to 93 years resulted in significant increases in strength and power, but only minimal improvements in functional ability.[51] Further research by this group showed that strength training sessions that included the practice of functional tasks and mobility produced substantial increases in balance, strength, flexibility and selected tests of functional mobility.[16] It may be that strength training to maintain function needs to be very specific. That is, training programmes should focus on movements that are used in activities of daily living and not just general movement.

Whereas strength training has been shown to have a positive influence on function in elderly women, there is still research to be done. It remains unclear whether other forms of exercise that are popular with elderly women – such as walking, stretching or pool exercises – will elicit the same improvements or maintenance of physical function as strength training. Clark suggested that walking 4–7 days a week may protect against lower body decline,[52] however other researchers have not been able to show improvements in strength, mobility or function with walking[53,54] or general land based or water based exercise programmes.[32] Kerchan *et al.* showed that an unvarying home based exercise programme may support greater agility, but does not yield enough force to improve muscle strength and postural stability in healthy, non-disabled, post-menopausal women.[55] However, general activity, although not improving physical function, may have a significant impact on the psychosocial health of elderly women.

Psychological benefits of exercise

In 1992 the International Society of Sports Psychology endorsed the position statements earlier issued by the American National Institute of Mental Health which described the link between regular exercise and psychological wellbeing.[56] A recent review of psychological wellbeing and physical exercise has suggested that there is a complex relationship between the two and certainly not a one-dimensional one as had been previously suggested.[57] Exercise has been shown to help reduce the effects of insomnia, stress, depression and chronic illness. It also plays a vital part in improved weight control, body image and, especially in the case of the elderly population, independence. Physical activity can also provide an alternative to alcohol and substance misuse and may help patients who have mild to moderate depression.[58] Rejeski in a

---

Box 6.2   Advantages of exercise

- In recent years researchers have begun to study the links between fitness and functional day to day abilities matching specific fitness variables to improving functional tasks
- There is compelling evidence of a significant positive relation between physical activity and psychological variables for the mentally healthy population; this relation is even stronger for patients with psychiatric illness
- Some research has shown that strength training exercise prevents or reduces the bone loss seen in elderly women who do not exercise

---

review of dose dependent relations between exercise and psycho-social outcomes reported that low to moderate levels of aerobic exercise are better than traditional demanding programmes in terms of enhancing mood and improving psychological function-ing.[59]

It is not known if an exercise programme will enhance psychological variables in women who are not experiencing defined mental health problems. Most research on the effects of exercise on mental health has used young and middle aged subjects or has been conducted in clinical settings. There is a paucity of research on the influence of exercise on the mental health of older healthy women. However, one study has shown that improvements in muscle strength as a result of strength training increased independence of the elderly and caused improvements in mental attitude. Bozoian and McAuley had 33 subjects, mean age 86.4 years, complete a 10 week activity program of either flexibility exercises or strength exercises.[60] They found that the strength group significantly increased strength in upper body compared to the flexibility group. Both exercise groups increased in positive effect and decreased in negative effect. The strength training group were significantly more satisfied with life than the flexibility subjects and also showed a significant improvement in their ability to carry out activities of daily living. Bravo *et al.* also showed that self perceived health increased with weight bearing exercise in 124 osteopenic women aged 50–70 years.[61]

Traditionally, women have had more barriers to physical activity than men – this is particularly true for elderly women. Many senior women were raised in an era where vigorous exercise was not recommended for women. As women entered puberty, physical activity dropped dramatically as it was thought that exercise was not ladylike and would harm the reproductive organs. Additionally, marital status, socio-economic status and health problems may discourage elderly women from participating in physical activity. As a result many elderly women have never taken part in a regular exercise programme. A strength training study had a group of women aged 65 to 75 years participate in a supervised strength training programme for 12 weeks.[33] The women then continued training on their own for a further 9 months, keeping log books of all of their workouts. All of the women completed the study and the attendance at the required number of workouts per week was close to 100% for all of the subjects. The study showed that with encouragement and support, older women can successfully maintain a strength training programme for many months without direct supervision.

The results of Bozoian and McAuley certainly suggest a positive impact of strength training in elderly people.[60] Furthermore, it seems that elderly women can maintain an exercise regimen over the long term.[33] More research is required to understand fully the interplay between regular physical activity, such as strength training, functional independence and psychological wellbeing.

Exercise and bone

One of the most important roles of exercise in elderly women is its potential to maintain bone integrity. This chapter is not meant to be a comprehensive review of the impact of ageing and exercise on bone mineral density or osteoporosis as this has been reviewed extensively elsewhere.[62,63] Instead, it is intended to highlight some of the issues concerning the impact of strength training on bone integrity in elderly women.

Osteoporosis affects one in four women over the age of 50 and nearly half by the age of 75 and may be inevitable in some women depending on their diet and exercise habits in their younger life.[64] Postmenopausal women are the group at highest risk for osteoporosis. Osteoporosis is a condition of low bone density such that susceptibility to low trauma fractures (typically wrist, vertebra and hip) is greatly increased. A comprehensive population study of hip fractures in two million Canadians indicated that there are about 20 000 hip fractures annually in Canada, with women accounting for 75% of the total.[65] This figure is increasing rapidly and will almost double in the next 20 years as the population ages. Debilitating osteoporotic fractures of the spine are also at epidemic proportions. The huge personal, social and economic costs of osteoporosis make it imperative that effective preventive and therapeutic strategies be developed.

The two main determinants of hip fractures are bone density and increasing falls. One of the most effective ways of combating the decline in bone density and decreasing the risk of falls in women who may be susceptible to the disease or already have it, is through weight bearing exercise. There is a tendency for fallers to be older and have lower muscular strength than non- or infrequent fallers.[66]

Relatively few studies examining the effect of weight bearing exercise on bone density have included older subjects and these have produced equivocal results, largely because of methodological problems such as small sample size. However, it has been clearly shown that immobilisation induces the greatest reported rate of bone loss, greater even than that caused by a total loss of oestrogen.[67] Furthermore, Alekel et al. found that the combined contribution of total body weight and lifetime physical activity to bone mineral density is much greater in postmenopausal women than premenopausal women, particularly for the proximal femur, indicating that activity is particularly important for postmenopausal women.[68]

Most researchers have been unable to prove that weight bearing exercise increases bone density in middle aged and elderly men and women; however, many have found that such exercise prevents or reduces the bone loss seen in those who do not exercise.[61,63,69-71] Martin et al. found that strength training resulted in an increase in bone mineral density of the lumbar spine and a trend towards improvement at the hip in women aged 65 to 75 years.[72] Also Rhodes et al.[73] and Ryan et al.[74] have shown that upper body strength significantly increased by 29–65% and 20–55%, respectively after training. Muscular strength of the leg press and quadriceps curl were significantly associated with bone mineral density of the L2-L4, femoral neck, Wards' triangle and the greater trochanter (range of $r = 0.31$ to 0.84; $P < 0.05$). Both studies concluded that a resistive training programme maintains bone mineral density and improves muscular strength in healthy, older women. This is important in the prevention of negative health outcomes associated with age related loss of bone density.

Exercise prescription for elderly people has typically focused on cardiovascular training and stretching. However, aerobic activities such as walking or running lack lateral and twisting movements and may not induce high enough strain levels sufficiently to maintain bone density.[63] Further research is required to determine if an aerobically based exercise programme can be designed to include sufficient bone loading. At the present time, however, strength training appears to be the exercise mode of choice for maintaining bone integrity in elderly women.

Considerations when designing exercises for elderly women

Although adherence to continual physical activity is low for most of society's population, elderly women often report the lowest frequency of exercise of all demographic groups.[75] Furthermore, little research exists to explain adequately factors that determine exercise adherence among older women.[76] At present, findings from adherence research in younger and middle aged populations often have to be generalised to older people. However, several factors have been rather consistently cited and associated with continued physical activity among elderly people, even though more sophisticated and standardised research parameters are required in future. For example, demographic factors such as education and socioeconomic standing positively correlate with physical activity among all age groups.[77] Also, social cognitive frameworks like self efficacy theory,[78] the theory of planned behaviour,[79] and the stages of change in exercise behaviour[80] have successfully shown applicability among older subjects. Social factors such as perceived social support,[81] and encouragement by doctors[82] may account for significant variance in activity adherence among older women. However, barriers to continued activity may provide considerable influence over an older adult's decision to adhere to exercise,[83] while perceived physical frailty and poor health may provide elderly people's greatest barrier to physical activity.[84] Programme factors such as the exercise setting and leadership are cited as influential factors for physical activity but supportive research is scarce for any population.[85] Finally, intervention efforts, although indicative of an increase in continued physical activity,[86] require more systematic attempts to reflect theory and research based constructs with randomised controlled designs to understand how individual variables and techniques influence exercise behaviour among older women.

Furthermore, when we consider increased physical activity in elderly people, the number of injuries may increase.[87] It is a paradox for exercise prescription for elderly people that the types of exercise such as strength training that have been shown to result in the greatest gains in strength, function, and maintenance of bone integrity are also the type most likely to cause fractures and injury. The development or exacerbation of joint symptoms with exercise is obviously a potential barrier to strength training in elderly women. Both clinicians and patients commonly believe that weight bearing exercise produces joint symptoms, however existing evidence suggests that well regulated exercise does not produce or exacerbate these problems.[88] In a study by Powell et al. that examined rates of injury in commonly performed activities, the population aged between 18–44 years experienced more injuries in

---

Box 6.3   Benefits of regular exercise

- Increase in exercise capacity, muscle strength, and flexibility
- Decrease in mortality from cardiovascular disease
- Decrease in resting heart rate and blood pressure
- Decrease in bone loss through weight bearing exercise
- Improved lipid profile
- Decreased percentage of body fat
- Improved carbohydrate metabolism
- Weight control
- Increase in perceived wellbeing and self image
- Improved cognitive function and reaction time
- Decreased anxiety, insomnia and depression

Adapted from Rohan.[89]

---

weight lifting than those aged over 45.[90]

Although elderly women may have potential limitations for exercise and although there is a potential increased risk of injury with increased activity, the benefits of regular exercise far outweigh the potential drawbacks. The positive influence of physical activity is apparent for all age groups, but the most dramatic differences in functional ability and psychological health are seen within older people. Sherman *et al.* found that women aged 75 years or older who were more active were more independent and lived longer than their inactive counterparts.[91] More research is needed into frequency of injury and techniques for the prevention of injury in strength training in elderly people.

There are several strategies available for targeting less active people, including elderly women within the population. These include:

- Setting physical activity targets for particular groups who are at higher risk of a sedentary lifestyle
- Planning facilities, schedules and other aspects of the social and physical environment to minimise potential barriers to increased participation
- Encouragement of women in their middle years to become and remain highly active; this offers long term protection against osteoporosis and cardiovascular disease and can significantly reduce the national healthcare bill for older adults
- Targeting older women, especially those who live alone as a result of widowhood, divorce, or separation; women may live longer

115

than men but they experience more limitations
- Consider low cost and accessible physical activity opportunities and facilities for individuals within lower income and educational brackets.[89]

Box 6.4   Future research needs

- Elderly women have been shown to be able to maintain exercise programmes long term but more research needs to be done regarding resistances and barriers to physical activity as well as factors which facilitate compliance
- Older women, especially those at greatest risk of low activity, should be targeted for specific exercise research programmes
- Further research needs to be done to see if other modes of exercise besides specific strength training can elicit improvements in bone integrity and functional independence

---

Summary

Many healthy elderly women are at, or near to, functionally important strength related thresholds and so have either lost or are in danger of losing the ability to perform some important everyday tasks.[92] There is much research still to be done on the influence of exercise on strength, function, bone mineral density and psychological health in elderly women. Current research in the topic has shown that there are many advantages to strength training with elderly women. The most important of these are the maintenance of bone mineral density (and the consequent reduction of hip fractures) and functional independence. However, the long term effectiveness of strength training on these parameters has yet to be established. Additionally, further research is required to determine if there are other modes of exercise that can elicit the same improvements in functional dependence and bone integrity as seen with strength training.

Barriers to physical activity are still a problem for many elderly women. They need to be identified and strategies to overcome them must be put into place. Continuing physical activity is so important to older women, not only because they make up a significant portion of the elderly population, but because the decline in physical activity and the subsequent increase in incidence of chronic illnesses are much more apparent in this population.

1 Gill TM, Williams CS, Tinetti ME. Assessing risk for the onset of functional dependence among older adults: the role of physical performance. *J Am Geriatr Soc* 1995;**43**:603–9.

2 Manton KG, Corder LS, Stallard E. Estimates of change in chronic disability and institutional incidence and prevalence rates in the US elderly population from the 1982, 1984 and 1989 national long term care survey. *J Gerontol* 1993;**48**:s153–66.

3 Katz S, Brach LG, Branson MH *et al*. Active life expectancy. *N Engl J Med* 1983;**309**:1218–24.

4 Kemper P. The use of formal and informal home care by the disabled elderly. *Health Serv Res* 1992;**27**:421–51.

5 Spector WD, Katz S, Murphy JB, Fulton JP. The hierarchical relationship between activities of daily living and instrumental activities of daily living. *J Chronic Dis* 1987;**40**:481–9.

6 Fitness Directorate Health Canada. *Active living and health: benefits and opportunities*. FDHC, 1994.

7 Shephard RJ. *Physical activity and ageing*. London: Croom Helm, 1978: 268–91.

8 Anderson SF. An historical overview of geriatric medicine: definition and aims. In: Pathy MSJ, ed. *Principles and practice of geriatric medicine*. London: Wiley, 1985: 7–13.

9 Ashworth JB, Reuben DV, Benton LA. Functional profiles of healthy older persons. *Age Ageing* 1994;**23**:34.

10 Evans A, Meredith B. Exercise and nutrition in the elderly. In: Munro HN, Danford DE, eds. *Nutrition, ageing and the elderly*. New York: Plenum Press, 1989: 89–128.

11 Brooks SV, Larsson L, Woledge R, Schultz AB. Impairments in the structure and function of skeletal muscle with ageing. *Med Sci Sports Exerc* 1994;**26**:s27.

12 Weir LT, Jackson AS, Ayers GW, Stutevill JE. Determinates of male and female longitudinal changes in $\dot{V}O_2$MAX. *Med Sci Sports Exerc* 1994;**26**:s35.

13 Nadel ER, DiPietro L. Effects of physical activity on functional ability in older people: translating basic science findings into practical knowledge. *Med Sci Sports Exerc* 1995;**25**:s36.

14 Van Den Hambergh CEJ, Schouten EG, Van Staveren WA, Van Amelsvoort LG, Kok FJ. Physical activities of noninstitutionalized Dutch elderly and characteristics of inactive elderly. *Med Sci Sports Exerc* 1995;**27**:334–9.

15 Green H, Milne A, Rauta I, Eldridge J, Wilmot A, Levy G. *General household survey* 1986. HMSO, 1989.

16 Skelton DA, McLaughlin AW. Training functional ability in old age. *Physiotherapy* 1996;**82**:159–67.

17 Foster VL, Hume GJ, Byrnes WC *et al*. Endurance training for elderly women:moderate vs low intensity. *J Gerontol* 1989;**44**:M184–8.

18 Denh MM, RA Bruce. Longitudinal variations in maximal oxygen intake with age and activity. *J Appl Physiol* 1972;**33**:805–7.

19 Nakamura E, Moritani T, Kanetaka A. Biological age versus physical fitness age. *Eur J Appl Physiol* 1989;**58**:778–85.

20 Brown WF, Strong MJ, Snow R. Methods for estimating number of motor units in biceps-brachialis muscle and losses of motor units with ageing. *Muscle Nerve*

1988;**11**:423–32.

21 Hicks AL, Cupido CM, Martin J, Dent J. Muscle excitation in elderly adults: the effect of training. *Muscle Nerve* 1992;**15**:87–93.

22 Piscopo J. *Fitness and ageing.* New York: Wiley, 1985: 96–151.

23 Vandervoort AA, McComas AJ. Contractile changes in opposing muscles of the human ankle joint with ageing. *J Appl Physiol* 1986;**61**:361–7.

24 Aniansson A, Sperling L, Rundgren A, Lehnberg E. Muscle function in 75-year-old men and women: a longitudinal study. *Scand J Rehab Med Suppl* 1983;**90**:92–102.

25 Cook PN, Smith-Exton AN, Brocklehurst JN, Lempert-Barber SM. Fractured femurs, galls and bone disorders. *J R Coll Physicians Lond* 1982;**16**:45–9.

26 Young A. Exercise physiology in geriatric practice. *Acta Medica Scandinavica* 1986;**711**(suppl):227–32.

27 Sipila S, Suominen H. Knee extension strength and walking speed in relation to quadriceps muscle composition and training in elderly women. *Clin Physiol* 1994;**14**:433–42.

28 Rantanen T, Sipila S, Suominen H. Muscle strength and history of heavy manual work among elderly trained women and randomly chosen sample population. *Eur J Appl Physiol* 1993;**66**:514–7.

29 Voorips LE, Lemmink KAP, Van Heuvelen MJG, *et al.* The physical condition of elderly women differing in habitual physical activity. *Med Sci Sports Exerc* 1993;**25**:1152–7.

30 Simonsick EM, Lafferty ME, Phillips CL, *et al.* Risk due to inactivity in physically capable older adults. *Am J Public Health* 1993;**83**:1443–50.

31 Klitgaard H, Mantoni M, Schiaffino S, *et al.* Function, morphology and protein expression of ageing skeletal muscle: a cross-sectional study of elderly men with different training backgrounds. *Acta Physiol Scand* 1990;**140**:41–54.

32 Taunton JE, Rhodes EC, Wolski LA, *et al.* The effect of land-based and water-based fitness programs on the cardiovascular fitness, strength and flexibility of women aged 65–75 years. *Gerontology* 1996;**42**:204–10.

33 Rhodes EC, Martin AD, Taunton JE, *et al.* Effects of one year of resistance training on strength and bone density in elderly women. *Med Sci Sport Exerc* 1995;**27**:s21.

34 Morganti C, Nelson M, Fiatarone M, Crawford B, Economos C, Evans W. Strength improvement with progressive resistance training in older women. *Med Sci Sports Exerc* 1994;**26**:s31.

35 Pyka G, Lindenberger E, Charette S, Marcus R. Muscle strength and fiber adaptations to a year-long resistance training program in elderly men and women. *J Gerontol* 1994;**49**:M22–27.

36 Hunter GR, Treuth MS, Weinsier RL, *et al.* The effects of strength conditioning on older women's ability to perform daily tasks. *J Am Geriatr Soc* 1995;**43**:756–60.

37 Connelly DM, Vandervoot AA. Improvement in knee extensor strength of institutionalized elderly women after exercise with ankle weights. *Physio Can* 1995;**47**:15–23.

38 Kovanen V, Sipila S, Elorinne M, Alen M, Suominen H. Effects of intensive physical training on muscle fiber characteristics in elderly women. *Med Sci Sports Exerc* 1994;**26**:s115.

39 Fiatarone, MA, EC Marks, ND Ryan, CN Meredith, LA Lipsitz, WJ Evans. High-intensity strength training in nonagenarians. *JAMA* 1990;**263**:3029–34.

40 Laforest S, St-Pierre DMM, Cyr J, Gayton D. Effects of age and regular exercise on muscle strength and endurance. *Eur J Appl Physiol* 1990;**60**:104–11.

41 Aloia JF, Cohn AH, Ostuni JA, Cane R, Ellis K. Prevention of involutional bone loss by exercise. *Ann Intern Med* 1978;**89**:356–8.

42 Rikli R and Busch S. Motor performance of women as a function of age and physical activity level. *Med Sci Sports Exerc* 1986;**41**:645–9.

43 Cauley JA, Petrini AM, LaPorte RE *et al*. The decline of grip strength in the menopause: relationship to physical activity, estrogen use and anthropometric factors. *J Chronic Dis* 1987;**40**:115–20.

44 Baylor AM, Spirduso WW. Systematic aerobic exercise and components of reaction time in older women. *J Gerontol* 1988;**43**:121–6.

45 Spirduso WW. Reaction and movement time as a function of age and physical activity level. *J Gerontol* 1975;**30**:435–40.

46 Spirduso WW, Clifford P. Replication of age and physical activity effects on reaction and movement time. *J Gerontol* 1978;**33**:26–30.

47 Chapman EA, Vries HA, Swezey R. Joint stiffness: effects of exercise on young and old men. *J Gerontol* 1972;**27**:218–21.

48 Buchner DM, Wagner EH. Preventing frail health. *Clin Geriatr Med* 1992;**8**:1–17.

49 Fiatarone MA, O'Neill EF, Ryan ND, *et al*. Exercise training and nutritional supplementation for physical frailty in very elderly people. *N Engl J Med* 1994;**330**:1769–75.

50 Sauvage LR, Myklebust BM, Crow-Pan J, *et al*. A clinical trial of strengthening and aerobic exercise to improve gait and balance in elderly male nursing home residents. *Am J Phys Med Rehabil* 1992;**71**:333–42.

51 Skelton DA, Young A, Greig DA, Malbut KE. Effects of resistance training on strength, power and selected functional abilities of women aged 75 and over. *J Am Geriatr Soc* 1995;**43**:1081–7.

52 Clark DO. The effect of walking on lower body disability among older blacks and whites. *Am J Public Health* 1996;**86**:57–61.

53 MacRae PG, Asplund LA, Schnelle JF, *et al*. A walking program for nursing home residents: effects on walk endurance, physical activity, mobility and quality of life. *J Am Geriatr Soc* 1996;**44**:175–80.

54 Duncan JJ, Gordon NF, Scott CB. Women walking for health and fitness: how much is enough? *JAMA* 1991;**266**:3295–9.

55 Kerchan K, *et al*. Functional impact of unvarying exercise program in women after menopause. *Am J Phys Med Rehab* 1998;**10**:326–32.

56 International Society of Sport Physiology. Physical activity and psychological benefits: a position statement. *Sport Psychol* 1992;**6**:199–204.

57 Scully D, *et al*. Physical exercise and psychological wellbeing: a critical review. *Br J Sports Med* 1998;**32**:111–20.

58 Taylor CB, Sallis JF, Neelde R. The relation of physical activity and exercise to mental health. *Public Health Rep* 1985;**100**:195.

59 Rejeski WJ. Dose-response issues from a psychosocial perspective. In: Bouchard C, Shepard RJ, Stephen T, eds. *Physical activity, fitness and health*. Champaign, Illinois: Human Kinetics, 1994:1040–55.

60 Bozoian S, McAuley E. Strength training effects on subjective well-being and physical function in the elderly. *Med Sci Sports Exerc* 1994;**26**:s156.

61 Bravo G, Gauthier P, Roy PM *et al*. Impact of a 12-month exercise program on the physical and psychological health of osteopenic women. *J Am Geriatr Soc* 1996;**44**:756–62.

62 Martin AD. Osteoporosis: a geriatric public health issue. *Top Geriatr Rehabil* 1995;**10**:1–11.

63 Martin AD and Houston CS. Osteoporosis, calcium and physical activity: a review. *Can Med Assoc J* 1987;**136**:587–93.

64 Armstrong AL, Wallace WA. The epidemiology of hip fractures and methods of prevention. *Acta Ortho Belgica* 1994;**60**:85–101.

65 Martin AD, Silverthorn KG, Houston CS, *et al*. The incidence of fracture of the proximal femur in two million Canadians from 1972 to 1984. *Clin Orthop* 1991;**266**:111–8.

66 Dalsky GP, Fehling PC, Fenster J, Judge J, King M. Balance testing and falls in healthy older adults. *Med Sci Sports Exerc* 1994;**26**:s61.

67 Mazess RB, Whedon GD. Immobilization and bone. *Calcif Tissue Int* 1983;**51**:105–10.
68 Alekel L, Clasey J, Fehling P, Lee K, Stillman R. Regional bone mass in pre vs post menopausal women: contribution of body weight and lifetime activity. *Med Sci Sports Exerc* 1994;**26**:s158.
69 Grove KA, Londeree BR. Bone density in postmenopausal women high impact versus low impact exercise. *Med Sci Sports Exerc* 1992;**24**:1190–4.
70 Michel BA, Lane NE, Bloch DA, Jones HH, Fries JF. Effect of changes in weight bearing exercise on lumbar bone mass after age fifty. *Ann Med* 1991;**23**:397–401.
71 Peterson SE, Peterson MD, Raymond G, Gilligan C, Checovich MM, Smith EL. Muscular strength and bone density with weight training in middle-aged women. *Med Sci Sports Exerc* 1991;**23**:499–504.
72 Martin AD, Rhodes EC, Willis S, *et al*. Effect of progressive strength-training on bone mineral density of elderly women. *Med Sci Sports Exerc* 1995;**27**:s220.
73 Rhodes EC, Martin AD, Taunton JE, Donelly M, Elliot J. Effects of one year of resistance training on the relationship between muscular strength and bone density in elderly women. *Med Sci Sport Exerc* 1995;**27**:21.
74 Ryan AS, Trenth MS, Hunter GR, Elahi D. Resistive training maintains bone mineral density in postmenopausal women. *Calcif Tissue Int* 1998;**62**:295–9.
75 Casperson CJ, Merritt RJ, Stephens T. International physical activity patterns: a methodological perspective. In: Dishman RK, ed. *Advances in exercise adherence*. Champaign, Illinois: Human Kinetics, 1994.
76 Williams P, Lord SR. Predictors of adherence to a structured exercise program for older women. *Psychology Aging* 1995;**10**:617–24.
77 Stephens T, Craig CL. *The well-being of Canadians: highlights of the 1988 Campbell's soup survey*. Ottawa: Canadian Fitness and Lifestyle Research Institute, 1990.
78 McAuley E. Self-efficacy and the maintenance of exercise participation in older adults. *J Behav Med* 1993;**16**:103–113.
79 Courneya, KD. Understanding readiness for regular physical activity in older individuals: an application of the theory of planned behavior. *Health Psychol* 1995;**17**:80–7.
80 Gorely T, Gordon S. An examination of the transtheoretical model and exercise behavior in older adults. *J Sport Exerc Psychol* 1995;**17**:312–24.
81 Chogahara M, O'Brien C, Wankel LM. Social influences on physical activity in older adults: a review. *J Aging Physical Activity* 1998;**6**:1–17.
82 O'Brien Cousins S. Social support for exercise among elderly women in Canada. *Health Prom Int* 1995;**10**:273–82.
83 Shephard RJ. Determinants of exercise in people aged 65 years and older. In: Dishman RK, ed. *Advances in exercise adherence*. Champaign, Illinois: Human Kinetics, 1994:343–60.
84 Wolinsky FD, Stump TE. Antecedents and consequences of physical activity and exercise among older adults. *Gerontologist* 1995;**35**:451–62.
85 Willis JD, Campbell LF. *Exercise Psychology*. Champaign, Illinois: Human Kinetics, 1992.
86 Dishman RK. Increasing and maintaining exercise and physical activity. *Behav Ther* 1991;**22**:345–78.
87 Caspersen CJ, Kriska AM, Dearwater SR. Physical activity epidemiology as applied to elderly populations. *Baillieres Clin Rheumatol* 1994;**8**:7–27.
88 Coleman EA, Buchner DM, Cress ME, *et al*. The relationship of joint symptoms with exercise performance in older adults. *J Am Geriatr Soc* 1996;**44**:14–21.
89 Rohan I. Benefits and risks of exercise in elderly patients. *Can J Cont Med Ed* 1994;**9**:49–62.
90 Powell KE *et al*. Injury rates from walking, gardening, weightlifting, outdoor bicycling and aerobics. *Med Sci Sports Exerc* 1998;**30**:1246–9.

91 Sherman SE, D'Agostino RB, Cobb JL, Kannel WB. Does exercise reduce mortality rates in the elderly? Experience from the Framingham heart study. *Am Heart J* 1994;**128**:965–72.
92 Canadian Fitness and Lifestyle Research Institute. *Progress in Prevention: Popular physical activities.* CFLRI, 1996.

Multiple choice questions

1 According to the authors, what may represent the greatest barrier for the elderly to engage in regular exercise?
(a) Perceived lack of time
(b) Perceived physical frailty
(c) Perceived lack of access to exercise facilities
(d) Perceived lack of knowledge towards physical activity

2 What possible determinant of older adult exercise adherence has not been substantially researched for any population?
(a) Social support
(b) Exercise barriers
(c) The exercise setting and programme leadership
(d) Social-cognitive theories

3 Which one of the following statements about the relationships between exercise and function has proven to be false by research to date?
(a) Impaired balance and decreased lower extremity strength are important risk factors for the loss of physical function
(b) Moderate to high activity levels reduce the likelihood of developing limitations in doing heavy housework.
(c) Popular exercises like walking, stretching and pool exercises have proven to be as effective as strength training in improving physical functioning
(d) Stair climbing can be improved by strength conditioning in frail elderly subjects

4 Which of the following statement(s) are correct?
(a) Females are weaker than males in overall body strength at all ages
(b) Older individuals do not respond positively to strength training regimens
(c) Many strength training studies have focused on males with very little research on females
(d) Some researchers have shown strength improvements in the

elderly after only 8 weeks of training

5 A well designed strength training study in elderly subjects cannot:
(a) Improve bone mineral density of the lumbar spine
(b) Significantly improve strength in the 20–50% range
(c) Significantly improve cardiovascular fitness
(d) Prevent the negative outcomes associated with age-related loss of bone density

Answers are on p. 363.

7 Exercise and hypertension

M A van Baak

Introduction

In 1986 the World Health Organisation (WHO) and the International Society of Hypertension (ISH)[1] stated very tentatively that "increased physical activity is likely to reduce the risk of cardiovascular disease and is appropriate in mildly hypertensives". In 1991 a consensus document entitled *Physical exercise in the management of hypertension* was published by the World Hypertension League, which concluded that exercise programmes can contribute to the management of hypertension, enhance the sense of wellbeing and may improve life expectancy.[2] In 1992 the WHO/ISH recommended lifestyle interventions such as weight reduction in the overweight, reduction of alcohol consumption, regular mild exercise in sedentary subjects, and salt restriction in the primary prevention of hypertension.[3] In 1993 this was followed by a memorandum of the WHO/ISH, which stated that "it appears reasonable to advise that efforts to lower blood pressure by lifestyle modifications, including exercise, should normally precede any decision about the necessity of drug treatment and mild hypertension".[4] At about the same time the United States Joint National Committee on the Detection, Evaluation and Treatment of High Blood Pressure stated that physicians should vigorously encourage their hypertensive patients to adopt lifestyle modifications, including increased physical activity.[5] The American College of Sports Medicine recommended endurance exercise to reduce the incidence of hypertension in susceptible individuals and as the initial treatment strategy for individuals with mild to moderate hypertension.[6] Since then, regular exercise has been widely advocated as an effective tool in the non-pharmacological treatment of hypertension and as an adjunct to its pharmacological treatment.

Nevertheless, the evidence on which this view is based is sometimes challenged.[7,8] In this chapter I will try to summarise the evidence for the role of exercise in the treatment of hypertension and also point out areas that are still uncertain.

Hypertension, cardiovascular risk, and treatment

Cardiovascular risk and blood pressure are positively correlated: the higher the blood pressure, the higher the risk of both stroke and coronary events.[9] The current dividing line between normotension and hypertension lies at the level of blood pressure above which intervention has been shown to reduce the risk.[4] The operational classification of hypertension by the World Health Organisation/International Society of Hypertension is shown in table 7.1.

The worldwide prevalence of hypertension is high. In most countries 15–25% of the adult population have raised blood pressure at screening. In most of these individuals blood pressure is mildly increased.[4] Lowering of blood pressure in patients with hypertension by pharmacological treatment significantly reduces the risk of stroke and myocardial infarction.[10] The reduction of mortality from myocardial infarction is, however, less than predicted from observational studies. There is considerable suspicion that some of the drugs used may have adverse effects which partly counteract the benefits of the blood pressure reduction.[8] Non-pharmacological blood pressure reduction—for instance, by regular exercise—therefore seems an attractive alternative. However, no prospective randomised trials have been performed to show that exercise training reduces cardiovascular morbidity and mortality in hypertensive patients.

The evidence that regular exercise has hypotensive efficacy comes from both epidemiological and intervention studies.

Table 7.1   Classification of hypertension by resting blood pressure level

Detail	SBP (mm Hg)		DBP phase V (mm Hg)
Normotension	< 140	and	< 90
Mild hypertension	140–180	and/or	90–105
subgroup: borderline	140–160	and/or	90–95
Moderate and severe hypertension	≥ 180	and/or	≥ 105
Isolated systolic hypertension	≥ 140	and	< 90
subgroup: borderline	140–160	and	< 90

Reproduced from ref 4.

Hypotensive efficacy of exercise

Evidence from epidemiological studies

Two large epidemiological studies in the United States (Harvard Alumni Study and Aerobics Center Longitudinal Study) seem to suggest that normotensive individuals with a low level of physical activity or fitness have an increased risk of developing hypertension in the future.[11,12] On the other hand, the results from epidemiological studies that have prospectively studied the association between changes in physical activity or physical fitness and changes in blood pressure are inconsistent, with the majority finding no attenuation of the increase in blood pressure in those who improved their fitness or increased their physical activity.[7] Several, but not all, large epidemiological studies have reported an inverse relation between blood pressure and level of physical activity or physical fitness.[6,13]

Thus, although there is some evidence from epidemiological studies that regular exercise is associated with lower blood pressure, the evidence is by no means very strong. This may be inherent to this type of study in which level of physical activity is very difficult to measure reliably and many confounding factors, such as diet and body weight, may play a part.

Evidence from intervention studies

In the 1990s a number of meta-analyses and reviews of controlled intervention studies on the effects of regular exercise on blood pressure have been published.[13–18] A summary of their results is shown in table 7.2. The picture that emerges from these meta-analyses is quite clear: aerobic exercise training reduces resting systolic and diastolic blood pressure. The range of mean blood pressure reductions in the meta-analyses including only randomised trials[15,17] tends to be smaller than in meta-analyses with less stringent inclusion criteria (4–5/3–4 mm Hg v 3–10/3–8 mm Hg).[13,14,16] In only one of the approximately 50 reviewed studies was an increase in (diastolic) blood pressure found. It has been shown that a reduction in diastolic blood pressure of 5–6 mm Hg by pharmacological treatment is associated with a 42% reduction in the incidence of stroke and a 14% reduction in coronary heart disease.[10]

Ambulatory blood pressure is more closely related to hypertension-related target organ damage than casual resting blood

Table 7.2   Meta-analyses of the effects of regular exercise training on resting blood pressure

Author(s)	No of studies included	Blood pressure effect	
		SBP (mm Hg)	DBP (mm Hg)
Arroll and Beaglehole (1992)[14]	13	− 6	− 7
Fagard (1993)[13]	36	− 10	− 8 (HT)
		− 6	− 7 (BHT)
		− 3	− 3 (NT)
Kelley and McClellan (1994)[15]	9*	− 7	− 6 (HT)
		− 3	− 3 (control)
Hagberg and Brown (1995)[16]	47	− 10.5	− 8.6 (HT)
Halbert et al. (1997)[17]	27*	− 4.0	− 3.6 (HT)
		− 4.8	− 3.1 (NT)
Kelley (1997)[18]	9†	− 4.6	− 3.8

*Only randomised controlled aerobic exercise studies. †Only randomised controlled dynamic resistance studies. HT = hypertensive; NT = normotensive; BHT = borderline hypertensive.

pressure.[19] Fagard reviewed the studies in which the effect of exercise training on ambulatory blood pressure was studied.[20] Since ambulatory blood pressure measurement is a relatively new technique, the number of studies is small (10). Fagard concluded that daytime systolic and diastolic blood pressure seemed to be reduced in subjects with initially raised blood pressures. Night-

Box 7.1   Evidence for the hypotensive efficacy of exercise

- Although there is some evidence from epidemiological studies that regular exercise is associated with lower blood pressure, the evidence is not strong. This may be inherent to this type of studies, where level of physical activity is difficult to measure reliably and many confounding factors, such as diet and body weight, may interfere
- Meta-analyses of controlled intervention studies on the effects of regular exercise on blood pressure consistently show that aerobic exercise training reduces resting systolic and diastolic blood pressure. The magnitude of this reduction is 4–5/3–4 mm Hg in the meta-analyses with the most stringent inclusion criteria
- Considerable heterogeneity in hypotensive efficacy of exercise between studies is reported. Factors that may contribute to this heterogeneity are blood pressure, age, ethnicity, and type and duration of exercise training

> **Box 7.2   Evidence for cardiovascular risk reduction by exercise in people with hypertension**
>
> - There is no direct evidence that regular exercise reduces cardiovascular risk in patients with hypertension
> - The Aerobics Center Longitudinal Study by Blair *et al.* shows that mortality is lower in people with a high fitness and a combination of two or more cardiovascular risk factors (smoking, high serum cholesterol, raised blood pressure) than in people with a low fitness without any of these risk factors
> - Small reductions in blood pressure, such as found during exercise training in patients with hypertension, may reduce the risk of stroke and other cardiovascular events considerably
> - Apart from lowering blood pressure, regular exercise also favourably affects other cardiovascular risk factors, such as dyslipidaemia, insulin resistance, body weight, arterial compliance, left ventricular hypertrophy, or impaired cardiovascular reflex control

time blood pressure in general did not change significantly. Hagberg and Brown stated that the reductions in ambulatory blood pressure tended to be smaller and less consistent than those for casual blood pressure but thought that this was not surprising in view of the inherent variability in ambulatory blood pressure recordings.[16]

All the meta-analyses in table 7.2 report considerable heterogeneity in hypotensive efficacy between studies. A large number of known and unknown individual and environmental factors probably contribute to this heterogeneity. It is the challenge for the future to be able to predict which subjects under what environmental conditions will benefit from exercise intervention.

Level of blood pressure

It is not entirely clear whether the hypotensive effect of exercise training is different in hypertensive and normotensive subjects. Although a more pronounced blood pressure reduction by aerobic exercise in hypertensives is suggested by the analyses of Fagard[13] and Hagberg and Brown,[16] this finding was not confirmed by Halbert *et al.*[17] On the other hand, in studies where normotensive and hypertensive subjects followed the same training programme, the blood pressure change was always greater in the hypertensive subjects than in the normotensive subjects.[13]

127

Age, sex, and ethnicity

The effects of age, sex, and ethnicity on the blood pressure reducing efficacy of exercise training have been reviewed by Hagberg and Brown.[16] They conclude that middle-aged hypertensives may reduce their blood pressure more with exercise training than both their younger and their older counterparts. In addition, they reported that Asians and Pacific Islanders may be more responsive than white people. There are still insufficient data in Africans and African Americans to assess the hypotensive efficacy of exercise in these populations. Hagberg and Brown did not find evidence for a sex difference in responsiveness.[16]

Aerobic or resistance exercise training

The blood pressure lowering efficacy of dynamic resistance exercise training was examined in the meta-analysis by Kelley.[18] The number of studies (9) with resistance exercise training as the only training modality is still much smaller than those using aerobic exercise. The number of studies in hypertensive subjects (3) is even more limited. Nevertheless, the analysis showed reductions of resting systolic and diastolic blood pressure with dynamic resistance training comparable with those with aerobic exercise. In none of the reviewed studies was an increase in blood pressure found.

Exercise modality

The aerobic exercise studies included in the above analyses used walking, jogging, cycling, or a combination of these as training modalities. Guidelines for exercise training in the management of hypertension often mention other aerobic exercise forms such as swimming and cross country skiing.[2–4] These recommendations have been extrapolated from the effects of other aerobic exercise forms and are not based on scientific evidence. There have been reports that blood pressure is increased in swimmers and cross country skiers compared with other athletes.[21,22] A recently published study by Tanaka et al. fortunately shows that swimming training also lowers blood pressure in hypertensive individuals: a change of $-6/-5$ mm Hg in supine blood pressure was found in the swimming group ($P < 0.05$) compared with a change of $-2/-3$ mm Hg in the control group (NS).[23] For cross country skiing such data are not available.

Long term hypotensive efficacy

The duration of the studies varied between 4 and 52 weeks. The meta-analysis by Hagberg and Brown suggests that most of the blood pressure reduction is already obtained within the first 10 weeks (or even more rapidly) of training, but that there may be a small additional effect (2–2.5 mm Hg) with more prolonged duration of the exercise programme.[16] Although there are no controlled studies lasting more than 1 year, there are also no indications that the hypotensive efficacy of exercise training gradually decreases.

Exercise intensity, frequency, and duration

Fagard showed in his meta-analysis that weekly frequency, time per session, and exercise intensity did not contribute significantly to the variance in blood pressure response to training.[13] Halbert et al. also found no difference between programmes with training intensities of $\geq 70\%$ and $< 70\%$ $\dot{V}O_2$MAX or > 3 and ≤ 3 sessions per week. However, these authors indicate that the absence of a difference may be due to the limited heterogeneity of the included studies. Hagberg and Brown, on the other hand, who included more studies in their meta-analysis, did find a difference when studies with training intensities $< 70\%$ and $\geq 70\%$ $\dot{V}O_2$MAX were compared (9.5/7 v 6.8/6.8 mm Hg).[16] However, it is doubtful whether a clear picture can be derived form these meta-analyses because other programme-related or group-related factors may bias the results. In studies in which low and high intensity training programmes have been directly compared, the lower intensity programmes were either more effective[24-26] or as effective[27,28] as the higher intensity programmes. It is worth while to study the relation between exercise intensity and blood pressure reduction in more detail since low intensity training is associated with better adherence and lower musculoskeletal and cardiovascular risks and is easier to implement.

Mechanism of blood pressure lowering effect of exercise

Several mechanisms have been proposed for the hypotensive efficacy of regular exercise. Studies by Japanese investigators suggest that the blood pressure reduction is initiated by volume depletion, induced by activation of the renal kallikrein-kinin, dopamine, and prostaglandin systems.[29,30] A subsequent reduction in sympathetic activity might be involved in the maintenance of the blood pressure reduction.[30] Jennings,[31] on the other hand, suggests that in white people the primary events are an improvement of endothelium mediated vasodilation[32] and an increase in systemic arterial compliance in large vessels,[33,34] although increases in arterial compliance are not always found.[35] This changes the afferent input to the arterial baroreceptors.[36] The result could be a reduced sympathetic outflow to the renal bed,[37] which could counterbalance any tendency to an increase in blood volume and thus blood pressure. It is quite possible that the antihypertensive mechanism of exercise training differs among populations depending on the underlying hypertensive mechanism.

Kouamé et al. suggest that an attenuation of the cardiopulmonary baroreflex control of skeletal muscle vascular resistance after training at 70% $\dot{V}O_2\text{MAX}$ compared with training at 50% $\dot{V}O_2\text{MAX}$ may contribute to the less pronounced hypotensive efficacy of higher intensity training compared with lower intensity training.[38]

In addition to the direct effects of regular exercise on blood pressure described above, exercise training may also affect other factors that influence blood pressure such as diet, body weight, smoking, and alcohol consumption.

Exercise and cardiovascular risk reduction in hypertension

The ultimate goal of a recommendation of regular exercise to hypertensive subjects must be to reduce morbidity and mortality associated with hypertension. As stated above, to date there have been no prospective randomised trials to show that exercise training indeed reduces cardiovascular morbidity and mortality in hypertensive patients, and it is conceivable that other exercise induced effects offset the blood pressure lowering benefit of exercise in patients with hypertension.[7] An important study in this respect, which at least suggests that hypertensives benefit from regular exercise, is the Aerobics Center Longitudinal Study by Blair and coworkers.[39] In this study over 25 000 men and over 7000 women aged 20–88 years were followed for an average of 8 years. Men and women were categorised into three cardiorespiratory fitness levels based on the outcome of a maximal exercise test at baseline: low (least 20%), moderate (next 40%), and high (most fit 40%). High fitness men with a systolic blood pressure ≥140 mm Hg had a 32% lower all cause mortality rate than low fitness men.

An even larger difference (81%) was found in women. However, no inverse gradient across fitness categories was seen for cardio-vascular mortality in men with a systolic blood pressure of $\geq$ 140 mm Hg. In women the number of deaths from cardiovascular origin was too small to do this analysis. A raised blood pressure often clusters with other risk factors for cardiovascular disease. Blair *et al.* showed that high fitness men with a combination of two or three risk factors (smoking, high serum cholesterol, raised blood pressure) had a 15% lower death rate than low fitness men without one of these risk factors.[39] The difference in women with 50% was even more pronounced. Assuming that the level of cardio-respiratory fitness is, at least partly, related to the level of exercise, these results indicate that hypertensive subjects may also benefit from regular exercise, although a direct reduction of mortality from cardiovascular diseases could not be shown in this study.[39]

It also remains unclear to what extent a reduction of blood pressure contributes to the beneficial effect of regular exercise in hypertension. Regular exercise is also known to affect other cardiovascular risk factors favourably, such as dyslipidaemia, insulin resistance, body weight, arterial compliance, left ventricular hypertrophy, or impaired cardiovascular reflex control.[40,41] On the other hand, even relatively small reductions of blood pressure such as those found during exercise training in hypertensive subjects may reduce the risk of stroke and other cardiovascular events considerably.[3,9,10]

Risks of exercise in hypertension

Exercise has benefits but also risks. Fortunately the risk of the most serious complication of exercise—sudden death—is very low in the general population: estimations vary between 0 and 2 deaths per 100 000 hours of exercise,[42] although the risk increases in the presence of heart disease.[43] It has been suggested that hypertension increases the risk of sudden death or exercise induced myocardial ischaemic events.[7] On the other hand, regular exercise protects against sudden death or other cardiovascular events during exercise.[7] It is therefore generally believed that the benefits of regular exercise exceed the risks even in patients with cardiovas-cular disease, especially when individuals are encouraged to avoid sudden high intensity exercise.[6,43] Patients with hypertension are usually discouraged from participating in high intensity resistance training because of the excessive rise in blood pressure that may accompany such exercise.[44] However, an increased risk associated with high intensity resistance training in hypertensive subjects has not been documented.[6] The 26th Bethesda Conference of the American College of Sports Medicine and the American College of Cardiology recommends that the presence of mild hypertension in the absence of target organ damage or concomitant heart disease should not limit the eligibility for any competitive sports, whether dynamic or static.[45]

A pre-exercise screening is often recommended for hypertensive patients.[2,7,43] In patients with more than mildly raised blood pressure, drug treatment to reduce blood pressure will usually be initiated before the start of an exercise programme.[6]

Combination of pharmacological treatment and exercise

In patients with mild hypertension in whom non-drug lifestyle interventions do not result in adequate blood pressure reduction, and in patients with more severe hypertension, drug treatment will often be combined with an exercise advice.[4,6] Several publications have reviewed the interaction between exercise and antihypertensive drug treatment.[6,46-49]

There is convincing evidence that β adrenoceptor blocking agents impair endurance exercise performance considerably; an average reduction of 40% is found with β_{1+2} adrenoceptor blocking agents and a reduction of 20% with β_1 adrenoceptor blockers.[47] Subjective exertion is also increased during exercise in hypertensive patients treated with β blockers.[47] Treatment with β adrenoceptor blocking agents is therefore not attractive for physically active patients with hypertension, although some exercising patients may tolerate β_1 selective agents well. Other antihypertensive agents such as calcium antagonists, ACE inhibitors, and α adrenoceptor blocking agents usually have no significant effect on exercise performance. If significant effects are found, they always tend to be negative.[48,50,51] The effects of diuretics on exercise performance have not been studied very well. Diuretics may induce arrhythmias during exercise in the presence of hypokalaemia.[46,49]

There is very little information on the combined effects of drug treatment and exercise on blood pressure and results have been inconsistent.[5,46,47,49] It has been suggested that the reduction in blood pressure resulting from regular exercise may lead to lower doses of antihypertensive drugs to control blood pressure,[6] but in the literature very few data can be found to support this suggestion. Another important question is whether regular exercise still exerts its other beneficial effects such as increase in fitness, improvement of insulin sensitivity, and lowering of blood lipids, in combination with drug treatment. This is an area where further studies are badly needed to provide a scientific basis for the combination of drug treatment and exercise training in hypertension.

Exercise recommendations

The recommendations for exercise in hypertensive individuals follow those for the general public:[6,43,52] frequency 3–5 times a week; intensity 50–85% $\dot{V}O_2MAX$; duration 20–60 minutes of continuous activity; mode of activity that uses large muscle groups and is rhythmic and aerobic in nature; resistance exercise (minimum of 2 days a week, 8–12 repetitions of the major muscle groups) is recommended as an integral part of each programme. In 1993 the American College of Sports Medicine added that exercise with an intensity of 40–70% $\dot{V}O_2MAX$ seems to lower blood pressure as much as, or even more than, higher intensity exercise. Resistance exercise was not recommended as the only form of exercise for hypertensive individuals but rather as part of a well rounded fitness programme.[6] Since then recommendations have further emphasised the effectiveness of low to moderate activity[43] and the value of relatively short lasting activities (intermittently, as short as 8–10 minutes at a time) amounting to a total of 30 minutes or more over the course of most (and preferably all) days of the week outside formal exercise programmes.[53]

Summary

Regular exercise is recommended in the non-pharmacological treatment of hypertension. Intervention studies show that regular exercise lowers blood pressure. The average reduction of blood pressure in several meta-analyses of studies on the effects of aerobic exercise training in hypertensive patients ranges from 4 mm Hg to 10 mm Hg. The smaller reductions are reported for the better designed studies. Individual (level of blood pressure, ethnicity) and environmental factors (type of exercise programme) may influence the hypotensive effectiveness of exercise programmes. Several hypotheses have been put forward to explain the reduction in blood pressure resulting from regular exercise. It is possible that the mechanism differs across populations because of differences in the underlying hypertensive condition. There are no long term studies showing that regular exercise lowers the risk of cardiovascular morbidity and mortality in hypertensive individuals. Nevertheless, epidemiological data suggest that a high fitness level protects against the influence of risk factors for cardiovascular mortality such as a raised blood pressure.

In many patients regular exercise will be advised as an adjunct to drug treatment. Data on the hypotensive effectiveness of exercise in such combinations are limited. Moreover, the interaction between antihypertensive agents and other potentially beneficial effects of regular exercise is often not known.

Despite the fact that a number of uncertainties with respect to the optimal exercise programme and the combined effects of drug treatment and exercise exist, there is sufficient direct and indirect evidence to encourage sedentary hypertensive patients to become more active to improve their health and fitness.

1 Memorandum from the WHO/ISH. Guides for the treatment of mild hypertension. *Hypertension* 1986;**8**:957–61.
2 World Hypertension League. Physical exercise in the management of hypertension: a consensus statement by the World Hypertension League. *J Hypertens* 1991;**9**:283–7.
3 WHO/ISH Guidelines Committee. Prevention of hypertension and associated cardiovascular disease: a 1991 statement. *Clin Exp Hypertens (A)* 1992;**14**:333–41.
4 Guidelines Sub-Committee of the WHO/ISH Mild Hypertension Liaison Committee. 1993 guidelines for the management of mild hypertension: memorandum from a World Health Organization/International Society of Hypertension Meeting. *J Hypertens* 1993;**11**:905–18.
5 Joint National Committee on Detection, Evaluation, and Treatment of High Blood Pressure. Report V. *Arch Intern Med* 1993;**153**:154–84.
6 American College of Sports Medicine. Physical activity, physical fitness, and hypertension. *Med Sci Sports Exerc* 1993;**25**:i–x.
7 Puddey IB, Cox K. Exercise lowers blood pressure – sometimes? Or did Pheidippides have hypertension? *J Hypertens* 1995;**13**:1229–33.
8 Chalmers J. The treatment of hypertension. *Br J Clin Pharmacol* 1996;**42**:29–35.
9 MacMahon S, Peto R, Cutler J, *et al.* Blood pressure, stroke and coronary heart disease. Part 1: Prolonged differences in blood pressure: prospective observational studies corrected for the regression dilution bias. *Lancet* 1990;**335**:765–74.
10 Collins R, Peto R, MacMahon S, *et al.* Blood pressure, stroke and coronary heart disease. Part 2: Short-term reductions in blood pressure; overview of randomised drug trials in their epidemiological context. *Lancet* 1990;**335**:827–38.
11 Paffenbarger RS, Wing AL, Hyde RT, *et al.* Physical activity and incidence of hypertension in college alumni. *Am J Epidemiol* 1983;**117**:245–57.

12 Blair SN, Goodyear NN, Gibbons LW, *et al.* Physical fitness and incidence of hypertension in healthy normotensive men and women. *JAMA* 1984;**252**:487–90.

13 Fagard RH. Physical fitness and blood pressure. *J Hypertens* 1993;**11**(suppl 5):47–52.

14 Arroll B, Beaglehole R. Does physical activity lower blood pressure? A critical review of the clinical trials. *J Clin Epidemiol* 1992;**45**:439–47.

15 Kelley G, McClellan P. Antihypertensive effects of aerobic exercise. A brief meta-analytic review of randomized controlled trials. *Am J Hypertens* 1994;**7**:115–9.

16 Hagberg JM, Brown MD. Does exercise training play a role in the treatment of essential hypertension? *J Cardiovasc Risk* 1995;**2**:296–302.

17 Halbert JA, Silagy CA, Finucane P, *et al.* The effectiveness of exercise training in lowering blood pressure: a meta-analysis of randomized controlled trials of 4 weeks or longer. *J Hum Hypertens* 1997;**11**:641–9.

18 Kelley G. Dynamic resistance exercise and resting blood pressure in adults: a meta-analysis. *J Appl Physiol* 1997;**82**:1559–65.

19 Pickering TG, Devereux RB. Ambulatory monitoring of blood pressure as a predictor of cardiovascular risk. *Am Heart J* 1987;**114**:925–8.

20 Fagard RH. The role of exercise in blood pressure control: supportive evidence. *J Hypertens* 1995;**13**:1223–7.

21 Marti B. Physische Aktivität und Blutdruck. Eine epidemiologische Kurzreview des primärpräventiven Effekts von körperlich-sportlicher Betätigung. *Schweiz Rundschau Med* 1992;**81**:473–9.

22 Jennings GLR. Exercise and blood pressure: walk, run or swim? *J Hypertens* 1997;**15**:567–9.

23 Tanaka H, Bassett Jr DR, Howley ET, *et al.* Swimming training lowers the resting blood pressure in individuals with hypertension. *J Hypertens* 1997;**15**:651–7.

24 Hagberg JM, Montain SJ, Martin WH, *et al.* Effect of exercise training on 60–69-year-old persons with essential hypertension. *Am J Cardiol* 1989;**64**:348–53.

25 Matsusaki M, Ikeda M, Tashiro E, *et al.* Influence of workload on the antihypertensive effect of exercise. *Clin Exp Pharmacol Physiol* 1992;**19**:471–9.

26 Rogers MW, Probst MM, Gruber JJ, *et al.* Differential effects of exercise training intensity on blood pressure and cardiovascular responses to stress in borderline hypertensive humans. *J Hypertens* 1996;**14**:1369–75.

27 Roman O, Camuzzi AL, Villalon E, *et al.* Physical training program in arterial hypertension: a long-term prospective follow-up. *Cardiology* 1981;**67**:230–43.

28 Tashiro E, Miura S, Koga M, *et al.* Crossover comparison between the depressor effects of low and high work-rate exercise in mild hypertension. *Clin Exp Pharmacol Physiol* 1993;**20**:689–96.

29 Arakawa K. Antihypertensive mechanism of exercise. *J Hypertens* 1993;**11**:223–9.

30 Miura S, Tashiro E, Sakai T, *et al.* Urinary kallikrein activity is increased during the first few weeks of exercise training in essential hypertension. *J Hypertens* 1994;**12**:815–23.

31 Jennings GLR. Exercise and blood pressure: walk, run or swim? *J Hypertens* 1997;**15**:567–9.

32 Kingwell BA, Sherrard B, Jennings GL, *et al.* Four weeks of cycle training increases basal production of nitric oxide from the forearm. *Am J Physiol* 1997;**272**:H1070–7.

33 Cameron JD, Dart AM. Exercise training increases total systemic arterial compliance in humans. *Am J Physiol* 1994;**266**:H693–701.

34 Wijnen JAG, Kuipers H, Kool MJF, *et al.* Vessel wall properties of large arteries in trained and sedentary subjects. *Basic Res Cardiol* 1991;**86**:(suppl 1):25–9.

35 Wijnen JA, Kool MJ, Kooman JP, *et al.* Vessel wall properties of large arteries and endurance training. *J Hypertens* 1993;**11**(suppl 5):88–9.

36 Kingwell BA, Cameron JD, Gillies KJ, *et al.* Arterial compliance may influence baroreflex function in athletes and hypertensives. *Am J Physiol* 1995;**258**: H411–18.

37 Meredith IT, Friberg P, Jennings GL, *et al.* Exercise training lowers resting renal but not cardiac sympathetic activity in human. *Hypertension* 1991;**18**:575–82.

38 Kouamé N, Nadeau A, Lacourcière Y, *et al.* Effects of different training intensities on the cardiopulmonary baroreflex control of forearm vascular resistance in hypertensive subjects. *Hypertension* 1995;**25**:391–8.

39 Blair SN, Kampert JB, Kohl III HW, *et al.* Influences of cardiorespiratory fitness and other precursors on cardiovascular disease and all-cause mortality in men and women. *JAMA* 1996;**276**:205–10.

40 Gilders RM, Dudley GA. Endurance exercise training and treatment of hypertension. *Sports Med* 1992;**13**:71–7.

41 Jennings GLR. Mechanisms for reduction of cardiovascular risk by regular exercise. *Clin Exp Pharmacol Physiol* 1995;**22**:209–11.

42 Fletcher GF, Balady G, Blair SN, *et al.* Statement on exercise: benefits and recommendations for physical activity programs for all Americans. A statement for health professionals by the Committee on Exercise and Cardiac Rehabilitation of the Council on Clinical Cardiology, American Heart Association. *Circulation* 1996;**94**:857–62.

43 Fletcher GF, Balady G, Froelicher VF, *et al.* Exercise standards. A statement for health care professionals from the American Heart Association. *Circulation* 1995;**91**:580–615.

44 MacDougall JD, Tuxen D, Sale DG, *et al.* Arterial blood pressure response to heavy resistance exercise. *J Appl Physiol* 1983;**58**:785–90.

45 Kaplan NM, Devereux RB, Miller Jr HS. Systemic hypertension. *Med Sci Sports Exerc* 1994;**26**(suppl):268–70.

46 Chick TW, Halperin AK, Gacek EM. The effect of antihypertensive medications on exercise performance: a review. *Med Sci Sports Exerc* 1988; **20**:447–54.

47 Van Baak MA. β-Adrenoceptor blockade and exercise: an update. *Sports Med* 1988;**4**:209–25.

48 Van Baak MA. Hypertension, β-adrenoceptor blocking agents and exercise. *Int J Sports Med* 1994;**15**:112–15.

49 Peel C, Mosberg KA. Effects of cardiovascular medications on exercise responses. *Phys Ther* 1995;**75**:387–96.

50 Van Baak MA, Mooij JM, Wijnen JA, *et al.* Submaximal endurance exercise performance during enalapril treatment in patients with essential hypertension. *Clin Pharmacol Ther* 1991; **50**:221–7.

51 Tomten SE, Kjeldsen SE, Nilsson S, *et al.* Effect of α_1-adrenoceptor blockade on maximal VO_2 and endurance capacity in well-trained athletic hypertensive men. *Am J Hypertens* 1994;**7**:603–8.

52 American College of Sports Medicine. The recommended quantity and quality of exercise for developing and maintaining cardiorespiratory and muscular fitness in healthy adults. *Med Sci Sports Exerc* 1990;**22**:265–74.

53 Pate RR, Pratt M, Blair SN, *et al.* Physical activity and public health. A recommendation from the Centers of Disease Control and Prevention and the American College of Sports Medicine. *JAMA* 1995;**273**:402–7.

Multiple choice questions

1 Epidemiological studies on the relation between physical activity and blood pressure show that:

(a) A low level of physical activity is associated with an increased risk of future hypertension in normotensive individuals

(b) An increase in physical activity is associated with a reduction of blood pressure

(c) There is a negative relation between blood pressure and level of physical activity

(d) An increase in physical activity lowers the risk of cardiovascular morbidity and mortality in hypertensive individuals

2 Exercise intervention studies show that regular exercise:

(a) Reduces systolic blood pressure but not diastolic blood pressure

(b) Reduces systolic blood pressure by 15 mm Hg or more in hypertensive individuals

(c) Reduces blood pressure in hypertensive but not in normotensive individuals

(d) Reduces daytime ambulatory blood pressure more than resting blood pressure

3 Which of the following statements about the hypotensive effectiveness of regular exercise are correct?

(a) Women are less responsive than men

(b) Older individuals are less responsive than younger individuals

(c) Swimming increases blood pressure

(d) Normotensive individuals are more responsive than hypertensive individuals

4 Low to moderate intensity, high repetition resistance training:

(a) Increases blood pressure during exercise

(b) Is contraindicated in hypertensive individuals

(c) Has similar hypotensive effects as aerobic exercise training

(d) Is recommended as part of any exercise programme

5 The recommendations for exercise in hypertensive individuals are

(a) The same as in normotensive individuals

(b) A minimal exercise intensity of 70% $\dot{V}O_2MAX$

(c) A frequency between 3–5 times a week but preferably daily

(d) Continuous instead of intermittent exercise

Answers are on p. 364.

8   Diabetes and exercise

N S Peirce

The possible hypoglycaemic benefits of physical activity were originally observed by Aristotle, and later re-advocated as a mainstay of treatment by Allen and Joslin, in the early 1920s. Now widely considered as one of the three main cornerstones of diabetes management, there still remains relatively little guidance for the exercising diabetic. This is despite increasing evidence that many aspects of diabetes can be improved and possibly prevented by regular exercise. At present there are no United Kingdom recommendations for screening, exercise protocols, or treatment regimens, and the personal experience of many with diabetes, including elite athletes, has included frustration and a lack of support on issues of insulin dosage, nutrition, and the potential limits on performance and safety. This review aims to highlight the literature available, while examining the underlying physiology of exercise in diabetes, the benefits and risks of exercise, the strategies for minimising complications, and the potential limitations. The risks and strategies for the distinct population groups represented by type 1 and type 2 diabetes will be looked at separately.

Methods

This review was sourced through searches of Medline, BIDS, and SportDiscus from 1966 to 1998, using the terms "type 1" and "type 2 diabetes mellitus", "impaired glucose tolerance", "non-insulin" and "insulin dependent diabetes", "insulin sensitivity", "exercise", and "physical activity". Cross referencing was undertaken and the opinions of diabetologists and athletes on diabetes and exercise were considered.

Classification of diabetes mellitus

Diabetes is a group of chronic metabolic disorders characterised by hyperglycaemia resulting from a relative deficiency in insulin through either reduced insulin secretion or reduced insulin action or both. The subsequent chronic hyperglycaemia causes glycation of tissues, which almost inevitably leads to acute disturbances in metabolism and long term end organ damage and severe health complications. In the United States there are nearly 16 million reported cases and an estimated 6 million undiagnosed.[1] The worldwide prevalence of diabetes appears to be increasing, with estimates of 4.0% (135 million) in 1995 expected to rise to 5.4% (300 million) by the year 2025. Thus diabetes and its complications are set to be an increasing burden on health care budgets and already account for 30% of the Medicare budget in the United States.[2]

Almost all diabetes falls into two categories: type 1, an absolute deficiency of insulin production, and type 2, characterised by resistance to insulin and inadequate compensation. These were recently reclassified following a report by the expert committee on the diagnosis and classification of diabetes mellitus which has suggested removal of the terms "insulin dependent diabetes" and "non-insulin dependent diabetes", in use since 1979. Impaired glucose tolerance, gestational diabetes, and maturity onset diabetes of the young are among other conditions reclassified.[3]

Normal blood glucose control

At rest

Blood glucose concentrations must be maintained within narrow limits. This is essential to prevent the acute and chronic complications seen in diabetes mellitus[4] and is achieved through a balance between the processes that add and remove glucose from the normal circulation. In the fasting state, glucose is produced by the liver and closely balances the uptake and losses into body tissues, responding closely to the circulating plasma glucose concentrations. In the postprandial state, glucose is absorbed through the alimentary system, causing a rise in blood glucose concentrations. Insulin is released which reduces hepatic glucose production and increases the disposal of glucose in peripheral tissue, thus reducing blood glucose. Some 90% of this clearance occurs through increased uptake in skeletal muscle where glucose is transported into muscle by facilitated diffusion. This occurs through the translocation of a family of transporter proteins to the membrane surface, almost all of which are the GLUT4 transporter (fig 8.1). A limited number of GLUT5 transporters are also present which allow relatively slow fructose transport.

During exercise

During exercise the large changes in energy utilisation require fine adjustments of glucose and non-esterified fatty acid concentrations within the blood. During the first 5–10 minutes of moderate intensity exercise, glycogen provides the major fuel source for skeletal muscle, but as exercise duration is prolonged, the contribution of plasma (blood borne) glucose and non-esterified fatty acid predominates. To match this increased demand, a

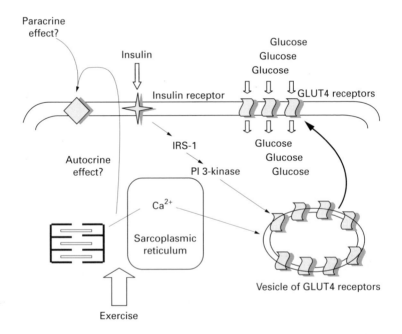

Fig 8.1 Glucose uptake in skeletal muscle. Insulin and exercise independently facilitate glucose transport across the mitochondrial membrane through promotion of GLUT4 transporters from the vesicles. The action is also cumulative producing enhanced glucose uptake/sensitivity during and after exercise. IRS-1, insulin receptor substrate 1; PI 3-kinase, phosphatidylinositol 3-kinase. Modified from Goodyear.[147]

complex hormonal and autonomic response allows an increase in hepatic glucose production and tissue uptake while increasing mobilisation of non-esterified fatty acid from adipose tissue deposits. This is produced both by a fall in circulating insulin concentrations and a wide variety of "counter-regulatory" hormones, increased secretion of which counters the hypoglycaemic action of insulin (fig 8.2). Elevations in the blood concentrations of these hormones, which include adrenaline, glucagon, cortisol, and growth hormone, promote both increased glucose production and mobilisation of non-esterified fatty acids from adipose storage sites. In addition, production of new glucose in the liver (gluconeogenesis) from substrates such as lactate is enhanced. Direct sympathetic stimulation of the pancreas and liver after muscle contraction may also bypass initial hormonal control, and additional fuel supplies

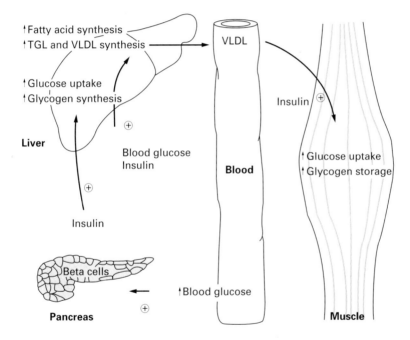

Fig 8.2 Actions of insulin. Insulin secretion from β cells in the pancreas reduces hepatic glucose production while increasing glucose uptake in skeletal muscle. Lipid and glucose storage (as liver and muscle glycogen) is enhanced while lipolysis and ketone formation are suppressed. In type 1 and 2 diabetes the secretion and actions are reduced respectively. VLDL, very low density lipoprotein; TGL, triacylglycerol. Modified from Brooks et al.[148]

are provided by ketone formation and mobilisation of lactate from inactive muscle glycogen.

Glucose transport into muscle is again provided by the transporter protein GLUT4, but the protein is recruited to the membrane surface in large quantities in contracting muscle, independently of insulin (fig 8.1). Together these changes maintain the increased fuel supply for exercising muscle and prevent hypoglycaemia from excessive utilisation.

After exercise

At the end of exercise the body in essence enters a fasted state in which glycogen stores in muscle and liver are low and hepatic glucose production is accelerated. The counter-regulatory hormone levels may remain elevated for some considerable time and there is a concomitant hyperglycaemic and hyperinsulinaemic response. Glycogen resynthesis in the muscle occurs at first largely as a result of increased GLUT4 transport and insulin sensitivity and without the need for insulin. At a variable time point later, as homoeostasis is reached and glycogen, glucose, and hormone levels return to normal, insulin may be required to produce additional glucose uptake and glycogen resynthesis in muscle and liver. In the insulin deficient or resistant state, storage of glucose may therefore be impaired within muscle because of incomplete transport and decreased glycogen synthase activity.

Type 1 diabetes

In type 1 diabetes there is autoimmune destruction of the pancreas leading to a failure to secrete insulin. Although trials are underway to explore the prevention of this process, it is at present a relentless and chronic disorder. It represents the most common endocrinological disease of childhood affecting as many as 1 in 500 children under 18, and the incidence would appear to be increasing.[1] Exogenous insulin is essential in the treatment of this condition and represents the only available treatment for approximating normal physiology. Since the introduction of insulin in the 1920s, when treatment was aimed at preventing ketoacidosis, the process of insulin administration has become more elaborate with increasing varieties and techniques. The aims of treatment for a diabetic now include mimicry of normal insulin levels throughout the day, achieving tight control, and prevention of microvascular and macrovascular complications.

Blood glucose control

Ambient insulin concentrations are vital in normal glucose homoeostasis both during exercise and in recovery. In type 1 diabetes the normal mechanism is lost and must be approximated using exogenous insulin, with consequent problems of excessive or insufficient insulin administration.

Excess insulin prevents normal hepatic glucose production and mobilisation of non-esterified fatty acids. In addition, whole body glucose disposal increases through facilitated muscle glucose uptake with the subsequent risk of exercise induced hypoglycaemia,[5,6] exacerbated in turn if inappropriately injected into exercising muscle.[7] The uptake of glucose into skeletal muscle can occur independently of insulin, but, because of the increase in insulin sensitivity after exercise and reduced liver and glycogen stores, glucose production cannot meet the excessive uptake, and thus hyperinsulinisation will also increase the risk of post-exercise hypoglycaemia.

Despite the independent glucose uptake that occurs in skeletal muscle with exercise, a relative deficiency in the insulin dosage can result in hyperglycaemia, hyperlipidaemia, and possible ketosis. This can eventually lead to ketoacidosis and coma. Once exercise commences, this condition will deteriorate, with a further increase in the production of counter-regulatory hormones, especially glucagon and adrenaline, producing elevated hepatic glucose production and impaired muscle glucose uptake and therefore further rises in blood glucose. Ketosis may also increase as lipolysis will be more pronounced.[8,9] This exaggerated hyperglycaemia and ketosis occurs despite rising blood glucose concentrations and appears to be correlated with the initial ketotic state of the person. Berger et al.,[10] in 1980, showed the importance of the pre-exercise state. Increases in pre-exercise values above the normal blood levels of non-esterified fatty acid (1173 μmol/l), glucose (18 mmol/l), ketone bodies (2.13 mmol/l), and branched chain amino acids (0.74 mmol/l) proved critical before three hours of cycling at 30–40% $\dot{V}O_2MAX$. Exaggerated glucagon and cortisol levels were observed which in turn promoted hyperglycaemia and ketosis. Conversely exercise below these starting concentrations allowed an appropriate fall in blood glucose during the exercise period.[10] However, these starting values are variable between subjects, and some trial and error may be required to establish them, which equally applies to intense exercise of shorter duration. Interestingly lactate production also appears to be higher in type 1 diabetes, which is possibly related to the increased production of counter-regulatory hormones.

Risks of exercise in type 1 diabetes

The major risks to the exercising type 1 diabetic are potentially life threatening metabolic disturbances and the associated morbidity and mortality of microvascular and macrovascular complications.

Despite the best precautions, hypoglycaemia can occur, and, although moderate exercise itself may not mask hypoglycaemic responses in patients with type 1 diabetes, during vigorous activity this feedback may be impaired,[11] with additional orthostatic hypotension, impaired thermoregulation, and neuropathy confusing the hypoglycaemic symptoms.[12] These may be worse in the morning,[13] and all patients with type 1 diabetes should carry rapidly absorbable high glycaemic carbohydrates/drinks, glucagon, or "Hypostop". The normal alcohol consumption that occurs after a game in many sports can also pose additional risks of exercise induced hypoglycaemia with a failure to recognise the warnings, occasionally seen as a problem in subaqua divers where "nitrogen narcosis" and exercise induced hypoglycaemia produce interchangeable symptoms.

Post-exercise hypoglycaemia and delayed onset hypoglycaemia can occur up to four and 24 hours after exercise respectively. The increased insulin sensitivity and depleted glycogen stores conspire to produce profound hypo, most commonly nocturnal.[14] This neuroglycopenia has been suggested to disturb sleep patterns, alter recovery, and therefore affect physical performance the following day and carries significant morbidity and mortality. Recent studies in this department have shown that one hour of nocturnal hypoglycaemia reduces the sense of wellbeing and increases subjective determinants of fatigue but produces no alterations in the hormonal, glucose, and lactate response to exercise. Interestingly, cerebral, cardiovascular, and physical performance also show no objective alterations.[15] For the person concerned, nocturnal hypoglycaemia nevertheless remains an alarming risk, and an evening snack or reduced evening dose of insulin after activity may be warranted. Hyperglycaemia as discussed above produces both acute and long term consequences, increasing the risks of cardiovascular disease, sudden death, reduced exercise capacity, hypertension, retinopathy, nephropathy, and neuropathy, which can all significantly worsen with impaired control. These complications will be discussed below.

There are a large number of significant physical and psychological benefits of exercise which demand regular physical activity where possible. Unfortunately the evidence for improvements in glycaemic control in type 1 diabetes are not well established. Only a handful of studies, often relatively small, have provided mixed evidence for improvements in glycaemic control. Several have shown reduced insulin secretion and hypoglycaemia but little reduction in HbA1c,[16–18] although when activity was stratified according to participation, metabolic control was significantly better among diabetic subjects participating frequently (at least 11 of 13 sessions), regardless of the type of activity.[19] More recently a study of 61 subjects with type 1 diabetes showed that modest changes in exercise and diet were sufficient to improve measures of glycaemic control and lipoprotein mediated risk of coronary heart disease.[20] In addition, some evidence suggests that the timing of exercise is an important factor, with regular postprandial exercise improving long term blood glucose control.[21]

Aims of treatment

The diabetes control and complications trial and more recently the UK prevention of diabetes study have both shown conclusively that tight control helps to prevent the development of macrovascular and microvascular complications. Thus the aims of treatment should be to keep blood glucose concentration between 4 and 7.2 mmol/l and to prevent large and significant swings either below 3.0 mmol/l, leading to symptomatic hypoglycaemia, or above 8–10 mmol/l, increasing the immediate and long term complications. However, with extremely tight control, there is a potential for an increased risk of hypoglycaemia during exercise. Thus personalised insulin regimens and nutritional strategies in advance of physical activity need to be adapted.

Insulin regimens

Insulin regimens should be tailored to each patient. One to one education and establishing self empowerment have been shown to significantly improve glycaemic control but, unfortunately, a degree of trial and error is necessary for all patients with type 1 diabetes taking up any new activities.

Insulin regimens for most patients range between 0.5 and 1.0 U/kg/day. This dose may be reduced in lean subjects, athletes, and during the honeymoon period, which can be prolonged in diabetic athletes. In these groups insulin doses are between 0.2 and 0.6 U/kg/day. Traditionally, regimens sought to provide a basal insulin presence by injection of intermediate or long acting insulin once or twice a day, administered in the morning and evening and amounting to 50% of the daily insulin dose. Additional fast acting regular insulins were then introduced and given with breakfast, lunch, and sometimes dinner. Unfortunately the presence of longer acting insulins produces a significant risk of hypoglycaemia during the midmorning or afternoon and at night, which is exaggerated in the exercising diabetic.

To improve tight control, intensive insulin regimens with regular self monitoring of glucose are now used widely by exercising patients with type 1 diabetes. These intensive multiple component regimens include regular mealtime injections of short acting insulin analogues (onset of action 15–30 minutes), such as Lispro, or regular insulins (onset 30–60 minutes), with a lower dose of intermediate acting insulin once or twice a day to provide a low basal insulin presence. In the exercising diabetic this may be best served by a low dose intermediate acting insulin injection in the evening only, to prevent hypoglycaemia during the day, although this may promote increased blood glucose levels during the following day. Some studies report common exercise induced hypoglycaemia,[6,22] but an intensive education programme in 700 subjects[23] showed that large reductions in exercise induced hypoglycaemia can be achieved by careful planning.

Moderate exercise

Any physical activity including household chores may reduce daily insulin requirement. If it is only 20–30 minutes duration and less than 70% $\dot{V}O_2MAX$, minimal adjustments may need to be made. If early morning physical activity is to be performed, the basal insulin provided by an evening injection of intermediate to long acting insulin may need to be reduced by 20–50% with checking of the morning blood glucose. Increases of more than 7–8 mmol/l may compromise long term control, although levels below 10–12 mmol/l will allow safe exercise. Conversely, levels below 6 mmol/l may increase the risk of hypoglycaemia even if the exercise intensity is likely to be moderate (50–70%). The morning regular acting insulin dose will also need to be reduced by 30–50% before breakfast or even omitted if exercise is taken before food. Insulin should otherwise be taken 30–60 minutes before the meal as usual. Depending on the intensity and duration of the initial activity and the likelihood of further activity, a similar reduction of 30–50% may need to be made with each subsequent meal. After exercise, hyperglycaemia will occur. However, insulin doses should still be reduced by 25–50%.

If exercise is unexpected, then adjustment of insulin dosage will be impossible. Instead supplementing with 20–30 g carbohydrate – that is, a carton of orange juice or an energy bar – at the onset of exercise and every 30 minutes thereafter may prevent hypoglycaemia.

Elite athletes and intense activity

The elite athlete provides both a unique challenge and a unique resource. As a possible role model they provide a focus for diabetics throughout their home country. In the United Kingdom, Gary Mabbut and Steven Redgrave (fig 8.3) are household names and have contributed to normalising attitudes towards exercise and diabetes. Many doctors find it remarkable that people with type 1 diabetes can compete at the highest level. Despite this attention, however, most athletes even now find most information to be vague, limited, and often of little relevance, and some have even put these thoughts in print in the hope of helping others.[13,24]

It is extremely important for an elite athlete to establish habitual training programmes that mimic competition. If the exercise intensity is sufficiently high or competitive, insulin may even be

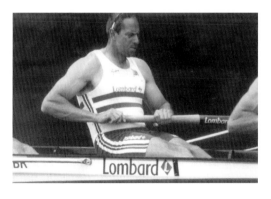

Fig 8.3   Steven Redgrave.

omitted at the beginning of competition, although the recom-mendations need careful individual attention. A reduction of 70–90% is more likely to be appropriate in such situations, which applies equally to extremely intense prolonged exercise, such as is encountered in marathons and triathlons,[25] and vigorous team sports with interrupted activity such as rugby, football, and hockey. Additional carbohydrates may need to be taken on board and blood sugar checked at changeovers/half time, if necessary. A reduction of 50–70% in insulin administered the night before may also be necessary to prevent long acting insulins from increasing hypoglycaemia during early morning exercise and may also be required for 24–36 hours after intense exercise.

Both elite and recreational diabetic athletes can also learn to identify hyperglycaemia (>14 mmol/l glucose) which may be manifested as poor concentration, dehydration, or even under confidence. In the period after exercise, hyperglycaemia can arise from continued glucose production and reduced disposal, and an increase in insulin dose may be necessary. Care should be taken with this dose, which will need to be relatively low, as the risk of post-exercise hypoglycaemia is increased because of enhanced insulin sensitivity and low glycogen stores. Consideration must also be given to any additional medication that may promote hypogly-caemia or hyperglycaemia, and one must also be alert to the possible use of anabolic agents such anabolic steroids and stimulants which may all worsen hyperglycaemia.

With regular attention and simple strategies (table 8.1), it is possible to achieve both adequate control and high intensity

---

Box 8.1   Type 1 diabetes

- Programmes of intensive individual education allow a person to be self empowered and reduce the risk of complications. Small teams of health professionals working closely with an individual are essential to improve a person's understanding of his or her condition
- Exercise improves many aspects of health including cardiovascular risk factors and psychological wellbeing, but it is not clear whether glycaemic control and progression of disease is substantially improved
- Careful screening for many of the occult microvascular and macrovascular risk factors needs to be undertaken on an annual basis and allows for appropriate type and intensity of exercise participation to be determined

Table 8.1 Metabolic control in type 1 diabetes

Monitor	Action
Establish good control before exercise	If unstable avoid exercise until control established
Check nature of exercise, ambient conditions, changes in weight, hydration status	Adjust for cold/heat/winds/weight loss/intense game/activity
Blood glucose > 14 mmol/l (250 mg/dl) ketosis ($1-2^{++}$) urinalysis	Avoid exercise
Blood glucose >17 mmol/l (300 mg/dl)	Avoid exercise
Blood glucose <5.5–6.0 mmol/l (100 mg/dl)	Ingest extra carbohydrate and avoid vigorous or prolonged exercise unless established protocol
Monitor glucose before and after exercise	Establish routine and response to exercise, identify changes required before activity, identify symptoms of hypoglycaemia
Establish timing and quantity of food	Allow for delayed gastric emptying for glucose absorption and discomfort. Provide readily available and absorbable carbohydrate
Adjust insulin doses according to intensity of exercise	For moderate intensity exercise allow 50% reduction in insulin dosages. For high/prolonged intensity reduce dose by 70–90%

exercise. During periods of inactivity such as holidays or recovery from injury increased insulin requirements are to be expected.

Site of injections and glucose monitoring

Standard advice should include establishing a routine site and technique and avoiding injecting into the exercising leg,[26] although hypoglycaemia cannot be averted by simply altering the site. Care needs to be taken to avoid intramuscular injections,[7] and in hot or warm ambient conditions absorption may also be increased. The most common site used by athletes appears to be the abdomen as this allows ease of access at meal times and is least likely to affect performance.

Ideally, monitoring should be undertaken each morning, before and after exercise and before and after meals. Computer programs have also been suggested,[27] and athletes involved in potentially dangerous activities such as scuba diving should check blood glucose at 90, 30 and five minutes before exercise. This shows the direction of blood glucose changes, which should be stable. Blood glucose monitoring kits are now small and portable and should be kept within easy access at all times.

Insulin pumps

These have come into vogue and "pumpies" are increasingly using continuous subcutaneous insulin infusion pumps for treatment during elite sports participation. They have been in use for 20 years,[28] and increasing numbers of elite athletes are using the pumps to secure intensive insulin regimens, tight control, and increased flexibility. Studies on continuous subcutaneous insulin infusion have shown that reducing the action of the pump by 50% before exercise, similar to multiple component regimens, prevents hypoglycaemia.[29-31]

Lispro

Lispro is a rapid acting insulin analogue which has recently been developed, particularly for injection immediately before a meal. Its rapid absorption and short duration of action provide several advantages, and, although reports on Lispro and exercise are limited, the use of a shorter acting analogue will probably allow a greater degree of flexibility and the ability to accommodate short term planning or unexpected exercise.[32]

150

Box 8.2 Type 1 diabetes

- Exercise in people with type 1 diabetes has a risk of exercise induced and late onset hypoglycaemia up to 24 hours after an event. Increased blood glucose concentration before exercise and the presence of ketosis may promote hyperglycaemia especially with prolonged or vigorous activity
- Careful monitoring of glucose before, during, and after exercise and at night, accompanied by adjustments of insulin and carbohydrate intake, can considerably reduce the risk of these complications
- Planning of exercise and adjustment of insulin regimens for prevailing ambient conditions and exercise type, duration, and intensity with appropriate availability of rapidly absorbed carbohydrates is essential to allow safe physical activity in people with type 1 diabetes

Performance

Traditionally it has been felt that diabetics, especially over 35 years of age, cannot succeed at the highest level of athletic endeavour. However, there is now a sufficient number of professional athletes, Olympic gold medallists, and world champions with type 1 diabetes to make us question the limits of the disease process. Relatively few studies have investigated performance parameters in the elite type 1 diabetic population. Certainly patients with diabetic neuropathy may have an increased risk of falling and injuries secondary to instability and reduced muscle strength. People with type 1 diabetes have a greater proportion of type 2 muscle fibres under conditions of hyperinsulinaemia with a consequent reduction in absolute strength; however, they adapt normally to strength and endurance with appropriate increases in muscle fibre type. Other studies show reduced left ventricular function and maximal oxygen consumption in association with type 1 diabetes, but all show improvement with training. Even impaired secretion of endogenous opioids in type 1 diabetes has been suggested to alter performance.

Nutrition

The use of an intensive insulin regimen requires careful attention to nutrition. With delayed gastric emptying often present, adjustments in dietary regimens to suit personal preferences, such as

151

liquid supplements, may be required. Meals may also need to be taken between three and five hours before exercise. "Counting the carbohydrate" content of meals has become increasingly popular as a means of adjusting insulin doses and dietary calories. An individual ratio of 1 unit of insulin per 10 g carbohydrate is widely advocated, with adjustments made for the intensity or duration of exercise. Many athletes use programmes such as the "ex-carbs" and the "450 program" which have been formularised and advocated within athletic circles but have not been studied. A balanced diet needs to take into account energy requirements and should provide 60% of total energy expenditure as carbohydrates (5–10 g/kg/day depending on exercise intensity and duration) before, during, and after exercise. This should be accompanied by additional fluids and protein (0.6–1.2 g/kg/day) and a reduction in fat, less than 30–40 g a day.

Type 2 diabetes

Type 2 diabetes (formerly known as non-insulin dependent diabetes mellitus) occurs almost exclusively in the adult population and its main feature is insulin resistance, manifested as hyper-insulinaemia and hyperglycaemia. It is strongly correlated with obesity, physical inactivity, and family history and accounts for 90% of all diabetes. Typically as many as 80% are overweight and many are elderly. Not surprisingly the incidence of the disease is increasing in western societies.

Physiology of exercise and training in impaired glucose tolerance and type 2 diabetes

Many of the extreme changes in metabolism seen in type 1 diabetes are blunted. Instead, hyperinsulinism and hyperglycaemia are present concurrently because of the preservation of pancreatic β cell function and hepatic and skeletal muscle insulin resistance, with hypoglycaemia therefore relatively uncommon. The initial presentation of type 2 diabetes is as insulin resistance, an impaired response to endogenous insulin, and therefore impaired glucose tolerance. As with type 1 diabetes, exercise produces increased glucose uptake in skeletal muscle. Unlike in type 1 diabetes, however, those with type 2 diabetes are able to produce significant decreases in ambient blood glucose and insulin concentrations without increasing the risk of hypoglycaemia. This is due in part to reduced hepatic glucose production but mainly to increased muscle glucose uptake through increased delivery, oxidation, and storage of carbohydrates. In type 2 diabetes, this increased uptake appears to bypass the normal regulation at rest and promotes increased glucose uptake for up to several hours with a concomitant fall in glycaemia.[33] A single exercise bout has been shown to increase insulin sensitivity in liver and muscle for up to 16 hours[34] while prolonged exercise produces a fall in hyperglycaemia and hyperinsulinaemia.[35]

Initially athletes were noticed to have reduced plasma glucose and insulin concentrations in response to oral glucose loading,[36] with the suggestion that exercise improved insulin sensitivity.[37] The increase in insulin sensitivity with exercise has since been well established,[38–40] and controlled studies of exercise intervention/ training have resulted in improved insulin sensitivity,[41] increased carbohydrate oxidation, and reductions in body mass.[42] Hughes *et al.*[43] showed an improvement in insulin sensitivity with training at 50–70% $\dot{V}O_2$MAX, and many studies have reported immediate changes in total glucose disposal[34,44,45] and skeletal muscle uptake.[41,46,47] In subjects who trained vigorously, improvements in glucose disposal were double for up to 10 days.[48] These beneficial effects of training unfortunately appear to be transient, declining after seven days[49] and 10 days,[43,50,51] and are in part derived from increased GLUT4 transporter recruitment, which has also been shown to be higher in athletes[52] and after training.[43,53] In addition, exercise and training promote increased blood flow, insulin receptor, and oxidative and non-oxidative enzyme concentrations in muscle. Although aerobic training also promotes the transition to a greater percentage of type 1 and 2a muscle fibres, the importance of this is not fully understood. Instead the preservation of the lean body tissues, in particular muscle mass, and the reductions in fat mass appear to be significant contributors to improved insulin sensitivity.[47] Although the risks of hypoglycaemia in type 2 diabetes appear small, conflicting advice on concomitant exercise and treatment with sulphonylureas is still given. Caution when undertaking vigorous exercise should therefore be encouraged, as some reports of hypoglycaemia exist.[54–56] Metformin has also been linked with type B lactic acidosis and its use is probably inappropriate during intense exercise.[57]

However, do these immediate changes in the actions of insulin produce long term adaptive benefits?[58]

Epidemiology of physical activity and improved glycaemic control

Early studies indicated that prolonged bed rest was associated with impaired glucose tolerance.[49,59] Epidemiological evidence has strongly pointed to a number of correlates of physical inactivity promoting type 2 diabetes,[60] including lack of vigorous exercise, reduced energy expenditure, ageing, aerobic capacity, heart rate changes, and time spent exercising.[61,62] Importantly these studies also suggest that physical activity can reduce the risk of developing type 2 diabetes. In those individuals with impaired glucose tolerance[61,63–66] the relative risk over five years was approximately 0.70 (P = 0.0006) for participants who exercised vigorously in comparison with sedentary subjects.[60–62,67,68] In high risk groups such as those with a family history of diabetes mellitus or increased body mass index there is a beneficial outcome from regular physical activity, also shown in the large cohort studies of college alumni[61] and nurses. These studies show a 6% reduction in the prevalence of type 2 diabetes with each 2.09 MJ of estimated recreational activity.[65] The recent insulin resistance atherosclerosis study showed improved insulin sensitivity in both non-vigorous (< 6 metabolic equivalent levels; METS) and vigorous (> 6 METS) exercise.[69–71]

Exercise trials to prevent diabetes

Some 30–40% of people with impaired glucose tolerance progress to type 2 diabetes at a rate of 1–1.5% per year, and several large studies have explored the relation between exercise and the prevention of the onset of diabetes. The diabetes prevention study in Finland showed that simple lifestyle changes including diet and moderate exercise decreased two hour glucose (0.9 mmol) and insulin (22.5 U/ml) after an oral glucose tolerance test.[72] In China, the Da Quing impaired glucose tolerance study followed 577 subjects with impaired glucose tolerance for six years; a 31%, 46%, and 42% reduction in the risk of developing diabetes was associated with diet, exercise, and diet plus exercise respectively.[73] The Oslo diet and exercise study randomised 219 men and women to a one year participation in supervised exercise (aerobic exercise three times a week) and dietary changes (fish and reduced fat) and showed significant benefits in insulin sensitivity especially using the combined approach.[74]

The Malmo prevention study, first reported several years ago,[64,66] has shown, after 12 years follow up, reduced mortality in patients with impaired glucose tolerance (increased risk of both developing type 2 diabetes and premature death from ischaemic heart disease) and a reduction in type 2 diabetes by 50%.[75] The diabetic prevention project in Washington DC is at present examining impaired glucose tolerance; 855 patients have been randomised to taking troglitazone or metformin or lifestyle changes.

The potential to improve health in a population in which up to two out of every three adults are not regularly active at all[25,76] is staggering. However, considerable work is needed in many areas such as the benefits of educating children and the young,[36,48,77] the intensity of the exercise that is most beneficial,[78] and the most appropriate timing of any interventions, given the occult nature of diabetes and risk factors.[79]

Exercise benefits

The prescription of exercise for diabetic control should be considered for a variety of associated and independent health benefits. The full scope of these benefits can be seen in a number of reviews and include weight loss, weight loss maintenance, lipid profiles, blood pressure, psychological profile, and the constellation of symptoms that make up the metabolic/Reaven syndrome X.[80-82] It would appear that exercise and diet provide the first and possibly most effective interventions in improving cardiovascular risk,[83-86] with exercise intervention studies now showing reduced

---

Box 8.3   Type 2 diabetes

- Improvements in the glycaemic control of people with impaired glucose tolerance and type 2 diabetes seems to be established and maintained by physical activity, especially when associated with dietary measures and associated weight loss
- Exercise prescription programmes seem to be safe and to delay, even possibly prevent, the onset of symptoms especially when combined with lifestyle interventions. Compliance rates can be helped by group work and psychological support
- Occult cardiovascular and autonomic disease can predispose to silent myocardial ischaemia and sudden death in both type 1 and 2 diabetes. Careful screening before participation in exercise, including exercise stress testing when appropriate, needs to be considered in all patients before physical activity is undertaken

death rates (6.5 v 14.0; P = 0.009) in those with impaired glucose tolerance.[75]

It has become evident that possibly the most important role for exercise will be in weight loss and weight loss maintenance. A loss of 4.5 kg or more appears to be critical in preventing the development of covert diabetes and reducing blood pressure,[87] and evidence for the importance of exercise in increasing weight loss and helping maintain weight loss with subsequent improvements in type 2 diabetes is now overwhelming.

Exercise prescription

Once a patient has been screened and the risk factors and exercise capacity determined, regular exercise may then be considered. The typical patient with type 2 diabetes is sedentary, overweight, and middle aged or older.[88] In this group of patients, exercise may well be beneficial but needs to be carefully implemented. Guidelines issued jointly by the American Diabetes Association (ADA) and the American College of Sports Medicine (ACSM) suggest a gentle warm up period of 5–10 minutes, a period of stretching, and then an active cool down period of 5–10 minutes to allow gradual adjustment of heart rate and blood pressure.[89] The intensity, duration, and frequency of exercise necessary for good health has been adjusted from the 60–80% of maximal oxygen consumption outlined in the ACSM guidelines in 1976. Instead the target of an adult should be to achieve 30 minutes of continuous moderate activity, equivalent to brisk walking on five or six days a week,[60] with the flexibility of shorter bouts of more intense activity increasingly being considered important. Vigorous activity is widely implicated in health benefits and can be safely undertaken in diabetics provided that cardiovascular and hypertensive problems are taken into consideration. As no studies have accurately defined the most suitable exercise programme for diabetics, it is inappropriate to be too prescriptive and instead we should concentrate on adherence and compliance.[90] When ACSM guidelines are used, there is a drop out rate of 40–70% after 12–18 months despite an active intervention programme.[91] However, the recent guidelines have gained wider acceptance[92] and much greater success has been reported in the Malmo intervention studies[93] for relatively informal exercise programmes[94] with mixed high and low intensity exercise,[95] although exercise below 30% $\dot{V}O_2$MAX may have little benefit.[96] In general, exercise programmes appear to be safe, with a very low incidence of hypoglycaemia, a 12% incidence of musculoskeletal injuries, and 29% increase in proteinuria of unknown significance. In part because of autonomic neuropathy, heart rate may be an unreliable indicator of relative intensity of exercise and therefore the rating of perceived exertion scales may be a more useful predictor of 50–70% $\dot{V}O_2MAX$.[97]

Exercise prescription must also take into account patients' readiness to exercise, attitudes, and belief systems, while positively encouraging decisions to exercise. Support can be provided through a team of doctors, nurses, physiotherapists, lifestyle counsellors, and exercise consultants and even through health policy decision-making at government and local level.[98,99]

Screening

For safe participation in activity, patients of any age should have regular medical examinations to predict and prevent major complications. Exercise intensity and activities can then be planned accordingly. A routine examination should include the points outlined in table 8.2 and further specific tests initiated as appropriate.

Nephropathy

Nephropathy occurs in 20–40% of patients with type 1 and type 2 diabetes, and, when combined with hypertension, with which it is strongly correlated, it accounts for one fifth of all end stage renal disease. Nephropathy is classified according to urinary albumin excretion rates: <20 µg/min, normoalbuminuria; 20–200 µg/min,

Table 8.2 Evaluation of subject before exercise

Evaluation
History, age, duration of disease, family history
Examination
Cardiovascular
Blood pressure
Retinal examination (table 8.4)
Neuropathy (tables 8.5 and 8.6)
Vascular
Foot
Exercise stress test (table 8.3)
Blood HbA1c, lipid profile, renal function
Urinalysis, glycosuria, microalbumin, protein, ketones

incipient nephropathy; >200 μg/min, overt nephropathy.[100] Although exercise increases albumin excretion, there is no evidence that this hastens the progression of nephropathy, even though exercise induced albumin excretion was once used as a diagnosis of covert nephropathy. Instead improved glycaemic control and maintenance of normal blood pressure can help slow overall progression of macrovascular disease and mortality,[4,101] and, as exercise both raises blood pressure acutely and helps to reduce blood pressure chronically, the benefits are not clear cut. One small study showed no detriment to renal function after exercise,[102] but at present no guidelines exist on either the benefits or risks of exercise in the presence of nephropathy. The ADA/ACSM has suggested that participation may need to be limited, but has not defined this. However, it would appear sensible to consider the strong association of renal disease with associated risk factors of hypertension and microvascular and macrovascular complications, and therefore restrict those with overt nephropathy to moderate intensity activity. In addition, the presence of anaemia or uraemic myopathy and taking medications such as antihypertensive drugs (up to 30% of diabetics require triple antihypertensive treatment) may all reduce exercise capacity. In dialysis patients, exercise capacity is reduced but this can be increased by exercise training, dietary changes, erythropoietin administration, and ultimately renal transplant.[103]

Cardiovascular disease

Atherosclerosis, hypertension,[104] and cardiomyopathy[105] are more common in diabetes with the relative risk doubled for myocardial events and sudden death, especially in the young. Ischaemic heart disease is present in 50% of patients with type 2 diabetes at the time of initial diagnosis,[106] with early signs of cardiovascular disease and reduced performance capacity[107] predicting the likelihood of future cardiac events and ischaemic heart disease.[108] These are increased 2- and 4-fold in male and female patients with type 2 diabetes respectively[109] and 3–10-fold in those with type 1 diabetes.[110-115] Complications include reduced left ventricular function, higher resting heart rates, reduced cardiac reserve, reduced cardiac return, orthostatic hypotension, and coronary artery stenosis.[116-120] In addition, hypoglycaemia may promote prolongation of PR and QT intervals, promoting arrhythmias during exercise.

Hypertension is also more prevalent in type 1 and type 2 diabetes than in the background population, especially in younger patients.[65,101,121–124] Appropriate control is necessary, as systolic blood pressure rises may be higher during exercise;[123–125] however, blood pressure can be reduced by 5–10 mm Hg after 10 weeks training and this may be sufficient with concomitant weight reduction to establish normotension.[126] Treatment needs to consider potential reductions in performance and exercise induced systolic pressure, and ultimately participation will depend on an informed decision, with exercise above 70% $\dot{V}O_2$MAX and use of isometric contractions restricted. Protocols for resistance training can be found in the ACSM guidelines,[127] and appropriate references include the guidelines for prevention, detection, evaluation, and treatment of hypertension by the Joint National Committee VI.[87] In addition, recently the UK prevention of diabetes study has shown equal benefit from β blockers and angiotensin converting enzyme inhibitors for prevention of macrovascular complications.[101,122]

Table 8.3, adapted from ACSM/ADA, recommends pre-exercise screening, with stress testing for the cardiovascular risk stratification which should be considered as a minimum. Abnormal results may then demand appropriate management and planned intensity of exercise prescription.

Retinopathy

The presence of retinopathy should always be suspected in any diabetic patient and should form part of any routine assessment before participation in exercise. Some 98% of cases of type 1 diabetes and 78% of cases of type 2 diabetes will progress, resulting in detectable changes 15 years from diagnosis,[128] correlating with duration of disease, poor control, hypertension, hyperlipidaemia, fluid overload, and renal disease. Diabetic retinopathy can be

Table 8.3   Modified ACSM/ADA screening protocol

Cardiovascular risk factors demanding exercise stress testing[89]

Vigorous/elite activity
Type 2 > 10 years
Type 1 > 15 years
> 35 years of age
Any coronary artery disease risk factors
Any macrovascular disease
Any microvascular disease
Peripheral vascular disease

simplified as non-proliferative or proliferative, with the natural progression of the latter to blindness in approximately 3–5% of cases. Patients with proliferative diabetic retinopathy have abnormal haemodynamic responses of the cerebral and ophthalmic circulation both at rest and with exercise.[129] A reduced exercise capacity is seen with proliferative[117] and non-proliferative[130] diabetic retinopathy in type 1 diabetes. Vigorous physical activity, especially isometric contractions, produces significant increases in blood pressure and can accelerate proliferative diabetic retinopathy with significant risk of retinal and vitreal haemorrhage and detachment. Therefore caution should be considered when proliferative diabetic retinopathy is present, and guidelines have been provided by the ADA/ACSM that should form part of any recommendations for valsalva-like manoeuvres (table 8.4).

Autonomic neuropathy

Diabetic neuropathy presents in an occult manner in 17–40% of diabetics, with subclinical abnormalities in type 1 diabetes frequently found within a year of diagnosis.[131,132] It can present with somatic or autonomic changes (table 8.5) with a variety of different neuropathies possible, including amyotrophy, mononeuropathy, and entrapment syndrome.[25,131] The symptoms and signs may be subtle, necessitating careful examination with the aid of special tests (table 8.6). The autonomic nervous system is involved in all involuntary regulations, essential for unimpaired exercise capacity, and neuropathy can produce a wide variety of effects (table 8.5). The most important of these include silent myocardial ischaemia,

Table 8.4 Exercise guidelines in retinopathy

Level of diabetic retinopathy	Acceptable activities	Discouraged activities	Ocular re-evaluation months
None	★	★	12
Non-proliferative			
Mild	★	★	6–12
Moderate	★		4–6
Severe	★	Dramatic increase in BP e.g. weights, valsalva	2–4
Proliferative	Low impact, aerobic	Substantial inc. BP e.g. boxing, rowing. High impact, anaerobic, aerobic, racquet	1–2

★Dictated by medical status. Modified from ACSM/ADA guidelines.[89]

Table 8.5   Clinical signs of autonomic neuropathy

Signs

Cardiovascular
Hypotension during and after exercise (esp. vigorous activity)
Hypertension during exercise
Orthostatic hypotension (may be worse in the morning)
Cardiac denervation syndrome
   reduced maximal heart rate
   raised resting heart rate
Silent ischaemia
Impaired thermoregulation in hot and cold climate
Altered sweating
Altered cutaneous blood flow
Impaired proprioception (increased injury potential)
Impaired respiratory reflexes
Delayed gastric emptying
Diarrhoea
Impaired perception of hypoglycaemia
Pupillary

sudden death, hypertension and hypotension after exercise, delayed gastric emptying, and impaired sweating.[130,133–135] In the presence of peripheral neuropathy, 50% of patients are likely to have autonomic complications.[136,137]

Cardiac autonomic neuropathy also produces impaired blood pressure control and can result in cardiac denervation syndrome whereby heart rate cannot be increased in response to exercise.[138] Prolongation of the QT interval corrected for heart rate is more common than usual in diabetics, predisposing them to arrhythmias and sudden death,[139,140] and cardiac autonomic neuropathy

Table 8.6   Specific tests for autonomic neuropathy

Tests

Sensory
   Vibration, temperature
   Biothesiometer
   Reflexes
   Proprioception
Respiratory rate
Cardiac
   Resting heart rate > 100 beats/min raised
   R–R variation changes with respiration
   Valsalva manoeuvre
   Orthostatic response systolic
   Diastolic response to exercise
   QT interval corrected

appears to be associated with reduced cardiovascular function.[121] Formal cardiovascular stress testing may be prudent before the initiation of an exercise programme in such patients.[141] In addition, blunted adrenaline and noradrenaline responses may contribute to orthostatic impairment.[142]

Peripheral vascular disease and foot ulcers

The management of any exercising diabetic demands careful attention to the increased risk of foot ulceration and impaired vascular supply. Several reviews[2,143] highlight the fact that neuropathy and peripheral vascular disease can predict unnoticed foot injury. Footwear that relieves forefoot plantar pressure by up to 50% has been shown to be effective in preventing the recurrence of foot ulcers when worn for more than 60% of the day,[144] and it would appear that running shoes that protect the second and third metatarsal heads benefit patients significantly.[145]

Guidelines and resources

Even though ACSM and Sports Medicine Australia have determined that diabetes should be classified as a significant risk factor in any preparticipation physical examination,[89,146] it seems surprising that there are so few published guidelines on physical activity and diabetes. Only the ACSM/ADA[89] position statement with a recent outline from the International Sports Medicine Federation, not yet widely available in print, has attempted to address this.

In addition, there are relatively few definitive texts. The ADA provides significant resources, including the *Health professional guide to diabetes and exercise* and supports[25] the International Diabetic Athletes Association. This provides information and a forum for diabetic athletes to exchange ideas and techniques and has chapters in many countries.

Summary

As the understanding of the physiology of exercise and the treatment options in diabetes mellitus improve, the ability to combine tight control and normal exercise in type 1 diabetes appears increasingly possible. Exercise has not been shown definitively to improve glycaemic control in type 1 diabetes, but, with education and appropriate screening, it allows substantial physical and psychological rewards to be realised. In type 2 diabetes evidence for the role of exercise in the management of the disease is increasingly powerful and exercise may well be an important component of strategies for prevention and treatment. Further studies are required to determine what the exact nature of this exercise should be, but developments in the field of diabetes, such as the increasing evidence of genetic and cultural differences in insulin sensitivity, may change many aspects of our care. A more complete understanding of exercise and the health benefits that it can bring can only produce further improvements in the prevention, management, and treatment of diabetes.

I am grateful to Drs Peter Mansell, Siun Campbell, and Julie Lambourne for their support in the production of this review.

1 Landry GL, Allen DB. Diabetes mellitus and exercise. *Clin Sports Med* 1992;**11**:403–18.

2 Skyler JS. Prevention and treatment of diabetes and its complications. *Med Clin North Am* 1998;**82**:665.

3 Expert committee on the diagnosis and classification of diabetes mellitus. Report of the expert committee on the diagnosis and classification of diabetes mellitus. *Diabetes Care* 1997;**20**:1183–97.

4 Diabetes control and complications trial research group. The effect of intensive treatment of diabetes on the development and progression of long-term complications in insulin-dependent diabetes mellitus. *N Engl J Med* 1993;**329**:977–86.

5 Wasserman DH, Abumrad NN. Physiological bases for the treatment of the physically active individual with diabetes. *Sports Med* 1989;7:376–92.

6 Zinman B. Diabetes and exercise. *Postgrad Med* 1979;**66**:81–2.

7 Frid A, Ostman J, Linde B. Hypoglycaemia risk during exercise after intramuscular injection of insulin in the thigh of IDDM. *Diabetes Care* 1990;**8**:337–43.

8 Wasserman DH, Zinman B. Exercise in individuals with IDDM. *Diabetes Care* 1994;**17**:924–37.

9 Schneider SH, Vitug A, Ananthakrishnan R, *et al*. Impaired adrenergic response to prolonged exercise in type I diabetes. *Metabolism* 1991;**40**:1219–25.

10 Berger M, Assal JP, Jorgens V. Physical exercise in the diabetic. The importance of understanding endocrine and metabolic responses. *Diabete Metab* 1980;**6**:59–69.

11 Nermoen I, Jorde R, Sager G, *et al*. Effects of exercise on hypoglycaemic responses in insulin-dependent diabetes mellitus. *Diabete Metab* 1998;**24**:131–6.

12 Kilgour RD, Williams PA. Diabetes affects blood pressure and heart rate responses during acute hypothermia. *Acta Physiol Scand* 1998;**162**:27–32.

13 Berg K. The insulin-dependent diabetic runner. *Physician and Sportsmedicine* 1979;7:71–9.

14 Tattersall RB. A force of magical activity: the introduction of insulin treatment in Britain 1922–1926. *Diabet Med* 1995;**12**:739–55.

15 King P, Kong MF, Parkin H, *et al*. Well-being, cerebral function, and physical

fatigue after nocturnal hypoglycemia in IDDM. *Diabetes Care* 1998;**21**:341–5.

16 Zinman B, Zuniga-Guajardo S, Kelly D. Comparison of the acute and long-term effects of exercise on glucose control in type I diabetes. *Diabetes Care* 1984;**7**:515–19.

17 Stratton R, Wilson DP, Endres RK. Acute glycemic effects of exercise in adolescents with insulin-dependent diabetes mellitus. *Physician and Sportsmedicine* 1988;**16**:150–7.

18 Dunstan DW, Puddey IB, Beilin LJ, *et al.* Effects of a short-term circuit weight training program on glycaemic control in NIDDM. *Diabetes Res Clin Pract* 1998;**40**:53–61.

19 Huttunen NP, Lankela SL, Knip M, *et al.* Effect of once-a-week training program on physical fitness and metabolic control in children with IDDM. *Diabetes Care* 1989;**12**:737–40.

20 Perry TL, Mann JI, Lewis-Barned NJ, *et al.* Lifestyle intervention in people with insulin-dependent diabetes mellitus (IDDM). *Eur J Clin Nutr* 1997;**51**:757–63.

21 Rasmussen OW, Lauszus FF, Hermansen K. Effects of postprandial exercise on glycemic response in IDDM subjects: studies at constant insulinemia. *Diabetes Care* 1994;**17**:1203–5.

22 McDonald MJ. Post-exercise late-onset hypoglycaemia in insulin-dependent diabetic patients. *Diabetes Care* 1987;**10**:584–8.

23 Jorgens V, Grusser M, Bott U, *et al.* Effective safe translation of intensified insulin therapy to general internal medicine departments. *Diabetologia* 1993;**36**:99–105.

24 Blackett PR. Child and adolescent athletes with diabetes. *Physician and Sportsmedicine* 1988;**16**:133–49.

25 Devlin JT, Ruderman N, eds. The health professional's guide to diabetes and exercise. Alexandria, VA: American Diabetes Association, 1995.

26 Koivisto VA, Felig P. Effects of leg exercise on insulin absorption in diabetic patients. *N Engl J Med* 1978;**298**:77–83.

27 Salzsieder E, Fischer U, Stoewhas H. A model-based system for the individual prediction of metabolic responses to improve the therapy in type I diabetes. *Horm Metab Res* 1990;**24**(suppl):10–19.

28 Trovati M, Carta Q, Cavalot F, *et al.* Continuous subcutaneous insulin infusion and postprandial exercise in tightly controlled type I (insulin-dependent) diabetic patients. *Diabetes Care* 1984;**7**:327–30.

29 Sonnenberg GE, Kemmer FW, Berger M. Exercise in type 1 (insulin-dependent) diabetic patients treated with continuous subcutaneous insulin infusion. Prevention of exercise induced hypoglycaemia. *Diabetologia* 1990;**33**:696–703.

30 Schiffrin A, Parikh S. Accommodating planned exercise in type I diabetic patients on intensive treatment. *Diabetes Care* 1985;**8**:337–42.

31 Edelmann E, Staudner V, Bachmann W. Exercise-induced hypoglycaemia and subcutaneous insulin infusion. *Diabet Med* 1986;**3**:526–31.

32 Anderson Jr JH, Koivisto VA. Clinical studies on insulin lispro. *Drugs of Today* 1998;**34**(suppl C):37–50.

33 Minuk HL, Vranic M, Marliss EB. Glucoregulatory and metabolic response to exercise in obese noninsulin-dependent diabetes. *Am J Physiol* 1981;**3**:E458–64.

34 Devlin JT, Hirshman M, Horton ED, *et al.* Enhanced peripheral and splanchnic insulin sensitivity in NIDDM men after single bout of exercise. *Diabetes* 1987;**36**:434–9.

35 Koivisto VA, DeFronzo RA. Exercise in the treatment of type II diabetes. *Acta Endocrinol* 1984;**105**:107–11.

36 Lohmann D, Liebold F, Heilmann W, *et al.* Diminished insulin and response in highly trained athletes. *Metabolism* 1978;**27**:521–4.

37 Bjorntorp P, Fahlen M, Grimsby G, *et al.* Carbohydrate and fat metabolism in middle-aged physically well trained men. *Metabolism* 1972;**21**:1037–44.
38 Bjorntorp P, Krotkiewski M. Exercise treatment in diabetes mellitus. *Acta Medica Scandinavica* 1985;**217**:3–7.
39 Horton ES. Exercise and decreased risk of NIDDM. *N Engl J Med* 1991;**325**:196–8.
40 Koivisto VA, Jantunen M, Sane T, *et al.* Stimulation of prostacyclin synthesis by physical exercise in type I diabetes. *Diabetes Care* 1989;**12**:609–14.
41 Holloszy JO, Schultz J, Kusnierkiewicz J, *et al.* Effects of exercise on glucose tolerance and insulin resistance. Brief review and some preliminary results. *Acta Medica Scandinavica* 1986;**220**(suppl).
42 Segal KR, Edano A, Abalos A, *et al.* Effect of exercise training on insulin sensitivity and glucose metabolism in lean, obese, and diabetic men. *J Appl Physiol* 1991;**71**:2402–11.
43 Hughes VA, Fiatrone MA, Fielding RA. Exercise increases muscle GLUT-4 levels and insulin action in subjects with impaired glucose tolerance. *Am J Physiol* 1993;**264**:E855–62.
44 Devlin JT. Effects of exercise in diabetes mellitus. *J Fla Med Assoc* 1986;**73**:602–3.
45 Mikenes KJ, Sonne B, Farrell PA, *et al.* Effect of physical exercise on sensitivity and responsiveness to insulin in humans. *Am J Physiol* 1988;**254**:E248–59.
46 Richter EA, Ploug T, Galbo H. Increased muscle glucose uptake after exercise. No need for insulin during exercise. *Diabetes* 1985;**34**:1041–8.
47 Ivy JL. Role of exercise training in the prevention and treatment of insulin resistance and non-insulin-dependent diabetes mellitus. *Sports Med* 1997;**24**:321–36.
48 Heath GW, Gavin JR, Hinderliter JM, *et al.* Effects of exercise and lack of exercise on glucose tolerance and insulin sensitivity. *J Appl Physiol* 1983;**55**:628–34.
49 King H, Kriska AM. Prevention of type II diabetes by physical training: epidemiological considerations and study methods. *Diabetes Care* 1992;**15**:1794–9.
50 King AC, Blair SN, Bild DE. Determinants of physical activity and interventions in adults. *Med Sci Sports Exerc* 1992;**24**(suppl 6):S221–36.
51 Oshida Y, Yamanouchi K, Hayamizu S, *et al.* Long-term mild jogging increases insulin action despite no influence on body mass index or $\dot{V}O_2MAX$. *J Appl Physiol* 1989;**66**:2206–10.
52 Andersen PH, Lund S, Schmitz O, *et al.* Increased insulin-stimulated glucose uptake in athletes: the importance of GLUT4 mRNA and GLUT4 protein and fibre type composition of skeletal muscle. *Acta Physiol Scand* 1993;**149**:393–404.
53 Dela F, Ploug T, Handberg A, *et al.* Physical training increases muscle GLUT4 protein and mRNA in patients with NIDDM. *Diabetes* 1994;**43**:862–5.
54 Riddle MC, Mcdaniel PA, Tive LA. Glipizide-GITS does increase the hypoglycemic effect of mild exercise during fasting NIDDM. *Diabetes Care* 1997;**20**:992–4.
55 Gudat U, Bungert S, Kemmer F, *et al.* The blood glucose lowering effects of exercise and glibenclamide in patients with type 2 diabetes mellitus. *Diabet Med* 1998;**15**:194–8.
56 Kemmer FW. Prevention of hypoglycemia during exercise in type I diabetes. *Diabetes Care* 1992;**15**:1732–5.
57 De Fronzo RA, Goodman AM. The multi-centre metformin study group: efficacy of metformin in patients with non-insulin dependent diabetes. *N Engl J Med* 1995;**333**:541–9.
58 Regensteiner JG, Shetterly SM, Mayer EJ, *et al.* Relationship between habitual physical activity and insulin levels among non-diabetic men and women: the

San Luis Valley Diabetes Study. *Diabetes Care* 1995;**18**:490–7.

59 Lipman RL, Raskin P, Love T. Glucose intolerance during decreased physical activity in man. *Diabetes* 1972;**21**:101–7.

60 Physical acitivity and health. A report of the Surgeon General. Pittsburg: US Department of Health and Human Services, 1996.

61 Helmrich SP, Ragland DR, Leung RW, *et al.* Physical activity and reduced occurrence of non-insulin-dependent diabetes mellitus. *N Engl J Med* 1991;**325**:147–52.

62 Manson JE, Nathan DM, Krolewski AS, *et al.* A prospective study of exercise and incidence of diabetes among US male physicians. *JAMA* 1992;**268**:63–7.

63 Kaye SA, Folsom AR, Sprafka JM, *et al.* Increased incidence of diabetes mellitus in relation to abdominal adiposity in older women. *J Clin Epidemiol* 1991;**44**:329–34.

64 Eriksson KF, Lindgarde F. Prevention of Type 2 (non-insulin-dependent) diabetes mellitus by diet and physical exercise. The 6-year Malmo feasibility study. *Diabetologia* 1991;**34**:891–8.

65 Manson JE, Rimm EB, Stampfer MJ, *et al.* Physical activity and incidence of non-insulin-dependent diabetes mellitus in women. *Lancet* 1991;**338**:774–8.

66 Pan X, Li G, Hu Y. Effect of dietary and/or exercise intervention on incidence of diabetes in 530 subjects with impaired glucose tolerance from 1986–1992. *Diabetologia* 1995;**34**:891–8.

67 NIH consensus development panel on physical activity and cardiovascular health. Physical activity and cardiovascular health. *JAMA* 1996;**276**:241–6.

68 Manson JE, Nathan DM, Krolewski AS, *et al.* Exercise and incidence of diabetes among U.S. male physicians. *Ann Intern Med* 1992;**118**(suppl 1).

69 Mayer-Davis EJD, Agostino Jr R, Karter AJ, *et al.* Intensity and amount of physical activity in relation to insulin sensitivity: the Insulin Resistance Atherosclerosis Study. *JAMA* 1998;**279**:669–74.

70 Fukimoto WY. A national multicentre study to learn whether type 2 diabetes can be prevented. The Diabetes Prevention Program. *Diabetes Care* 1997;**15**:13–15.

71 Wing RR, Venditti E, Jakicic JM, *et al.* Lifestyle intervention in overweight individuals with a family history of diabetes. *Diabetes Care* 1998;**21**:350–9.

72 Bloomgarden ZT. American Diabetes Association. *Diabetes Care* 1997;**20**:1913–17.

73 Pan X, Li G, Hu Y, *et al.* Effect of diet and exercise in preventing NIDDM in people with impaired glucose tolerance. *Diabetes Care* 1997;**20**:537–44.

74 Torjesen PA, Birkeland KI, Anderssen SA, *et al.* Lifestyle changes may reverse development of the insulin resistance syndrome. *Diabetes Care* 1997;**20**:26–31.

75 Eriksson KF, Lindgarde F. No excess 12-year mortality in men with impaired glucose tolerance who participated in the Malmo Preventive Trial with diet and exercise. *Diabetologia* 1998;**41**:1010–16.

76 Anonymous. Summary of the surgeon generals report addressing physical activity and health. *Nutr Rev* 1996;**54**:280–4.

77 Miller WJ, Sherman WM, Ivy JL. Effect of strength training on glucose tolerance and post-glucose insulin response. *Med Sci Sports Exerc* 1984;**16**:539–43.

78 Pate RR, Pratt M, Blair SN, *et al.* Physical activity and public health: a recommendation from the Centers for Disease Control and Prevention and the American College of Sports Medicine. *JAMA* 1995;**273**:402–7.

79 Zimmet PZ. Kelly West Lecture 1991. Challenges in diabetes epidemiology: from West to the rest. *Diabetes Care* 1992;**15**:232–52.

80 Reaven GM. Role of insulin resistance in human disease. *Diabetes* 1988;**37**:1595–607.

81 Hjermann I. The metabolic cardiovascular syndrome: syndrome X, Reaven's

syndrome, insulin resistance syndrome, atherothrombogenic syndrome. *J Cardiovasc Pharmacol* 1992;**20**(suppl 8):S5–10.

82 Bierman EL. Atherogenesis in diabetes. *Arterioscler Thromb* 1992;**12**:647–56.

83 Paffenbarger Jr RS, Hyde RT. Exercise as protection against heart attack. *N Engl J Med* 1980;**302**:1026–7.

84 Paffenbarger Jr RS, Hyde RT, Wing AL, *et al*. Physical activity, all-cause mortality, and longevity of college alumni. *N Engl J Med* 1986;**314**:605–13.

85 Leon AS. Effects of exercise conditioning on physiologic precursors of coronary heart disease. *J Cardiopulm Rehab* 1991;**11**:46–57.

86 Blair SN, Kohl III HW, Paffenbarger Jr RS, *et al*. Physical fitness and all-cause mortality: a prospective study of healthy men and women. *JAMA* 1989;**262**:2395–401.

87 Sheps SG, Dart RA. New guidelines for prevention, detection, evaluation, and treatment of hypertension: joint national committee VI. *Chest* 1998;**113**: 263–5.

88 Blair SN, Kohl IH, Barlow CE, *et al*. Changes in physical fitness and all-cause mortality: a prospective study of healthy and unhealthy men. *JAMA* 1995;**273**:1093–8.

89 Anonymous. ADA/ACSM: diabetes mellitus and exercise. Joint position paper. *Med Sci Sports Exerc* 1997;**29**:1–6.

90 Blair SN, Powell KE, Bazzarre TL, *et al*. Physical inactivity: workshop V. *Circulation* 1993;**88**:1402–5.

91 Klesges RC, Klesges LM, Haddock CK, *et al*. Longitudinal analysis of the impact of dietary intake and physical activity. *Am J Clin Nutr* 1992;**55**:818–22.

92 Weyer C, Linkeschowa R, Heise T, *et al*. Implications of the traditional and new ACSM physical activity recommendations on weight reduction in dietary treated obese subjects. *Int J Obes* 1998;**22**:1071–8.

93 Eriksson KF, Lindgarde F. No excess 12-year mortality in men with impaired glucose tolerance who participated in the Malmo Preventive Trial with diet and exercise. *Diabetologia* 1998;**41**:1010–16.

94 Wallberg-Henriksson H, Gunnarsson R, Henriksson J, *et al*. Increased peripheral insulin sensitivity and muscle mitochondrial enzymes but unchanged blood glucose control in type I diabetics after physical training. *Diabetes* 1982;**31**:1044–50.

95 King AC, Haskell WL, Taylor CB, *et al*. Home-based exercise training in healthy older men and women. *JAMA* 1991;**266**:1535–42.

96 Maehlum S, Dahl-Jorgensen K, Meen HD. Physical activity and diabetes mellitus. *Tidsskr Norsk Laegeforen* 1980;**100**:840–4.

97 Noble BJ. Preface to the symposium on recent advances in the study and clinical use of perceived exertion. *Med Sci Sports Exerc* 1982;**14**:377–81.

98 Fox KR. Promoting physical activity in people with diabetes. *Practical Diabetes International* 1998;**15**:146–50.

99 Mittleman MA, Maclure M, Tofler GH, *et al*. Triggering of acute myocardial infarction by heavy physical exertion. *N Engl J Med* 1993;**329**:1677–83.

100 Dahlquist G, Aperia A, Carlsson L, *et al*. Effect of metabolic control and duration on exercise-induced albuminuria in diabetic teenagers. *Acta Paediatr Scand* 1983;**72**:895–902.

101 United Kingdom prospective diabetes study group. UK prospective diabetes study X: urinary albumin excretion over 3 years in diet-treated type 2 (non-insulin-dependent) diabetic patients, and association with hypertension, hyperglycaemia and hypertriglyceridaemia. *Diabetologia* 1993;**36**:1021–9.

102 Matsuoka K, Nakao T, Atsumi Y, *et al*. Exercise regime for diabetics with diabetic nephropathy. *J Diabetes Complications* 1991;**5**:98–100.

103 Sacco RL, Gan R, Boden-Albala B, *et al*. Leisure-time physical activity and ischemic stroke risk: the Northern Manhattan stroke study. *Stroke* 1998;**29**:380–7.

104 Goldstein D. Clinical applications for exercise. *JAMA* 1989;**17**:83–93.
105 Vered Z, Battler A, Segal P, *et al.* Exercise-induced left ventricular dysfunction in young men with asymptomatic diabetes mellitus (diabetic cardiomyopathy). *Am J Cardiol* 1984;**54**:633–7.
106 Margolis JR, Kannel WB, Feinlab M. Clinical features of unrecognised myocardial infarction: silent and symptomatic. Eighteen year follow up: The Framingham Study. *Am J Cardiol* 1973;**32**:11–17.
107 Bruce RA, Hossack KF, Doroun TA, *et al.* Enhanced risk assessment for primary coronary heart disease events maximal exercise testing: 10 years' experience of Seattle Heart Watch. *J Am Coll Cardiol* 1983;**2**:565–75.
108 Rubler S, Gerber D, Reitano J, *et al.* Predictive value of clinical and exercise variables for detection of coronary artery disease in men with diabetes mellitus. *Am J Cardiol* 1987;**59**:1310–13.
109 Schneider SH, Amorosa LF, Khachadurian AK, *et al.* Studies on the mechanism of improved glucose control during regular exercise in type 2 (non-insulin-dependent) diabetes. *Diabetologia* 1984;**26**:355–60.
110 Regensteiner JG, Sippel J, McFarling ET, *et al.* Effects of non-insulin-dependent diabetes on oxygen consumption during treadmill execise. *Med Sci Sports Exerc* 1995;**27**:874–81.
111 American Diabetes Association. Concensus statement: detection and management of lipid disorders in diabetes. *Diabetes Care* 1996;**19**(suppl 1):S96–102.
112 Krolewski AS, Kosinski EJ, Warram JH. Magnitude and determinants of coronary artery disease in juvenile-onset, insulin-dependent diabetes mellitus. *Am J Cardiol* 1987;**59**:750–5.
113 Krolewski AS, Warram JH, Valsania P. Evolving natural history of coronary artery disease in diabetes mellitus: the Finnish studies. *Am J Med* 1991;**90**(suppl 2A):56S–61S.
114 Panzram G. Mortality and survival in type 2 (non insulin-dependent diabetes) diabetes mellitus. *Diabetologia* 1987;**30**:123–31.
115 Moss SE, Klein R, Klein BE. Cause-specific mortality in a population based study of diabetes. *Am J Public Health* 1991;**81**:1158–62.
116 Naka M, Hiramatsu K, Aizawa T, *et al.* Silent myocardial ischemia in patients with non-insulin-dependent diabetes mellitus as judged by treadmill exercise testing and coronary angiography. *Am Heart J* 1992;**123**:46–53.
117 Estacio RO, Regensteiner JG, Wolfel EE, *et al.* The association between diabetic complications and exercise capacity in NIDDM patients. *Diabetes Care* 1998;**21**:291–5.
118 Nesto RW, Phillips RT, Kett KG, *et al.* Angina and exertional myocardial ischemia in diabetic and nondiabetic patients: assessment by exercise thallium scintigraphy. *Ann Intern Med* 1988;**108**:170–5.
119 Langer A, Freeman MR, Josse RG, *et al.* Detection of silent myocardial ischemia in diabetes mellitus. *Am J Cardiol* 1991;**67**:1073–8.
120 Kannel WB. Lipids, diabetes, and coronary heart disease: insights from the Framingham study. *Am Heart J* 1985;**110**:1100–7.
121 Hypertension in diabetes study group. HDS 1: prevalence of hypertension in newly presenting type 2 diabetic patients and the association with risk factors for cardio-vascular and diabetic complications. *J Hypertens* 1993;**11**:309–17.
122 United Kingdom prospective diabetes study group. UK prospective diabetes study 23: risk factors for coronary artery disease in non-insulin dependent diabetes. *BMJ* 1998;**316**:823–8.
123 Hypertension in diabetes study group. HDS 2: increased risk of cardio-vascular complications in hypertensive type 2 diabetic patients. *J Hypertens* 1993;**11**:319–25.
124 United Kingdom prospective diabetes study group. UK prospective diabetes study 30: diabetic retinopathy at diagnosis of type 2 diabetes and associated risk factors. *Arch Ophthalmol* 1998;**116**:297–303.

125 Schneider SH, Morgado A. Effects of fitness and physical training on carbohydrate metabolism and associated cardiovascular risk factors in patients with diabetes. *Diabetes Reviews* 1995;**3**:378–407.

126 Blackburn H. Physical activity and hypertension. *J Clin Hypertens* 1986;**2**:154–62.

127 Butler RM, Goldberg L. Exercise and prevention of coronary heart disease. *Primary Care* 1989;**16**:99–114.

128 Davies MD. Diabetic retinopathy: a clinical overview. *Diabetes Care* 1992;**15**:1844–74.

129 Albert SG, Gomez CR, Russell S, *et al.* Cerebral and ophthalmic artery hemodynamic responses in diabetes mellitus. *Diabetes Care* 1993;**16**:476–82.

130 Margonato A, Gerundini P, Vicedomini G, *et al.* Abnormal cardiovascular response to exercise in young asymptomatic diabetic patients with retinopathy. *Am Heart J* 1986;**112**:554–60.

131 Greene DA, Pfeifer MA. In: Olefsky JM, Sherwin RS, eds. *Diabetes mellitus.* New York: Churchill Livingstone, 1985.

132 Young R, Ewing D, Campbell B. Nerve function and metabolic control in diabetes. *Diabetes* 1983;**32**:142–7.

133 Karlefors T. Exercise test in male diabetes. *Acta Medica Scandinavica* 1966;**180**(suppl 449):3–8.

134 Hilsted J, Galbo H, Christensen NJ. Impaired responses of catecholamines, growth hormone, and cortisol to graded exercise in diabetic autonomic neuropathy. *Diabetes* 1980;**29**:257–62.

135 Hilsted J, Galbo H, Christensen NJ, *et al.* Haemodynamic changes during graded exercise in patients with diabetic autonomic neuropathy. *Diabetologia* 1982;**22**:318–23.

136 Rubler S, Chu DA, Bruzzone CL. Blood pressure and heart rate responses during 24-hour ambulatory monitoring and exercise in men with diabetes mellitus. *Am J Cardiol* 1985;**55**:801–6.

137 Ewing D, Campbell I, Clarke B. The natural history of diabetic autonomic neuropathy. *Quarterly Medical Journal* 1980;**49**:95–108.

138 Ewing D, Campbell I, Clarke B. Heart rate changes in diabetes mellitus. *Lancet* 1981;**i**:183–6.

139 Kahn JK, Sisson JC, Vinik AI. QT interval prolongation and sudden cardiac death in diabetic autonomic neuropathy. *J Clin Endocrinol Metab* 1987;**64**:751–4.

140 Ferrari AU. Modulation of parasympathetic and baroreceptor control of heart rate. *Cardioscience* 1993;**4**:9–13.

141 Broadstone VL, Roy T, Self M, *et al.* Cardiovascular autonomic dysfunction: diagnosis and prognosis. *Diabet Med* 1991;**8**(symposium):S88–93.

142 Sundkvist G, Bergstrom B, Manhem P, *et al.* Blunted epinephrine response following exercise in autonomic neuropathy. *Diabetologia* 1995;**38**(8):1003.

143 Conti SF, Chaytor ER. Steps to healthy feet for active people with diabetes. *JAMA* 1995;**23**:71–2.

144 Chantelau E, Kushner T, Spraul M. How effective is cushioned therapeutic footwear in protecting diabetic feet? *Diabet Med* 1990;**7**:355–9.

145 Kastenbauer T, Sokol G, Auinger M, *et al.* Running shoes for the relief of plantar pressure in diabetic patients. *Diabet Med* 1998;**15**:518–22.

146 Norton K, Olds T, Bowes D, *et al.* Applying the sports medicine Australia pre-exercise screening procedures: who will be excluded? *J Sci Med Sport* 1998;**1**:38–51.

147 Goodyear LJ. Exercise, glucose transport, and insulin sensitivity. *Annu Rev Med* 1998;**49**:235–61.

148 Brooks GA, Fahey TD, White TP. *Exercise physiology.* 2nd ed. Mount View, CA: Mayfield Publishing Co., 1996:56.

Multiple choice questions

1 For glucose uptake which of the following are true?
   (a) Training permanently improves insulin sensitivity in non-insulin dependent diabetes mellitus
   (b) Exercise can augment insulin stimulated glucose uptake in diabetes
   (c) Insulin increases hepatic glucose production
   (d) Insulin increases muscle and liver glycogen production
   (e) In type 2 diabetes hypoglycaemia occurs commonly because of enhanced insulin sensitivity

2 In hypoglycaemia which of the following are true?
   (a) Symptoms are likely to be masked by moderate intensity exercise
   (b) 1–5 g of carbohydrate at the onset of symptoms will alleviate most hypoglycaemic attacks
   (c) Diving is contraindicated in diabetes
   (d) Delayed onset hypoglycaemia occurs up to 4 hours after activity
   (e) Intensive education can reduce the risk of hypoglycaemia

3 In patients with insulin dependent diabetes mellitus which of the following are true?
   (a) There is an increased risk of retinal detachment during exercise
   (b) There is an increased incidence of silent myocardial ischaemia
   (c) A shortened QTc (corrected) interval is seen on electrocardiography
   (d) Reduced carbohydrate diets are needed to prevent hyperglycaemia during exercise
   (e) Resistance training is contraindicated

4 Which of the following are true for exercise programmes?
   (a) Gentle "warm up" increases risk of hypoglycaemia
   (b) Vigorous activity is always contraindicated in insulin dependent diabetes mellitus and non-insulin dependent diabetes mellitus
   (c) Motivation and compliance is low in non-insulin dependent diabetes mellitus

(d) They can reduce the relative risk of developing non-insulin dependent diabetes mellitus in those with impaired glucose tolerance by as much as 60%

(e) They are contraindicated in those with sensory neuropathy

Answers are on p. 364.

9 Fatigue and underperformance in athletes: the overtraining syndrome

R Budgett

Introduction

When athletes fail to recover from training they become progressively fatigued and suffer from prolonged underperformance. They may also suffer from frequent minor infections (particularly respiratory infections). In the absence of any other medical cause, this is often called the overtraining syndrome, burnout, staleness, or chronic fatigue in athletes.[1-3] The condition is secondary to the stress of training but the exact cause and pathophysiology is not known. Many factors may lead to failure to recover from training or competition.

Definition

"The overtraining syndrome is a condition of fatigue and underperformance, often associated with frequent infections and depression which occurs following hard training and competition. The symptoms do not resolve despite two weeks of adequate rest, and there is no other identifiable medical cause."

This contrasts with the definition of chronic fatigue syndrome, for which symptoms must last at least 6 months.[1]

Normal response to training

All athletes, in any sport, must train hard to improve. Initial hard training causes underperformance but if recovery is allowed there is supercompensation and improvement in performance.[4] Training is designed in a cyclical way (periodisation) allowing time for recovery with progressive overload. During the hard training/ overload period, transient symptoms and signs and changes in diagnostic tests may occur; this is called overreaching.[5]

Responses to the profile of mood state (POMS) questionnaire can indicate reduced vigour and increased tension, depression, anger, fatigue, and confusion.[6] Muscle glycogen stores are depleted and resting heart rate rises. The testosterone:cortisol ratio is reduced as the result of lower testosterone and higher cortisol concentrations. Microscopic damage to muscle also leads to raised creatine kinase concentrations if there is eccentric exercise.[7]

All these changes are physiological and normal if recovery occurs within 2 weeks. Overreaching is a vital part of training for improved performance.[5]

Abnormal response to training

In some athletes there is underrecovery as the result of excessively prolonged and/or intense exercise, stressful competition, or other stresses. This leads to progressive fatigue and underperformance. The reaction to this underperformance is often an increase in training rather than rest.[8]

Intensive interval training, in which 1 to 6 minutes of hard exercise is repeated several times with a short rest, is most likely to precipitate the overtraining syndrome. There may also be a history of a sudden increase in training, prolonged heavy monotonous training, and commonly some other physical or psychological stress. Nevertheless, however hard the training, most athletes will recover fully after 2 weeks of adequate rest. The cyclical nature of most training programmes (periodisation) allows this recovery and full benefit from hard exercise.[9] Figure 9.1 summarises the responses to training.

Eventually fatigue becomes so severe that recovery does not occur despite 2 weeks of relative rest. At this stage a diagnosis of the overtraining syndrome can be made.

Symptoms

The main complaint is of underperformance. Athletes will often ignore fatigue, heavy muscles, and depression until performance is chronically affected.[10] Sleep disturbance occurs in over 90% of

173

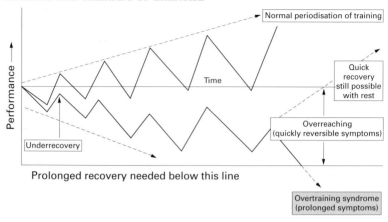

Fig 9.1 Overtraining or underrecovery, leading to the overtraining syndrome.

cases with difficulty in getting to sleep, nightmares, waking in the night, and waking unrefreshed.[11] There may also be loss of appetite, weight loss, loss of competitive drive and libido, and increased emotional ability, anxiety, and irritability. The athlete may report a raised resting pulse rate and excessive sweating. Upper respiratory tract infections or other minor infections frequently recur every time an athlete tries to return to training when they have not fully recovered. This gives an apparent cycle of recurrent infection every few weeks (figure 9.2).[1]

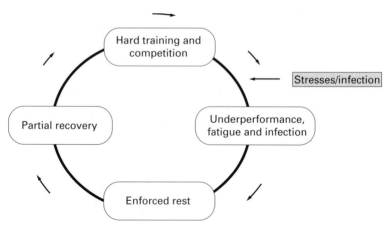

Fig 9.2   Cycle of recurrent minor infections.

Signs

Reported signs are often caused by associated illness and are inconsistent and generally unhelpful in making the diagnosis. Cervical lymphadenopathy is very common. There may be an increased postural fall in blood pressure and postural rise in heart rate, probably related to the underlying pathophysiology.[12] Physiological testing may show a reduced maximum oxygen consumption and maximum power output and an increased submaximum oxygen consumption and pulse rate, with a slow return of the pulse rate to normal after exercise.[11]

Prevention and early detection

Overtraining for one athlete may be insufficient training for another. Athletes tolerate different levels of training, competition, and stress at different times, depending on their level of health and fitness through the season. The training load must therefore be individualised and reduced or increased, depending on the athlete's response. Other stresses such as exams need to be taken into account.[13]

In practice it is very difficult to distinguish between overreaching and the overtraining syndrome. Researchers have attempted to follow blood parameters such as haemoglobin, packed cell volume, and creatine kinase but these do not help. Mood state profiling on a regular basis can give useful guidance.[14]

Many athletes monitor their heart rate. This is non-specific but can provide objective evidence that something is wrong.[15] Other prevention strategies are a good diet, full hydration, and rest between training sessions. It is more difficult for athletes who have a full time job and other commitments to recover quickly after training.

Because it is difficult to predict which athletes will slip into an overtrained state during a period of prolonged overreaching, it is prudent to allow full recovery at least every 2 weeks. Many sports scientists and coaches are advising alternate day hard and light training within the normal cyclical programme.[9]

Training intensity and spacing of the training are the most important factors in optimising performance and minimising the risk of overtraining. Morton used a complex mathematical model to optimise periodisation of athletic training.[16] In this he suggested intensive training on alternate days over a 150 day season, with a build up over the first half tapering off over the second half. This was more effective than moderate training throughout the whole year.

Clinical investigations

Athletes presenting with chronic fatigue and underperformance are often looking for a specific diagnosis and expert investigations. There is no diagnostic test available, so the aim of clinical investigations must be to exclude other causes of chronic fatigue and reassure the athlete that there is no serious pathology. The range of any test depends on a sensible approach to clinical possibilities, guided by the history and examination. A routine haematological screen may be all that is necessary, but occasionally more extensive investigations are justified to exclude serious disease such as viral myocarditis and arrhythmia.

A history of recurrent upper respiratory tract infections may represent allergic rhinitis or exercise induced asthma, in which case lung function tests are needed.[8] Creatine kinase levels are often very high in athletes, and the rise is proportional to the intensity, volume, and type of exercise (particularly eccentric work).[12] Unfortunately, creatine kinase cannot be used to indicate who will fail to recover from hard training. Many athletes also have a low packed cell volume and relatively low haemoglobin concentration. This athletic anaemia is physiological; it is due to haemodilution and does not affect performance.

The history may suggest a postviral illness. To make a firm diagnosis, viral titres must be shown to rise. There may also be reactive lymphocytes, and a positive result on Paul-Bunnell test is highly suggestive of Epstein-Barr viral infection.

Many athletes use supplements, but these do not seem to offer any protection from chronic fatigue. Trace elements and minerals such as magnesium have been investigated, but there is no proved link to the overtraining syndrome.[5]

Box 9.1

Overtraining is a condition of fatigue and underperformance caused by underrecovery from hard training and competition. There is no diagnostic test but other causes of fatigue must be excluded.

Pathophysiology

Training and psychology

Fry *et al.* tried to induce overtraining by short, near maximum, high intensity exercise but failed, suggesting that this is a safe regimen.[17] This may be because of the frequent long periods of rest between efforts and supports our observations that sprinters and power athletes do not suffer from the overtraining syndrome.

Other researchers have shown a fall in the "lactate:rating of perceived exertion" ratio with heavy training.[18] Thus, for a set lactate level the perceived exertion is higher, but this may represent glycogen depletion causing lower lactate levels rather than the overtraining syndrome.

The POSM questionnaire was used on a group of collegiate swimmers in the United States by Morgan *et al.*[14] Training was increased whenever the mood state improved and reduced whenever it deteriorated. The incidence of burnout, which was previously around 10% a year, was reduced to zero.

The mood state is most significant if it does not improve during tapering in the lead up to a competition, but unfortunately it may then be too late to prevent underperformance. The advice is therefore to taper and recover regularly throughout the season to enable regular monitoring of recovery.

At the British Olympic Medical Centre we have shown that both performance and mood state improve with 5 weeks of physical rest. Low level exercise has also been shown to speed recovery from chronic fatigue syndrome.[11]

Hormonal changes

The role of hormones in the overtraining syndrome is still not fully understood. Concentrations of stress hormones, such as adrenaline and cortisol, are higher in overtrained athletes compared with controls. Salivary cortisol concentrations (reflecting free cortisol concentrations) in a group of swimmers were significantly higher in stale underperforming athletes, and this correlated with the depressed mood state.[19]

A low testosterone:cortisol ratio has been suggested as a marker of the overtraining syndrome, reflecting a change in the balance of anabolism to catabolism. This ratio also falls in response to overreaching, so only a very low ratio is useful. In some athletes there is no significant change, despite all the symptoms of the overtraining syndrome.[19] There is one report of the (prohibited)

177

use of anabolic steroids to treat the overtraining syndrome.[20]

A reduced response to insulin induced hypoglycaemia was shown by Baron and Noakes and colleagues,[21] suggesting hypothalamic dysfunction.

Noradrenaline concentrations have been shown to be higher in overtrained swimmers than in controls, particularly during tapering, but concentrations were generally proportional to the training stress. There was no change in cortisol concentrations.[22] Plasma catecholamine concentrations and stress ratings (assessed by questionnaire) were a useful predictor of staleness, and a wellbeing rating questionnaire during tapering predicted performance.[23]

The rise in noradrenaline concentrations and fall in basal nocturnal plasma dopamine, noradrenaline, and adrenaline concentrations have been proposed as a method of monitoring overtraining. These concentrations correlate with symptoms.[24]

Central fatigue

The British Olympic Medical Centre has shown that overtrained athletes produce a lower peak power in 20 second Wingate sprint tests and weaker isometric and concentric quadriceps contractions than do controls. Superimposed tetanic stimulation produced a rise in isometric power. This suggests that there is central fatigue with a failure to activate fast twitch muscle fibres fully and is consistent with the history of an inability to lift the pace at the end of a race and to sprint for the line. Eccentric contraction was the same in controls and overtrained athletes so that the eccentric concentric ratio in overtrained athletes was almost 2:1 compared with the normal of 1.3:1.

Box 9.2 Monitoring for overtraining syndrome

- Performance
- Profile of mood state / questionnaires
- Lactate:rating of perceived exertion ratio
- Urea and creatine kinase
- Testosterone and cortisol ratio
- Noradrenaline / adrenaline concentrations
- Glutamine concentrations
- Eccentric:concentric power ratio

None are specific or sensitive. Awareness and experience of coach, athlete, and support staff is still most effective

---

Amino acids and central fatigue

The neurotransmitter 5-hydroxytryptamine (5HT, serotonin) may be important in tiredness and sleep. The amino acid tryptophan is converted in the brain into 5HT and competes with the branched chain amino acids for entry into the brain on the same amino acid carrier. Thus a decrease in levels of branched chain amino acids in the blood as a result of an increased rate of utilisation by muscle will increase the ratio of tryptophan to branched chain amino acids in the bloodstream and favour the entry of tryptophan into the brain. This may result in fatigue originating in the brain. Free tryptophan is further increased by a rise in plasma fatty acid concentrations. In endurance activity, non-esterified fatty acids increase and branched chain amino acids decrease. In rats it has been shown that this increases the concentration of 5HT in the hypothalamus and brainstem.[26]

5HT-containing cells are widespread in the central nervous system, and changes in 5HT levels could account for many of the symptoms of overtraining affecting sleep, causing central fatigue and loss of appetite, and inhibiting the release of factors from the hypothalamus that control pituitary hormones.[27,28]

Immunosuppression and glutamine

There is evidence that moderate regular exercise helps to reduce the level of infection in normal individuals. However, intense heavy exercise increases the incidence of infection.[29] Upper respiratory tract infections have been shown to be more likely with higher training distance[30] and after a marathon.[31] A number of factors probably contribute to this apparent immunosuppression, such as raised cortisol concentrations, reduced salivary immunoglobulin concentrations, and low glutamine concentrations. Glutamine is an essential amino acid for rapidly dividing cells such as lymphocytes. Low levels of glutamine have been found in overtrained athletes compared with controls, and levels are known to be lower after hard training.[32]

Glutamine intervention studies have been carried out, and there is some evidence that the incidence of infection after prolonged exercise in endurance athletes taking glutamine is reduced compared with those taking placebo.[33]

179

Box 9.3 Overtrained athletes are different from patients with chronic fatigue

- Present with underperformance
- Present earlier
- Less severely affected
- Recover more quickly
- Major stress (training and competition) can be eliminated
- Have to be restrained rather than encouraged to do rehabilitative exercise

---

Management

Athletes suffering from chronic fatigue and underperformance are different from sedentary individuals because they present earlier, they tend to recover more quickly, and there is an opportunity to alter the major stress in their lives (training and competition). Nevertheless, management is similar to that for any individual with chronic fatigue and requires a holistic approach. Rest and regeneration strategies are central to recovery.[1]

If told to rest, athletes will not comply. So they should be given positive advice and told to exercise aerobically at a pulse rate of 120–140 beats per minute for 5 to 10 minutes each day, ideally in divided sessions, and slowly build this up over 6–12 weeks. The exercise programme has to be individually designed and depends on the clinical picture and rate of improvement. The cycle of partial recovery followed by hard training and recurrent breakdown needs to be stopped. It is often necessary for athletes to avoid their own sports, and cross training should be used because of the tendency otherwise to increase exercise intensity too quickly. A positive approach is essential, with an emphasis on slowly building up volume, rather than intensity, to about 1 hour a day. Once this volume is tolerated, then more intense work can be incorporated above the onset of blood lactate accumulation.[18]

Very short (less than 10 seconds) sprints/power sessions with at least 3 to 5 minutes of rest are safe and allow some hard training to be carried out.

There have been no trials of the regeneration strategies widely used in the old Eastern bloc countries.[25] These include rest, relaxation, counselling, and psychotherapy. Massage and hydrotherapy are used, and nutrition is looked at carefully. Large quantities of vitamins and supplements are given, but there is no evidence that they are effective. Stresses outside sport are reduced as much as possible. Occasionally, depression may need to be treated with antidepressants but normally drugs are of no value, although any concurrent illness must be treated.

Athletes who have been underperforming for many months are often surprised at the good performance they can produce after 12 weeks of extremely light exercise. At this point, care must be taken not to increase the intensity of training too fast and to allow full recovery after hard parts of the training cycle. We recommend that athletes recover completely at least once a week.

Summary

The overtraining syndrome affects mainly endurance athletes. It is a condition of chronic fatigue, underperformance, and an increased vulnerability to infection leading to recurrent infections. It is not yet known exactly how the stress of hard training and competition leads to the observed spectrum of symptoms. Psychological, endocrinological, physiological, and immunological factors all play a part in the failure to recover from exercise.

Careful monitoring of athletes and their response to training may help to prevent the overtraining syndrome. With a very careful exercise regimen and regeneration strategies, symptoms normally resolve in 6–12 weeks but may continue much longer or recur if athletes return to hard training too soon.

1 Budgett R. The overtraining syndrome. *BMJ* 1994;**309**:4465–8.
2 Fry RW, Morton AR, Keast D. Overtraining syndrome and the chronic fatigue syndrome. *N Z J Sports Med* 1991;**19**:48–52.
3 Lehmann M, Foster C, Keull J. Overtraining in endurance athletes: a brief review. *Med Sci Sports Exerc* 1993;**25**:854–62.
4 Morton RH. Modelling training and overtraining. *J Sports Sci* 1997;**15**:335–40.
5 Budgett R. The overtraining syndrome. *Br J Sports Med* 1990;**24**:231-6.
6 Morgan WP, Costill DC, Flynn MG, *et al.* Mood disturbance following increased training in swimmers. *Med Sci Sports Exerc* 1988;**20**:408–14.
7 Costill DL, Flynn MG, Kirway JP, *et al.* Effects of repeated days of intensified training on muscle glycogen and swimming performance. *Med Sci Sports Exerc* 1988;**20**:249–54.
8 Smith C, Kirby P, Noakes TD. The worn-out athlete: a clinical approach to chronic fatigue in athletes. *J Sports Sci* 1997;**15**:341–51.
9 Fry RW, Morton AR, Keast D. Periodisation and the prevention of overtraining. *Can J Sports Sci* 1992;**17**:241–8.
10 Dyment P. Frustrated by chronic fatigue? *Physician and Sportsmedicine* 1993;**21**:47–54.
11 Koutedakis Y, Budgett R, Faulmann L. Rest in underperforming elite competitors. *Br J Sports Med* 1990;**24**:248–52.

12 Kindermann W. Das Ubertraining-Ausdruck einer vegetativen Fehlsteurung. *Deutsche Zeistchrift für Sportsmedizin* 1986;**37**:138–45.

13 Budgett R. The overtraining syndrome. *Coaching Focus* 1995;**28**:4–6.

14 Morgan WP, Brown DR, Raglin JS, *et al.* Psychological monitoring of overtraining and staleness. *Br J Sports Med* 1987;**21**:107–14.

15 Dressendorfer RH, Wade CE, Scaff JH. Increased morning heart rate in runners: a valid sign of overtraining? *Physician and Sportsmedicine* 1985;**13**:77–86.

16 Morton RH. The quantitative periodisation of athletic training: a model study. *Sports Medicine: Training Rehab* 1991;**3**:19–28.

17 Fry AC, Kramer WJ. Does short-term near-maximal intensity machine resistance training induce overtraining? *J Strength Conditioning Res* 1994;**8**:188–91.

18 Synder AC. A physiological/psychological indicator of overreaching during intensive training. *Int J Sports Med* 1993;**14**:29–32.

19 Flynn MG, Pizza FX, Boone JB, *et al.* Indices of training stress during competitive running and swimming seasons. *Int J Sports Med* 1994;**15**:21–6.

20 Kereszty A. Overtraining. In: Larson L, ed. *Encyclopedia of sports science and medicine.* New York: MacMillan, 1971:218–22.

21 Barron JL, Noakes TD, Levy W, *et al.* Hypothalamic dysfunction in overtrained athletes. *J Clin Endocrinol Metab* 1985;**60**:803–6.

22 Hooper SL, Mackinnon LT, Gordon RD, *et al.* Markers for monitoring overtraining and recovery. *Med Sci Sports Exerc* 1995;**27**:106–12.

23 Hooper SL, Mackinnon LT. Monitoring overtraining in athletes. *Sports Med* 1995;**20**:231–7.

24 Lehmann M, Dickhuth HH, Gendrisch E, *et al.* Training-overtraining. A prospective experimental study with experienced middle and long distance runners. *Int J Sports Med* 1991;**12**:444–52.

25 Koutedakis Y, Frishknecht R, Vrbová G, *et al.* Maximal voluntary quadriceps strength patterns in Olympic overtrained athletes. *Med Sci Sports Exerc* 1995;**27**:566–72.

26 Blomstrand E, Hassmen P, Newsholme EA. Administration of branched-chain amino acids during sustained exercise. *Eur J Appl Physiol* 1991;**63**:83.

27 Blomstrand E, Perrett D, Parry-Billings M, *et al.* Effect of sustained exercise on plasma amino acid concentrations and on 5-hydroxytryptamine metabolism in six different brain regions in the rat. *Acta Physiol Scand* 1989;**136**:473.

28 Rang HP, Dale MM. *Pharmacology.* London: Churchill Livingstone, 1987.

29 Nieman D. Exercise infection and immunity. *Int J Sports Med* 1994;**15**:S131.

30 Heath GW, Ford ES, Craven TE, *et al.* Exercise and the incidence of upper respiratory tract infections. *Med Sci Sports Exerc* 1991;**23**:152–7.

31 Nieman D, Johanssen LM, Lee JW, *et al.* Infection episodes before and after the Los Angeles marathon. *J Sports Med Phys Fitness* 1990;**30**:289–96.

32 Parry-Billings M, Budgett R, Koutedakis Y, *et al.* Plasma amino acid concentrations in the overtraining syndrome: possible effects on the immune system. *Med Sci Sports Exerc* 1992;**24**:1353–8.

33 Castell LM, Poortmans J, Newsholme EA. Does glutamine have a role in reducing infection during intensified training in swimmers. *Med Sci Sports Exerc* 1996;**28**:285–90.

Multiple choice questions

Which of the following statements are true or false?

1 The overtraining syndrome primarily affects sprinters and power athletes

2 A high creatine kinase concentration in the plasma is diagnostic of the overtraining syndrome
3 Low glutamine concentrations have been found in fatigued, overtrained athletes
4 Overreaching is an essential and normal part of training
5 High dose vitamins have been shown to prevent the overtraining syndrome

Answers are on p. 364.

10 Viral illness and sport

C R Madeley

Infections with viruses are common, so common that the comment by the doctor "It's probably a virus" excites little surprise and less anxiety in most patients. The implications are that the patient will recover fully without significant after effects and that there will be no specific treatment. Nevertheless, this is a simplistic view—there are serious, and even lethal, virus infections and there are an increasing number of antiviral drugs for use in specific circumstances. HIV (the cause of AIDS), Ebola, and rabies viruses are examples of viruses that can kill, with wide variations in the speed with which they do so, but the vast majority of common (often upper respiratory) infections are more of a nuisance than anything more sinister to the individual, although, collectively, they have economic importance to the community in lost work days. The perceived triviality of many virus infections means that confirmation of the involvement of a virus and its identification are rarely attempted except in hospital, and "It's probably a virus" usually terminates the investigation. To a professional virologist, this is both understandable and frustrating—we can identify viruses as infecting agents and would like to do so on every occasion but it is too difficult and usually too expensive outside the hospital context.

For athletes, viruses are important in two ways: firstly, as agents that may easily be spread among them, during competitive games in particular. In contact sports such as wrestling and rugby, skin infections such as herpes may be spread very readily ("herpes gladiatorum"), but other viruses may be transmitted by droplets during team talks or other forms of association. Secondly, viruses may be important to individual athletes who are training to a high level by interfering with training during the acute stage of an illness

---

Box 10.1   Virus infections are

- Very common
- Mostly, but not invariably, trivial, but
- May be important to athletes in knocking them off their peak of fitness
- May have longer term effects more difficult to pinpoint

---

and, in some, by leaving long term sequelae. Here there is a wide belief that viruses are directly involved, but hard data to underpin this belief are scanty and must be augmented if the aim is prevention.

Viruses differ in the body systems they infect and the extent of the damage they do. It is not sufficient just to confirm that a virus is involved; we need to know which one(s) if we want to do anything about it/them. Vaccines for viruses work well, and it is comparatively easy to develop an effective one to a virus that spreads systemically throughout the body during pathogenesis.

Whether an individual, athlete or not, is infected, or affected, by an infectious agent will be influenced by his or her immune status. Training, overtraining, and overreaching[1] will alter the parameters of immune function that we can measure and are therefore likely to affect the outcome, in the short term with respect to how quickly the agent is eliminated and in the long term with respect to how quickly previous levels of fitness and performance are regained. This recovery will also be influenced by any psychological effects of the episode. For example, postinfluenza depression[2] is not uncommon. Damage and recovery after a virus infection is a complex of interacting factors and any attempt to analyse and understand them will require a well planned and comprehensive prospective study. Is it important enough to put time, effort, and other resources into finding out? This question will be returned to later after the requirements to satisfy a virologist are outlined and a discussion of the issues from a virologist's point of view. Firstly, what does virus diagnosis and surveillance require?

Diagnosing a viral infection

These are the methods used for identifying specific virus activity, both during acute illness and afterwards. Diagnosis at the acute stage is essential if any long term effects are to be established.

185

> ## Box 10.2   Proof of a role for viruses
>
> - Needs to be scientific, not anecdotal
> - Needs a considerable investment by both athletes and investigators
> - Has to cover a wide variety of viruses
> - Cannot be provided by one catch all test
> - Has to cover both short and long term effects

Methods

The methods of diagnosis are treated in more detail by Halonen and Madeley.[3] Briefly, there are two arms to diagnosis. The first is isolating/identifying the virus and the second is monitoring the body's response to it, either by showing the appearance of specific antibodies in serum (and, increasingly, in saliva) or a lymphocyte response. The latter is confined in virology almost entirely to research laboratories, but documenting an antibody response (and, to a lesser extent, virus isolation/identification) is widely available in diagnostic virology laboratories and many microbiology ones.

Looking for an antibody reaction (serology) has significant disadvantages in the present context because it shows only what has happened after the event and does not define it accurately in time. To show whether a virus has affected an athlete's performance, it is necessary to pinpoint to the nearest day when the episode began. Serology is not precise enough for this. Moreover, it provides no information on which organs are involved. The effect on the respiratory system, for example, will not be the same as on the musculoskeletal system. Lastly, for technical reasons, serological tests are not available for every virus. Some viruses lack a group antigen and have too many serotypes for serology to be possible—for example, rhinovirus, the cause of the common cold, has over 100 serotypes. It would be impractical to test each serum over 100 times to get an answer. Although serological examination is cheap compared with isolation/identification, carrying out a full screen on all possible viruses would be a major undertaking in one individual and would be quite impractical in a study group large enough to draw useful statistical conclusions.

The alternative of looking directly for the virus (isolation or identification) has a number of advantages despite the greater cost. The first is that it links any associated illness to a narrow window in time and the diagnosis can be made at the acute stage. This is

Box 10.3   In diagnosing virus infections

- Identifying the specific virus is essential
- An antibody response:
  - Is too slow
  - Is too imprecise in time
  - Cannot identify the body system involved

illustrated in fig 10.1, which shows the profile of a typical acute infection with normal recovery. Virus is present at detectable levels during the early stage of the illness (usually for the first 5 days or so) while serum antibody does not appear until about a week after onset.

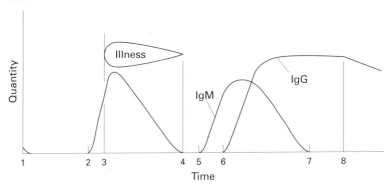

Fig 10.1   Typical acute virus infection. The x axis represents time but the numbers are events (1–8). The y axis represents quantity. The cycle begins with exposure to the virus (point 1), at which time a small amount of virus is theoretically detectable. Between points 1 and 3 is the incubation period, ending with the onset of illness. Shortly before this, the virus will reappear (point 2) but is rarely detected unless specifically sought. The curve of virus detectability rises to a peak as the patient develops symptoms and will, in most cases, decline to undetectable levels (point 4) after about 5 days. This period of detectability will vary considerably depending on the virus and the overall immune competence of the patient. It may persist for a considerable time and, in those who are seriously compromised, possibly for life. From about 1 week after the start of the illness (point 5), serum antibody becomes detectable, first IgM, followed by long term IgG (point 6). IgM antibody declines over about 1 month (to point 7) while IgG, after reaching a high level, will decline very slowly (from point 8) and may remain detectable for the rest of the patient's life. Individuals will show variations in this pattern but routine diagnosis is based on the assumption that the deviations are relatively minor; they usually are. Reprinted with permission from Halonen and Madeley.[3]

187

Table 10.1   Techniques commonly used to detect virus or viral components (no single technique is applicable to all viruses)

Method	Target	Time taken from receipt of specimen to diagnosis	Fragility of specimen*
Isolation	Infectious virus	2 days–3 weeks†	High
Immunofluorescence	Infected cells	2–3 hours	Moderate
Enzyme immunoassays	Viral antigen	2–3 hours	Low
Electron microscopy	Complete virus	15–30 minutes	Low
Genome amplification‡	Viral nucleic acid	Overnight	Moderate

*Rate of decay with time during transit to the laboratory.
†Depends on the amount of virus in the specimen and whether the virus grows quickly or slowly.
‡By polymerase chain reaction (PCR), nucleic acid sequence-based amplification (NASBA), ligase chain reaction (LCR), etc.

Table 10.1 illustrates the techniques commonly used to find virus or virus components at the acute stage. Isolation of virus in cell culture and electron microscopic examination of stool specimens have the advantages of being "catch all" techniques, which require no prior decisions on which viruses are being sought. A suitable cell type must be available for isolation or there must be enough virus present for microscopy.

Other methods require specific reagents and will detect a narrower range of viruses, often only a single type. They must therefore be repeated to search for a variety of viruses, thereby adding to the cost. Newer techniques such as the polymerase chain reaction (PCR) and other forms of nucleic acid (genome) amplification have the advantage of great sensitivity. This extra sensitivity may be useful in the follow up of acute infections (see below).

In neither serology nor isolation/identification is a single technique suitable for all viruses, and a combination is needed. Monitoring the infections of a group of athletes increases the work exponentially as more subjects are recruited and the net is cast wider. Cell culture is expensive to provide and labour intensive to use. Cells must be grown in defined medium and maintained in it for up to 3 weeks while small amounts of virus grow to detectable levels. Each culture has to be examined under a microscope every 2 to 3 days to see the effects of virus growth on the cells. Any putative viruses (and other material in the specimen that may be toxic for the cells in culture and can mimic virus induced degeneration closely) must then be identified by further tests, such as neutralisation and immunofluorescence. Not surprisingly, diagnosis by isolation, which to be adequately comprehensive requires inoculation of up to three different cell types, is expensive and, because the cultures have to be kept and regularly examined for longer, negative results are paradoxically more expensive than positive ones. Not only that, a negative result does not prove that no virus was present in the specimen, only that no virus grew. Hence, if the clinical picture is very "virus-like", it may be necessary to consider repeating the attempt at isolation from the original specimen.

Suitable specimens

It is trite but true that virus diagnostic methods are only as good as the specimens on which they are used. For isolation/identification, the specimen must contain sufficient virus or viral components for them to be found, and this raises two important aspects. The first is that it is easier to take a bad specimen than a good one—taking a good one is usually more uncomfortable for the patient. The second is that, to prove that a virus is *infecting* and therefore likely to be *affecting* a specific organ, it is more convincing to take the specimen from that organ. Unfortunately, not all parts of the body are readily accessible for specimen taking. While specimens may be taken easily from the skin—for example, to detect herpes simplex from cold sores—or with a little more difficulty from the nasopharynx—for example, for most upper respiratory infections—it is much more invasive to take specimens from muscle (relevant to the present discussion), the heart, or the lungs. It is not surprising that the evidence that viruses affect these organs is more scanty and indirect than for skin or the upper respiratory tract.

To grow and survive, viruses need suitable living cells—that is, cells that are respiring and metabolically active. Consequently, virus in any specimen will die off exponentially until it is put into culture, and therefore there is some urgency in getting it to the laboratory as quickly as possible. Cooling, but not freezing it, will slow the rate of decay. It is this fragility more than anything else that has inhibited virus diagnosis in general practice in the United Kingdom and elsewhere, except in rare circumstances when individual enthusiasm has overcome these obstacles. A delay in the specimen reaching the laboratory will cast doubt on the validity of a negative result, and respiratory viruses are particularly fragile.

Other components may be less fragile, but nothing in a virus is totally stable at room temperature. Viruses may be stored at $-70°C$ and below, but there are still significant losses during freezing and thawing, particularly in those viruses in which the outer coat is a lipid envelope (table 10.2).

Which viruses?

If all the different serotypes are included (and with some common viruses, such as rhinoviruses and enteroviruses, different serotypes are effectively different viruses in diagnostic terms), there are nearly a thousand viruses which either infect humans or can be transmitted from animals. Table 10.2 lists the common viruses circulating in temperate climes, such as the United Kingdom, with some of their distinguishing characteristics. A similar list for the tropics would have to be extended considerably to include insect transmitted (arbo-) viruses, such as dengue and Japanese encephalitis.

The viruses listed in table 10.2 are, mostly, associated with particular disease syndromes. The evidence that they cause disease is either direct (virus found in the lesions) or indirectly inferred from finding the virus regularly in other more accessible sites when the typical syndrome is present. Where viruses may be implicated as possible causes of damage to athletic performance, this may be too simple a concept. Because it is difficult to take a specimen from skeletal muscle, we know next to nothing about how frequently viruses invade muscle, and individual infections may be more or less extensive or persist for longer than we believe at present.

For example, a child with leukaemia died a few years ago with respiratory complications. At the postmortem examination the only pathogen isolated from his lung tissue was a rhinovirus, one of the causes of the common cold. Rhinoviruses may be recovered from the nasopharynx in a considerable number of upper respiratory tract infections but specimens from the lower tract (lower trachea, bronchi, bronchioles, and alveoli) are ethically inaccessible in a routine practice. How frequently do rhinoviruses invade the lower tract? Is it only in those who are more extensively affected? Is it inherently more likely in some individuals than others and, if so, is there anything we can measure to identify who they are? Is this relevant to infections in athletes?

Other agents

Viruses are not the only infectious agents that may affect physical performance. Bacteria, fungi, and parasites may contribute,

Table 10.2   Viruses primarily infecting humans[1]

Virus family	Members	No of serotypes	Lipid outer membrane	Stability
DNA viruses				
Herpesviruses	Herpes simplex★	2	Yes	Low
	Varicella zoster★	1	Yes	Low
	Cytomegalovirus	1	Yes	Low
	Epstein Barr virus★	1	Yes	Low
Adenoviruses		47	No	Moderate
Papovaviruses	Wart★	>60[2]	No	High
	BK	1	No	High?
	JC	1	No	High?
Hepatitis B★		Mutants[3]	No	High
Parvoviruses	Adenovirus-associated	?	No	?
Poxviruses	Vaccinia★	1	No	High
	Cowpox	1	No	High
	Molluscum contagiosum★	1	No	High
	Orf	1	No	High
	Pseudocowpox	1	No	High
RNA viruses				
Reoviruses		3	No	Moderate
Orthomyxoviruses★	Influenza A	Many[4]	Yes	Low
	Influenza B	Several[5]	Yes	Low
Paramyxoviruses	Parainfluenza★	4	Yes	Low
	Measles	1	Yes	Low
	Respiratory syncytial virus	1[6]	Yes	Low
Rotavirus		At least 5	No	High
Picornaviruses	Poliovirus	3	No	High
	Coxsackie A	23	No	High
	Coxsackie B★	6	No	High
	Echovirus	31	No	High
	Enterovirus	4	No	High
	Rhinovirus	>100	No	Moderate
Calciviruses		5	No	High
Small round structured viruses		>5	No	High
Retroviruses	HIV★	Many[7]	Yes	Low
	HTLV	2	Yes	Low
Hepatitis A		1	No	High
Hepatitis C★		~5	Yes	Low
Togaviruses	Rubella	1	Yes	Low

[1]Add to this list >200 viruses transmitted from animals to man by biting insects, those transmitted to man directly from animals, and many others confined to the tropics.
[2]Genotypes rather than serotypes.
[3]One basic serotype but an increasing variety of mutants.
[4]Appear sequentially, only 2–3 at any one time.
[5]Similar to influenza A but only one present at a time.
[6]Two subgroups, but very similar antigenically.
[7]Highly mutable but several subgroups.
★**Viruses more likely to be important in a sports context.**

separately, together or sequentially. Whooping cough, aspergillus, or malaria can all have significant consequences and should not be forgotten. Bacteria may infect secondarily the tissues already breached by viruses and prolong the pathology. Nevertheless, viruses, which often cause systemic infections, are probably responsible for most of the common and more important damage.

A prospective study

Given the difficulties of diagnosing virus infections from general practice—too difficult to carry out reliably and too expensive and too late to allow prevention or treatment—it will not be any easier from home, gymnasium, running track, or training ground. Is the information of sufficient value to justify making a special effort to collect it?

Much money is spent in training athletes and sending them to compete at venues all around the world. All the time, effort, and money can be wasted if a virus impairs performance or prevents competition. However, if the culprit can be identified, prevention or treatment can be considered in the future.

Attempts have been made to link viruses with longer term debility such as the chronic fatigue syndrome (CFS; also known as myalgic encephalomyelitis (ME) and the postviral fatigue syndrome (PVFS)). The role of viruses in these conditions in the general population and in other underperforming athletes is presumed, but often with only circumstantial evidence to back it up.

Good evidence of viral involvement in reducing physical performance, short or long term, would have wider implications than just for athletes. What would be needed to collect scientifically valid data? It would be necessary to recruit a group of athletes who were just starting serious training towards a specific event, and to follow their progress, measuring their developing fitness and changes in their immunological status, identifying any infectious episodes, and measuring their effects. This would require regular weekly assessments of their performance and weekly blood specimens for estimates of immune parameters (total and differential white cell counts, response to stimuli, including counts of CD4, CD8, and NK lymphocytes), interleukin levels, and antibody titres (at least weekly specimens for virology and other microbiology with increased frequency if an infection is detected).

It is now well accepted that moderate training produces

measurable improvements in immunological function,[4] but over-training can override this, as illustrated in fig 10.2. Within this overall pattern, individuals vary considerably,[4] such that average values may not be very helpful unless large numbers are included. For this reason, it may be more realistic to study a few individuals in depth, monitoring their experience(s) in detail. This is a conclusion supported by the number of assessments outlined below. The effort and cost required to study 100 or more subjects would be large compared with any likely resources.

A compromise number of about 10 athletes is probably the upper limit for carrying out even a pilot study. They should be following a course of training towards a high level of fitness, preferably with a defined goal such as a major athletic competition on a specific date. They would have to be willing not only to carry out the training regularly and conscientiously but also to keep records, to collect some specimens, and to allow others to be taken. As will be seen below, this is a major undertaking and a high level of both sports and scientific motivation would be needed.

The following regular assessments would have to be carried out

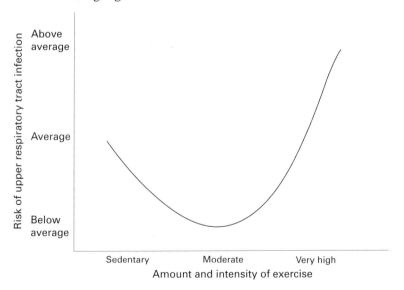

Fig 10.2 Approximate relation between the amount of exercise taken by individuals and the effects on their immune systems generally, reflected in their susceptibility to respiratory tract infection. Very high exercise levels may therefore increase susceptibility. Reproduced with permission from Nieman.[5]

to provide a baseline of fitness and immunological status and to identify the presence of potential pathogens before they cause problems:

- Fitness—This would be assessed weekly by a sports physiologist using standard methods appropriate to the sport in question. They would probably be no different from those performed routinely but would have to be recorded on a previously prepared assessment form.
- Virology—Weekly nose and throat swabs would need to be taken, placed in virus transport medium, and delivered to the virus laboratory early enough for culture that day. Faecal specimens would also be needed. The residual parts of the other specimens would be stored at $-70°C$ for reanalysis if necessary.
- Bacteriology, mycology, and parasitology—Weekly throat swabs and faeces would be taken as necessary to monitor the presence of throat and stool pathogens.
- Immunology—Not less than 50 ml heparinised whole blood would need to be taken weekly to cover all the relevant assessments of lymphocyte numbers, identity, and function, measurement of some lymphokine concentrations, provision of a sample of serum for virus antibodies, and for any possible future reassessments. The implications of this are discussed below under ethical considerations.
- Duration—The study would have to be over a complete training and competition season which, in the context of track and field athletics, would be a whole year. With other sports, the "season" is becoming longer and longer but may have a number of peak periods of competition which could make definition of the role of a virus more difficult. Whatever the sport, the essence would be to cover the training build up and the competitions/matches that follow.

If the longer term effects, if any, of viruses (or other agents) on athletes are to be documented and understood, further follow up of any infections is necessary. This is not as easy as it appears. With the standard techniques outlined above, virus is not usually detectable in an acute infection for longer than 5 days. If a virus continues to influence the performance of an individual, it must be interfering with a physiological process somewhere in the body. Which process, where, and how? In what form does the virus persist, in which organs (possibly elsewhere in the body as well as in this affected), and by what mechanism does it affect organ function? None of these questions is easy to answer.

Those patients unlucky enough to contract facial herpes know that the lesions return again and again. The recurrences are related to various factors, including sunlight, other infections, and physical and emotional stress. Between attacks, the virus lies inaccessibly dormant in the sensory root ganglia of the central nervous system but is readily detectable in the new skin lesions of a recurrence.

In longer term disability, such as the chronic fatigue syndrome, it is voluntary muscle that appears to be affected. Weakness has been documented by stimulation myography,[6] but this is more difficult to investigate virologically than, for example, the immediately accessible skin lesions of herpes simplex. Muscle biopsy would have to be performed to draw any valid conclusions, a procedure that few ethical committees would accept, especially if it meant taking several biopsy specimens, one in the acute phase and another about 6 months later. In theory, follow up biopsy samples would be taken only from those with persisting impairment, but these would not be known at the acute stage. Hence, all the subjects would have to have samples taken both at the acute stage and again later to provide normal controls. Even if, improbably, the subjects agreed to this assault, it seems very doubtful that any ethical committee would concur.

If it is not ethically acceptable to sample the affected organ it becomes difficult to answer any of the three questions posed above, except indirectly. However, demonstration of persistence anywhere in the body would be a start. Let us consider the implications of this approach with a candidate virus.

Coxsackie B (CB) viruses are linked with muscle infections. They are strongly associated with Bornholm disease (a very painful inflammation of the intercostal muscles) and have been recovered from cardiac muscle in fatal cases of cardiomyopathy.[7] These, however, are rare sequelae of a gut infection, which is itself very common, particularly in children, and which progresses only occasionally beyond the gut. CB viruses also cause aseptic meningitis and they may then be readily isolated from the cerebral spinal fluid. Infection of the gut is confirmed by isolating the virus from faeces but this does not prove muscle involvement.

It may be possible to increase the sensitivity of detection in faeces by using nucleic acid amplification techniques to show that small amounts of virus genomic material are still being excreted after complete virus can no longer be isolated. This, however, does not take us much further, and to understand how and in what form the virus is persisting would require gut biopsy, which is no more acceptable ethically. Nevertheless, examining easily acquired faeces in this way would, if results were positive, show that there was something else to investigate later. However, it would not tell us how to do it.

The genome of viruses is in the form of either DNA or RNA. CB viruses are among those with RNA, while others such as herpes use DNA. In the body, cells use DNA to store (genetic) information in the nucleus and it is therefore protected from degradation. RNA is used to transfer this information, as necessary, from the nucleus to the ribosomes to provide a template for protein production. Once it has been used, it is degraded so that the cell does not accumulate information that is not being used. Within a cell therefore RNA is essentially transient and, if the RNA of CB (or any other RNA-containing viruses) persists intracellularly, in what form does it do so? It is worth noting that one RNA virus known to persist, HIV, does so by carrying with it an enzyme, reverse transcriptase (RT), the function of which is to make a complementary DNA (cDNA) copy of the genome. This is integrated into the host cell genome and is then able to remain in a protected environment, probably for the rest of the patient's life. RNA-containing viruses do not, in general, have an RT and this enzyme is not found in human cells, only in some viruses. CB viruses are not among them.

A model of possibly greater relevance is provided by hepatitis C virus. It too is an RNA virus which persists and which has not been shown to possess RT. Virus activity has been shown in the liver,[8] but finding it does not explain how it persists. It may have a primary focus elsewhere, where low level continuing virus production repeatedly infects new liver cells. If this occurs with hepatitis C virus, it would be necessary to postulate a different mechanism for CB viruses, which cause an acute infection, producing large amounts of virus and cellular damage and releasing less virus. Invasion of another type of cell elsewhere in the body would be one explanation. Which cells? Where? Although follow up would be highly desirable, particularly of any individuals showing persisting effects, this would not be straightforward or easy.

Conclusions

The financial and emotional investment put by an individual into training to the highest level he or she can attain is immense. To find it effectively going to waste because an infection, often thought to be trivial, damages that performance must be very galling to athletes and coaches alike. We know little about the contribution of various viruses to these disappointments and even less to longer term problems such as the chronic fatigue syndrome. This syndrome is by no means confined to high class athletes but is very difficult to investigate retrospectively, especially as current definitions require it to be present for at least 6 months to qualify.[9]

A prospective study of highly motivated athletes would help to understand the syndrome in others and would therefore have wider implications. Such a study would be essential if any conclusions are to be valid, although the analysis in this review makes the problem plain. Athletes in training must be well motivated to achieve their best and they would have a personal and powerful interest in any factor that might deprive them of a medal. Peak training on the verge, or even over the edge, of overtraining will leave them vulnerable to infection in addition to the stress of reaching their peak on exactly the right day. Such highly motivated individuals would provide an appropriate study group, and there would be a high expectation that they would see it through.

Two obstacles would have to be overcome, however: cost and ethics. A proposal to do a similar study was costed in outline in 1997 and would have required at least £300 000 to carry out satisfactorily. This sum included all the reagents and cells necessary for culturing viruses, electron microscopy on stool specimens, serology, immunological assays for white cell counts, functional assays and interleukin levels, and bacteriology. It included a research fellow to monitor the regular collection of routine specimens and extra ones during any infective episodes and a part time nurse to take blood and other specimens. The part time services of a virologist, a microbiologist, and an immunologist would be needed, as well as the whole time services of an experienced technician. It did not include the cost of a coach/trainer, sports equipment to measure performance, nor any form of thank you to the athletes for allowing various forms of repeated assault.

Since a study like this would essentially be a "fishing expedition", it would face the same problem as any similar epidemiological study—"too open ended and too uncertain" of producing significant data. Nevertheless, the possibility of collecting valuable information that would also be applicable to those with the chronic fatigue syndrome should provide stronger impetus, if only to raise the possibility of a definite diagnostic test

197

for this condition.

The second obstacle is the ethical one already mentioned and may be even more difficult to overcome. A full investigation will, at the least, require regular and substantial samples of blood, which at 50 ml weekly could lead to anaemia in the study subjects if they were prepared to cooperate for up to a year. To add muscle biopsies would provoke most ethical committees into refusal.

Without a fully planned prospective study, only anecdotal evidence will remain, backed up by occasional data from biopsies, etc, carried out for other reasons. If the continuing concern, reinforced by pressure groups, to understand the chronic fatigue syndrome is to be satisfied, some scientifically valid studies, controlled as far as possible, are essential. Outlined above is one suggestion of how it might be tackled but is not the only possible one. Others may have different approaches, but the need for a prospective study seems clear. Given the variety of viruses that may be involved, improving on present anecdotal convictions should be the aim. There is scope for new approaches to this diagnostic challenge.

1 Budgett R. Fatigue and underperformance in athletes: the overtraining syndrome. *Br J Sports Med* 1998;**32**:107–10.
2 Christie AB. Acute respiratory infections. *Infectious diseases*. 4th ed. Edinburgh: Churchill Livingstone, 1987:413–74.
3 Halonen P, Madeley CR. The laboratory diagnosis of viral infections. In: Mahy BWJ, Collier L, eds. *Topley & Wilson's microbiology and microbial infections. Virology Vol 4*. 9th ed. London: Arnold, 1998:947–62.
4 Shephard RJ, Shek PN. Potential impact of physical activity and sport on the immune system: a brief review. *Br J Sports Med* 1994;**28**:247–55.
5 Nieman DC. Upper respiratory tract infections and exercise. *Thorax* 1995;**50**:1229–31.
6 Dickinson CJ. Chronic fatigue syndrome: aetiological aspects. *Eur J Clin Invest* 1997;**27**:257–67.
7 Melnick JL. Enteroviruses: polioviruses, coxsackieviruses, echoviruses and newer enteroviruses. In: Fields BN, Knipe DM, Howley P, eds. *Fields' virology*. 3rd ed. Philadelphia: Lippincott-Raven, 1996:655–712.
8 Houghton M. Hepatitis C viruses. In: Fields BN, Knipe DM, Howley P, eds. *Fields' virology*. 3rd ed. Philadelphia: Lippincott-Raven, 1996:1035–8.
9 Sharpe M. Chronic fatigue syndrome. *Psychiatr Clin North Am* 1996;**19**:549–73.

Multiple choice questions

1 Which of the following statements about viruses in humans are correct?
  (a) Virus infections are trivial (never life threatening)
  (b) Viruses infect only the respiratory tract

(c) Viruses are intracellular parasites

(d) Viruses can affect athletic performance

(e) The ribonucleic acid (RNA) of RNA-containing viruses persists intracellularly

2 In investigating the role of viruses in athletes, a satisfactory diagnosis of infection may be made by:

(a) Growing the virus from the affected organ

(b) Finding virus specific antibodies in the serum

(c) Amplifying viral genomic nucleic acid from the patient during the acute phase

(d) Recovering virus from a muscle biopsy

(e) Finding virus specific antibodies in the saliva

Answers are on p. 364.

11 Physical exercise and psychological wellbeing

D Scully, J Kremer, M M Meade, R Graham, K Dudgeon

Introduction

The positive role which physical exercise can have in the prevention and treatment of a range of medical conditions has received a great deal of attention over recent years, with numerous high profile reports supporting the popular message that exercise is good for you[1-3]. In addition, research has identified the long term protection which regular exercise affords against a plethora of somatic complaints, including coronary heart disease, hypertension, a number of cancers, diabetes and osteoporosis.[4,5] Following from these findings, recommendations for exercise regimes emphasise the physical benefits that accompany increased physical activity, for example, with the American College of Sports Medicine (ACSM) advocating that "Every US adult should accumulate 30 minutes or more of moderate-intensity physical activity on most, preferably all, days of the week".[6]

Unfortunately, while the somatic benefits associated with physical exercise are well documented, hard evidence to support an equivalent relationship between exercise and psychological wellbeing is less plentiful. Indeed, neither the ACSM guidelines nor many of the available international public policy documents on physical activity make specific recommendations concerning exercise and mental health. Of the 17 documents reviewed by Blair et al.,[7] only two make mention of the psychological benefits associated with physical activity.[8,9] This is true despite the fact that when asked about perceived health benefits of exercise, general practitioners are most likely to mention psychosocial benefits such as relaxation, increased social contact, promotion of self care and self esteem.[10]

The interview survey by Smith *et al.* bolsters a notion which has gained popularity both in the popular press as well as the academic community – namely, that the psychosocial benefits of physical exercise may equal if not surpass the physiological benefits.[10] In this chapter we examine the evidence presented in support of this contention and give practical recommendations on the prescription of exercise regimes for the treatment of a range of psychological problems.

Physical activity and psychological wellbeing

Over the past decade there have been several extensive reviews of the exercise psychology literature which together offer positive if guarded support for the role which exercise can have in the promotion of positive mental health.[11-13] This optimism is founded on growing numbers of controlled studies which have identified the positive effects of exercise, most often among clinical populations. At the same time, caution has been expressed both in relation to the direction of causality and in the use of reductionist arguments to interpret findings. In the words of Rejeski, "it is misguided to theorize that explanations for psychosocial outcomes will ultimately be reduced to some physiological system (e.g. cardiac-related cortical activity) or neurochemical activity".[14] Instead, what Rejeski and others maintain is that perceived psychosocial benefits may occur in the absence of clearly identifiable changes in physiological parameters, just as it is possible to establish physio-

---

Box 11.1

- Interest in the relation between physical exercise and psychological health has increased in recent years
- While the message from physiological research has extolled the general advantages of exercise in terms of physical health, the equivalent research from psychological specialties has revealed a more complex relation
- Evidence from research focuses on the association between physical exercise and depression, anxiety, self-esteem, response to stress, mood state, the premenstrual syndrome, and body image
- Exercise addiction and withdrawal has also been studied along with the implications for exercise prescription

---

logical changes in the absence of any perceived psychological benefits.

In a wide ranging literature review, McAuley considered the relationship between exercise and both positive and negative psychological health.[13] In common with other review articles, McAuley identifies the positive correlation between exercise and self-esteem, self-efficacy, psychological wellbeing and cognitive functioning, and the negative correlation between exercise and anxiety, stress and depression. While such information can be used to support the general benefits of exercise, it falls short of suggesting practical guidelines on how exercise may be used to alleviate particular symptoms and, just as significantly, which forms of exercise are likely to be most beneficial in which circumstances. In addition, establishing the direction of causality has proved difficult—that is, did psychological wellbeing precede, follow or operate independently from a particular exercise regime? With this in mind, it is unsurprising that reviewers remain critical of the methodological limitations of much of the exercise psychology literature (see Mutrie and Biddle[11]).

In a more innovatory critique of the literature, Rejeski attempted to frame the psychosocial outcomes of exercise in terms of a dose-response relation, a relation that had previously enjoyed popularity not in the exercise psychology but in the exercise physiology literature.[14] According to Shephard, one of the primary issues for exercise physiologists (alongside other healthcare professionals) centres on establishing the specific association between physical activity undertaken (a product of intensity, frequency and duration) and biological responses (assessed by improvement in aerobic fitness or health).[15] Despite unresolved concerns over the application of the research paradigm[15] many public policy initiatives continue to be based on recommendations derived from related research.

According to Rejeski, while the dose-response relationship may have heuristic value in relation to the physiology of exercise, in terms of psychological effects it fails to account for the cognitive and emotional experiences of the exerciser. Hence the complexity of the relationship, in terms of both dose (activity type, frequency, intensity and duration) and possible responses, makes it difficult to envisage research ever having the potential to move from description to prescription in relation to mental health.

Recent literature continues to urge caution in the extrapolation from the physiological to the psychological, and particularly as so few studies are exploring the dose-response relation between exercise and psychosocial outcomes. Rejeski reviews only four such studies, with the most significant conclusion derived from this work being that there appears to be a ceiling level in terms of psychosocial effects. More specifically, these studies have suggested that low to moderate levels of aerobic exercise are better than traditional, demanding (anaerobic) exercise programmes in terms of enhancing moods and improving psychological functioning.[16,17]

There is greater difficulty in establishing precise guidelines regarding the intensity and duration of exercise, partly because of methodological inconsistencies across studies reviewed, but also because of differences between the psychological functions being evaluated. At the level of general mental health, the literature therefore remains inconclusive as to the relation between exercise regimes and overall psychological wellbeing, and with this in mind, it is towards the specific effects of exercise on particular psychological functions and conditions that attention has turned.

In 1992, the International Society of Sport Psychology[18] endorsed the position statements earlier issued by the American National Institute of Mental Health[19] which described the link between regular exercise and psychological wellbeing. Briefly, these consensus documents posited that particular psychological dysfunctions, most notably depression, anxiety and stress, can benefit from involvement in physical activity. The evidence for a significant and positive relation between physical activity and psychological variables is taken as compelling for mentally healthy individuals[20,21] but is seen as even stronger for people with psychiatric problems.[22] This may not be unexpected—for example given that the normal population "score at the low end of depression scores and therefore, have relatively little room for improvement".[23] Much of the existing literature on exercise and mental health has focused on changes in anxiety, depression, mood, self-esteem and stress reactivity. Alongside these, we have also examined two less frequently cited areas of research—those dealing with exercise effects on premenstrual syndrome (PMS) and also the relation between exercise and body image.

Depression

Martinsen reviewed the literature dealing with the effects of exercise on patients diagnosed as suffering from clinical depression.[22] Initially, he found that such patients tended to be physically

---

Box 11.2

- There remains a paucity of substantial evidence to define a positive relation between exercise and psychological health
- The literature which does exist points to a positive correlation between exercise and self esteem, self efficacy, and cognitive functioning together with a negative correlation with anxiety, stress, and depression
- At the same time, practical guidelines as to which forms of exercise will alleviate which particular psychological symptoms is not yet available
- Low to moderate levels of aerobic exercise seem to be more successful in enhancing mood state and psychological functioning than anaerobic exercise, though precise levels of intensity and duration remain ill defined

---

sedentary and were characterised by a reduced physical work capacity compared with the general population. In itself this finding immediately provides an argument for the integration of physical fitness training into comprehensive treatment programmes for depression, while at the same time signaling the difficulties which may be involved in implementing an exercise regime with a population who are not predisposed towards exercise.

Although a number of studies stress the importance of using aerobic exercise in the treatment of clinical depression,[23] Martinsen found that the anti-depressant effects linked with non-aerobic exercise were equally effective. He also found that those who continued to exercise regularly after termination of a 1 year training programme were found to have lower depression scores than those who were sedentary. In addition, the patients themselves were found to be very much appreciative of the use of exercise as a form of treatment and, as Martinsen states, the patients ranked exercise as, "the most important element in comprehensive treatment programmes for depression".

In 1990, North et al. conducted a meta-analysis based on 80 studies conducted between 1969 and 1989 and included 290 effect sizes in their analysis.[24] The results provided positive support for a relation between physical exercise and depression. In particular, it was concluded that acute and chronic exercise effectively reduced clinical depression. All groups of participants, regardless of sex, age or health status, experienced the anti-depressant effects of exercise, with the greatest benefits noted among those receiving medical or psychological care. The mode and duration of exercise was also examined and it was found that both aerobic and non-aerobic exercise operated as effective anti-depressants. However, the authors concede that additional research should focus on the proposed psychotherapeutic benefits of non-aerobic exercise, given that numerous studies do not concur with this finding (for example, Folkins and Sime[25]; Sachs[26]). Finally, the authors also examined issues relating to length of exercise programme, number of sessions, as well as intensity and frequency of exercise. Insufficient data relating to the latter two elements yielded no firm conclusions but the meta-analysis did suggest that the greatest improvements in depression were found after 17 weeks of exercise (albeit that effects were found from 4 weeks onwards). Likewise, it was suggested that the greater the number of exercise sessions the greater the decrease in depression.

A narrative review criticised the meta-analysis of North *et al.* on methodological and interpretative grounds, urging that their conclusions and recommendations should be viewed with caution.[27] In contrast, Morgan[27] was sympathetic towards a monograph reviewing the psychological effects of aerobic fitness training.[28] Paradoxically, many of the conclusions of both studies are identical, in that depression was reduced following aerobic exercise for men and women, in all adult age groups, and across survey and experimental studies, and the effects were greatest among clinical samples.

Finally, a paper by Nicoloff and Schwenk attempted to integrate current research with a view to providing physicians with practical guidelines for exercise prescription as an adjunct to other forms of psychotherapy.[29] Despite acknowledging that no research-based guidelines exist for recommending exercise type, frequency, intensity and duration the authors invoke prescriptions suggested by Hill,[30] which basically concur with those proposed by ACSM.[98] Such programmes advocate aerobic exercise conducted at 60–70% of maximum heart rate, for 30–40 minutes, twice to five times per week.

In conclusion, on the basis of existing literature it seems safe to accept that physical exercise regimes will have a positive influence on depression, with the most powerful effects noted among clinical populations. Limited evidence would also suggest that aerobic exercise is most effective, including activities such as walking, jogging, cycling, light circuit training, and weight training, and that regimes extending over several months seem to yield the most positive effects.

Anxiety

To date, there have been over 30 published reviews dealing with the anxiolytic effects of exercise and physical activity. One review concludes that regardless of anxiety measures taken (trait or state, behavioural, self-report, physiological), or exercise regime invoked (acute versus chronic), the results point to a consistent link between exercise and anxiety reduction.[31] Furthermore, a meta-analysis specifically examining studies that distinguish between those who are coping with stress and those who are not, concluded that aerobic exercise training programmes were effective in reducing anxiety, particularly among those experiencing chronic work stress.[32] Their overall effect sizes were comparable to those found by other meta-analyses of the exercise-stress literature, as well as other forms of psychotherapy used to reduce anxiety.[33] Finally, more recent research in this area[34,35] has refuted criticisms of earlier studies which imply that anxiety reduction after exercise represents no more than a methodological artefact;[36] instead, the effect does seem to be real and substantial.

At the same time, explicating the variables that mediate the relation between exercise and anxiety reduction has proved problematic, a task made doubly difficult because so few studies specify levels of intensity, duration, and/or length of exercise programme. To date, it can be inferred that the majority of research studies have involved aerobic exercise, with the few studies examining non-aerobic activities (for example strength/flexibility training) actually revealing slight increases in anxiety. Although further research is obviously needed, it does seem that aerobic activity is more beneficial for anxiety reduction.

No consensus of opinion emerges from existing reviews and meta-analyses as regards the level of exercise intensity and its duration. For example, Landers and Petruzzello report conflicting results from a large number of studies.[31] Some suggest low intensity exercise (walking, jogging at 40-50% maximum heart rate) while others argue that moderately intensive exercise (50%–60% of maximum heart rate) is better, while yet others argue that high intensity activity (70–75% of maximum heart rate) is most beneficial.[37] Given this lack of consensus, a sensible compromise position in relation to prescription seems to be that originally proposed by Franks and Jette.[38] That is, for the individual to work with an adjustable level of intensity, chosen by him/herself in consultation with a physician. This solution is especially attractive in the light of the goal setting literature which argues that self selected goals receive greater commitment from the participant.

The duration of individual training sessions has been considered across individual studies, with somewhat surprising results. Research has shown that even a single, 5 minute exercise bout may be sufficient to induce an anxiolytic effect.[31,35,37] In terms of the length of training programmes, both clinical and non-clinical studies have revealed that the largest anxiolytic effects are noted when programmes have run from 10 to 15 weeks or even longer, with smaller effects observed for programmes lasting fewer than 9 weeks.

In conclusion, the literature unequivocally supports the positive effects of exercise on anxiety, with short bursts of exercise seemingly sufficient and in addition the nature of that exercise does not seem to be crucial. As with depression, the most positive effects are noted among those who adhere to programmes for several months.

Stress responsivity

Related literature has considered how exercise may protect against stress, although whether this should be regarded as psychological or physiological research is questionable. This aside, the available research suggests that increases in physical condition or improved fitness are likely to facilitate the individual's capacity for dealing with stress. In reviewing this work[39] a distinction has been made between research based on either cross sectional (categorising participants as "fit" or "unfit" and then observing differences between the groups) or longitudinal (using training and control groups) designs. Results derived from both procedures are best described as equivocal; while the majority do show that physical fitness correlates with a reduction in the physiological response to psychological stress, a smaller number of studies report negligible differences in stress reactivity between the physically fit and the less fit.

True experimental training studies remain rare, although more recent contributions are attempting firstly to manipulate levels of aerobic fitness experimentally and second, to correlate these fitness levels with stress responsivity. In addition, a number of studies have found that aerobic exercise does seem to influence stress responses.[40–42] In each of these studies, comparisons have been drawn between aerobic exercise and anaerobic strength training, with participants typically exercising at least three times a week at moderate intensity for 12 weeks. While the effect appears robust, other studies which have used a similar exercise paradigm and have used similar measures have failed to replicate these results.[43-45] As a consequence, discussion often revolves around methodological concerns, and definitive conclusions remain elusive.

In conclusion, while it may be that aerobically fit individuals do show a reduced psychosocial stress response, the part which exercise can play is probably best described as preventive rather than corrective, and the stress response itself remains only partially understood. Clearly, this work lies at the interface between physiology and psychology and hence raises a great many unanswered questions about the stress response itself and its relation with physiological and psychological symptoms. With these caveats in mind, it would appear that a regimen of aerobic exercise (continuous exercise of sufficient intensity to elevate heart rate significantly above resting pulse rate for over 21 minutes' duration) may significantly enhance stress responsivity, and in particular stress that is related to lifestyle or work.

Mood state

Numerous studies have investigated the mood-enhancing properties of exercise and have demonstrated that exercise can indeed have a positive influence on mood state. At the same time, the early optimism generated by studies of clinical samples has been tempered by the discovery that the effects of exercise on mood state may not be as pervasive as earlier thought. For example, Dishman[46] and Frazier and Nagy[47] have identified individuals who were not initially depressed or anxious, who failed to match after exercise mood enhancement as had been noted with clinical samples. On the other hand, it has also been demonstrated that individuals may self report an improvement in mood state without a corresponding improvement being detected by the psychometric test of mood.[48] These and other methodological concerns have been examined.[36] In particular, the fact that most studies examining exercise effects on mood have utilised the profile of mood states (POMS)[49] has been criticised because the test was initially validated for use in clinical populations and includes only one positive mood dimension (see LaFontaine et al.[23]). In the light of these and other criticisms[36] future reliance on the POMS as the primary measure of mood state in exercise research must be questioned.

A meta-analysis by McDonald and Hodgdon seemed to confirm a clear relation between exercise and positive moods, with significant effect sizes being revealed for all six sub-scales of the POMS.[28] However, more recent research suggests that this relation may be quite complex and demands further clarification. For example, Lennox et al. compared aerobic, anaerobic and waiting list control groups and found no significant improvements in long-term mood states among non-clinical samples.[50] By comparison, other studies found improvements in mood states of female exercisers.[51,52] Both of these latter studies examined chronic exercise over a similar duration to that used by Lennox et al., although the intensity of exercise was less pronounced. These studies highlight the possibility that gains in physical fitness may operate independently of mood and hence, it may be possible to show physical fitness gains in the absence of mood effects and vice versa. In comparison, acute aerobic exercise has been shown to be associated with significant positive mood changes.[53] Two studies examining the benefits of acute exercise have also found mood benefits associated with exercise.[54,55] Steinberg et al. compared different intensity (low-impact/high-impact) aerobic exercise of 25-minutes duration with a control group and found increases in positive moods and decreases in negative moods after exercise.[54] Another study adopting a slightly different approach set out to determine if a lengthy bout of acute aerobic exercise would attenuate the adverse mood effects induced by prescribed β blockers to normal healthy individuals.[55] Results showed that 1 hour of moderate (50% of maximum) treadmill walking was able to produce mood states comparable with those recorded for participants in placebo trials. The authors concluded that exercise prescription should be considered a highly desirable adjuvant therapy in cases where drug treatment is necessary.

Overall these results do indicate that various forms of exercise, both aerobic and anaerobic, can be associated with an elevation of mood state, particularly for clinical samples, although given the diversity of results it is likely that more than one underlying mechanism may be implicated. The nature of these mechanisms, whether psychosocial, psychological, psychopharmacological or psychophysiological, has yet to be understood.

Self esteem

In keeping with the other relationships already examined, a positive link between exercise and self esteem has been established and in turn this seems to be strongest among those whose self esteem is low.[13] However, the reported association is not without

209

criticism. For example, the majority of studies examine global self esteem, which is a relatively stable construct, rather than considering domain specific esteem.[56] Furthermore, few studies have explored changes in self esteem over time, with most focusing on differences between exercisers and non-exercisers at a given point in time.

According to an early review self esteem improved with participation in physical activity regardless of physical activity type.[57] However, a meta-analysis that focused solely on self esteem in young children found a greater effect size for aerobic activities.[58] A more recent review raised a number of methodological and conceptual concerns but also concurred with previous reviews in identifying a positive association between physical activity and self-esteem.[13] Recent work in this area has tended to focus on the development of valid and reliable measures of self esteem, which in turn is regarded as multifaceted. For example, Fox developed the physical self perception profile which distinguishes between global self esteem and physical self esteem and which in turn has been related to factors including body image and sports competence.[59] Subsequent work has been concerned with validation and in so doing has found further support for the notion that physical activity is associated with higher levels of self esteem in younger and older adult males and females.[60–62]

An emerging viewpoint suggests that the more specific sub-domains of self esteem, in particular perceived competence sports at physical condition, attractive body and strength, may be associated differentially with behaviour in various sports. For example, Sonstroem *et al.* found that exercise in adult female aerobic dancers was associated with positive evaluations of their physical condition but with negative evaluations of their bodies.[62] However, little can be said in terms of exercise prescription in the development of self-esteem or its subcomponents because so few studies have considered such changes over time. In fact, only one study appears to have considered this in middle aged males in the context of a 5 month walking programme.[56] The study showed a significant relation between improved aerobic capacity and a measure of physical esteem. Results indicate that the greatest degree of change over time was in the subdomain element of physical condition and the global level self esteem showed the smallest degree of change (although it was still significant).

While these associations are interesting, the literature provides little guidance as to which forms of exercise may be beneficial to which types of self esteem. That there is a relation is not questioned but the nature of that relation has yet to be explored.

Premenstrual syndrome

Despite anecdotal evidence pointing to a relationship between exercise and the premenstrual syndrome (PMS) and the fact that negative effect, depression and anxiety are commonly associated with PMS, only a small number of studies have considered the potential benefits of exercise. One such study investigated the impact of a 12 week training programme on symptom severity in relation to primary dysmenorrhea. Eighteen women with dysmenorrhea were assigned to a training programme which involved a 30 minute walking/jogging session three times a week for 12 weeks. Their symptoms were subsequently compared with a non-exercising control group, and it was concluded that this form of exercise had ameliorated symptoms.

This and other examples of early research on PMS has tended to confirm that exercise has a prophylactic effect on a range of symptoms both physiological and psychological.[64,65] More recently, Choi and Salmon monitored the effect of various frequencies of exercise on PMS in a self selected sample across one menstrual cycle.[66] Low exercise and sedentary groups showed no improvement in symptoms whereas the high exercising group experienced significantly fewer symptoms. Interestingly, competitive exercisers did not show improvements, perhaps indicating that strenuous exercise may be dysfunctional, and confirming earlier speculations[67–69] relating to the negative effects of competitive exercising on anxiety and mood state. Likewise, Cockerill *et al.* found that those who engaged in exercise more than four times a week reported higher tension, depression and anger, whereas those who exercised two to three times per week had healthier mood state profiles.[70]

As regards the type of exercise that appears most beneficial, a study that considered this looked at 23 premenopausal middle aged women engaged in either an anaerobic (strength training) or aerobic exercise programme which took place three times a week for 1 hour over a 12 week period.[71] Participants completed a menstrual symptom questionnaire during their luteal phase once before the start of the programme and once more at its conclusion. While both aerobic and anaerobic exercise were shown to reduce severity of premenstrual symptoms, aerobic exercise appeared to have a more significant effect on premenstrual depression.

This study, along with previous research,[72] suggests that it may not be necessary to reach aerobic capacity to alleviate negative effects as associated with PMS, and hence increased maximal oxygen consumption does not seem to be a causative factor. If this is the case then the question remains as to why exercise may be an effective treatment for PMS. Numerous explanations have been advanced, including the effect that exercise may have on the oestrogen-progesterone ratio. On the one hand, some research has indicated that sportswomen have lower levels of oestrogen than non-exercising women, while on the other hand, other studies have found no differences.[73–75] Rather than assuming a direct relation between exercise and lowered oestrogen levels, Wells has suggested that these levels reflect reduced body fat, since adipose tissue has been identified as a source of oestrogen.[76] An alternative explanation highlights improved glucose tolerance during this stage of the cycle, as the symptoms of poor glucose tolerance are similar to those often reported by women who experience PMS—namely, fatigue, depression, anxiety and increased appetite.[77] According to others, the elevation of endorphin levels prior to menstruation may be a significant factor, and regular exercise may stabilise or prevent extreme variation in endorphin levels and thus decrease the effects of PMS.[78,79]

In conclusion, although the evidence continues to point to the benefits of exercise for those who experience PMS, while less strenuous forms of non-competitive exercise appear most effective, the type of exercise, its duration, and length and in turn the reasons for improvement in symptoms still await clarification.

Body image

In prescribing activity for both physical and psychological benefit, due caution must be taken to ensure that risk factors are not introduced that may attenuate the process of exercise induced psychological health. The sex related factors of physical activity cannot be disregarded in this debate, for while men may enjoy a symbiotic relationship with sport, too often in the past, women's sport has been associated with sex role conflict and associated disorders. Fortunately, this picture may be changing rapidly but at the same time the relation between exercise and problems with body image should not be ignored, for either sex.

Despite significant gains in public acceptance and participation,[80] women are still more likely to engage in non-competitive activities such as aerobics and keep fit,[81–83] which in turn may serve to reinforce the cult of thinness and femininity. Franzoi has described a tendency among women to focus on their body as an aesthetic statement whereas traditionally men have been more likely to attend to the dynamic aspects of their bodies, such as coordination, strength and speed.[84] This emphasis on the female form in exercise settings may foster feelings of social-physique-anxiety (SPA), constrain enjoyment of the activity itself, and may even be exacerbated by the nature of the clothing required.[85] McAuley *et al.* reported that SPA correlates with self-presenta-tional motives for exercise such as weight control and attractiveness, and is higher among women.[86,87] Women con-sistently score higher than men on measures of self confidence with regard to their bodies and physical competence.[88,89] Biddle *et al.*, among others, have emphasised the need for exercise promoters to deal with this issue of poor self confidence among women and to think carefully about sporting venues and other contextual factors (for example, changing facilities) to make women feel more comfortable with their body image during exercise.[90]

Body image itself refers to a multidimensional construct consisting of a set of cognitions and feelings about one's physique. Research shows body image tends to be less positive among women[91] and is more closely linked to women's overall self esteem than men's.[92] For example, in a national survey of 803 women in the United States, over half reported globally negative evaluations of their body parts and a preoccupation with losing weight.[93] The implications of such findings are considerable given that distur-bances in body image have been so strongly implicated in the development of eating disorders[94] and clinical depression.[95] With-out doubt, physicians who advocate the adoption of exercise regimens must remain alert to these body related concerns when they prescribe forms of physical activity.

When training and diet regimes are overly stringent women in particular are susceptible to three distinct though interrelated disorders collectively referred to as the female athlete triad (FAT). Referring to disordered eating, amenorrhea and osteoporosis, FAT is the physical manifestation of a pathological adherence to exercise, often coupled with inappropriate diet.[96,97] In its position paper, the American College of Sports Medicine[98] maintains that the syndrome can cause morbidity and mortality, and notes in particular that women involved in sports that emphasise low body weight for performance or appearance—for example, gymnastics and dance—are most at risk. Nattiv has characterised the typical sufferer as someone driven to excel, who equates leanness with improved performance and who feels pressured to maintain a low body weight.[99] Nattiv has further outlined criteria for screening those at risk, based on interviewing and physical examination.

What is more, not only may exercise be associated with body dissatisfaction, once undertaken, it may actually be implicated in the perpetuation of eating disorders and weight control. Davis *et al.* have described the role that exercise may have in sustaining the cyclical, repetitious nature of eating disorders,[100] and have also outlined the manner in which exercise and self starvation may interact as mutual catalysts.[101] Disordered eating practices and a drive for thinness or leanness are often accompanied by psychopathological consequences observable in depressive symptoms such as low energy and poor self esteem.[102,103] With these thoughts in mind, caution is required in the recommendation of exercise practices which either may provide a link in the chain of disordered eating or which may represent a dysfunctional response to body dissatisfaction.

Exercise addiction and withdrawal

Within the literature on psychophysiology an emerging research focus is on the notion of exercise addiction[104,105] the contention being that the mood enhancing and analgesic properties associated with exercise are influenced by chemicals in the brain which are akin to opiates.[106] Until recently, support for the existence of exercise addiction was meagre and often anecdotal.[107-109] More

---

Box 11.3

- Exercise programmes, particularly comprising long term aerobic exercise, seem to have an ameliorative effect on depression, specifically clinical depression
- Various exercise programmes, both short and long term, have been shown to reduce anxiety and to improve mood state, whereas response to stress may be enhanced by aerobic exercise
- The literature remains rather equivocal in relation to the association between self esteem, the premenstrual syndrome (PMS), and exercise, though women who experience PMS do report positive effects associated with a range of exercise
- The relation between exercise and body image is complex, hence caution must be used when exercise is prescribed for those with problems associated with their body image

---

recent research has suggested strong links between exercise addiction and eating disorders.[110,111] For example, Davis *et al.* found a significant relation between exercise dependence, weight preoccupation and obsessive-compulsive personality traits in women with eating disorders.[110] Furthermore, the same study showed a significant relation between amount of physical activity and obsessive-compulsiveness in high-exercising women without eating disorders.

A related concept, that of withdrawal from habitual exercise, may also be relevant in the context of attempting to provide exercise prescription.[112] Morgan and colleagues speculate that cessation of regular physical activity could result in dysphoric states—for example, increased anxiety, depression, restlessness, guilt.[113] Indeed, a number of previous studies would concur with this speculation.[114-116] However, yet again, despite the intuitive appeal of anecdotal examples there is a limited amount of empirical research on the topic and comparison across studies is not possible given the methodological differences surrounding deprivation periods and behavioural measures.[113]

Whether the mechanism for supposed exercise addiction is based on psychological factors (for example, personality types), physiological mechanisms (for example, endorphin dependence) or an interplay between the two has yet to be established. A workshop concluded that much more systematic investigation needs to be conducted before definitive conclusions can be made about exercise prescription.[104] For example, a number of cautions were raised, including doubts about whether the syndrome of "exercise dependence" exists at all except as one facet of an eating disorder,[111] the danger of confusing exercise adherence with exercise dependence and exercise addiction,[117] and that the hypothesis for a "runner's high" – that is, that exercise releases endorphins which produce physiological dependence – is still only a hypothesis with little supportive evidence.[118]

Mental health and exercise prescription

Taken as a whole, the review posits that a range of exercise regimens may have a therapeutic role in relation to a number of psychological disorders. At the same time, the research evidence to date does not provide unqualified support for the efficacy of exercise, and enthusiasm must be tempered with an acknowledgment of the dangers associated with exercise. Certainly, the literature does not indicate that exercise should be treated as a panacea or snake-oil for psychological malaise of whatever kind. Instead, it does suggest that different forms of physical exercise may be palliative in relation to particular conditions. Whether that exercise be non-aerobic, aerobic or anaerobic, of short, medium or long term duration, competitive or non-competitive, team or individual, single or multi-session, is not always clear but there are suggestions that different psychological conditions respond differentially to alternative exercise regimens and recent attempts to develop taxonomies of physical activity and mental health may offer a realistic starting point in attempting to draw together some of the diverse recommendations.[30,119]

As to explanations of why more definitive conclusions cannot be reached at this stage, then three factors stand out. Firstly, the research base remains thin and primary data are not extensive. To overcome this problem there is a need for large scale, multi-dimensional experimental programmes, associated with multivariate analyses of covariance to clarify the complexities of the relationships between physical exercise and psychological health. Secondly, it is not yet clear how psychological and physiological processes and functions interact in the determination of outcomes. The grey areas of confusion are most apparent in the psychophysiological responses such as stress reactivity. Indeed, it could be that Cartesian notions of mind-body dualism continue to drive a wedge between the physiological and the psychological. Greater collaboration between the two disciplines would undoubtedly help. Thirdly, and in a related vein, the primary mechanisms that underlie the relation between exercise and psychological wellbeing remain poorly understood. It would also be fair to say that a great deal of the literature remains descriptive or atheoretical. That is, it is able to describe how exercise and psychological wellbeing interact but it has shied away from asking or exploring why the relationship is as it is. Here psychophysiologists have led the field in attempting to provide explanations, including consideration of the influence of catecholamines, body temperature and endorphins. Psychosocially, issues relating to lifestyle, boredom and "time-out" have also been implicated but how, when and where each factor may be involved is once more a matter for debate. In all likelihood, given the complexities of the relation between exercise and wellbeing outlined above, it is unlikely that any single theory, model or hypothesis will suffice. Instead, multiple perspectives must be used.

Finally, it is also important to recognise the difficulties associated with adherence to exercise regimens. No matter how beneficial such schemes may be, if there is no willingness to exercise voluntarily then the practical utility of exercise is diminished dramatically. Hence recommendations must be put in the context of adherence research. For example, it has been maintained that only 10% of the population is committed to physical activity; 20% will start but not adhere to exercise; 40% will promise to start an exercise programme; 20% need to be convinced to participate in exercise and 10% are not interested in any form of organised or recommended activity.[120] Such research highlights the deep rooted resistance to taking exercise among large sections of the population, sections that lead essentially sedentary lives, with inactivity rates of 25% and 15% recently recorded for American and British populations respectively,[6] and with the likelihood of even higher rates among those with psychological problems.

In exploring the population's apparent resistance to physical activity, a recent review has considered some of the theoretical models utilised in designing exercise interventions.[121] As with the arguments advanced earlier in relation to explanations for exercise induced mental health benefits, they conclude that no individual model can sufficiently explain exercise behaviour or how best to intervene. However, in proposing future directions, it is interesting to note that the authors draw on largely psychological components as offering promise for encouraging greater participation. Specific factors outlined include enhancing self efficacy, increasing enjoyment of the activity, enhancing social support and promoting the perceived benefits of exercise. While it is not within the scope of this chapter to explore public policy initiatives for exercise promotion further, we hope that a comprehensive review of the literature pertaining to exercise and mental health would assist in any future developments.

All these arguments aside, general practitioners remain the ideal mechanism by which to promote exercise regimens.[122,123] At the same time, recent surveys suggest that despite a generally favourable reception from general practitioners themselves, their role is not without problems, particularly in relation to the referral system, their lack of knowledge of exercise recommendations, and difficulty in evaluating community health promotion schemes.[124,125] Simultaneously, "exercise by prescription" schemes are gaining in popularity;[10] a newspaper article reported on one fundholding general practitioner in Warrington, Cheshire, who has invested

---

Box 11.4

- Exercise addiction, while not fully understood, probably depends on the complex interplay between both psychosocial and physiological factors
- While exercise regimens may be able to play a positive part in relation to certain psychological disorders, the type and duration of the most effective exercise programmes remains to be determined
- There is a need for large scale, multivariate, experimental research to clarify this relation and to begin to understand underlying psychological and physiological mechanisms
- Comprehensive theoretical explanations of the relation between exercise and psychological health must be able to accommodate multiple perspectives taken from a range of disciplines
- The role that general practitioners have and can have as promoters and prescribers of exercise is an issue that should be afforded immediate priority

---

practice funds in opening up a medical centre gym for his patients.[126]

This level of enthusiasm for exercise promotion makes it all the more important that researchers, physicians and exercise practitioners continue to work together to develop sound guidelines. This will be of practical benefit to the patient and will also advance our understanding of the interplay between exercise and wellbeing, allowing us to develop a firm foundation from which to make recommendations in the years to come. General recommendations are now commonly accepted as to the somatic benefits which accrue from exercise; the relation between exercise, fitness and general cognitive functioning is now also receiving closer scrutiny.[127] Alongside this research activity, now is the time to develop more specific guidelines relating to psychological benefits of exercise taking due cognisance of psychosocial variables—for example, sex, age, previous mental health, environment—and recognising that the picture which will be revealed will not be as unidimensional as previous work may have implied.

---

1 Department of Health. *Promoting better health*. London: HMSO, 1996.
2 Royal College of Physicians. *Medical aspects of exercise: benefits and risks*. London: RCP, 1991.

3 Allied Dunbar National Fitness Survey. *Main findings.* London: Sports Council and Health Education Authority, 1992.

4 Powell KE, Blair SN. The public health burdens of sedentary living habits: theoretical but realistic estimates. *Med Sci Sports Exerc* 1994;**26**:851–6.

5 Hillsdon M, Thorogood M. A systematic review of physical activity promotion strategies. *Br J Sports Med* 1996;**30**: 84–9.

6 Pate RR, Pratt M, Blair SN. Physical activity and public health: a recommendation from the Centers for Disease Control and Prevention and the ACSM. *JAMA* 1995;**273**: 402–7.

7 Blair SN, Booth M, Gyarfas I, *et al.* Development of public policy and physical activity initiatives internationally. *Sports Med* 1996;**21**:157–63.

8 Turner-Warwick MH, Petecost BL, Jones JH. Medical aspects of exercise. *J R Coll Physicians Lond* 1991;**25**:193–6.

9 Hardman AE, Blair SN. Physical activity, health, and well-being: a summary of the Consensus Conference. *Res Q Exerc Sport* 1995;**66**: ii.

10 Smith PA, Gould MM, See Tai S, *et al.* Exercise as therapy? Results from group interviews with general practice teams involved in an inner-London 'prescription for exercise' scheme. *Health Ed J* 1996;**55**: 439–46.

11 Mutrie N, Biddle SJH. Effects of exercise on non-clinical populations. In: Biddle SJH, ed. *European perspectives on exercise and sport psychology.* Champaign, Illinois: Human Kinetics, 1995:50–70.

12 Martinsen EW. Effects of exercise on mental health in clinical populations. In: Biddle SJH, ed. *European perspectives on exercise and sport psychology.* Champaign, Illinois: Human Kinetics, 1995:71–90.

13 McAuley E. Physical activity and psychosocial outcomes. In: Bouchard C, Shephard RJ, Stephens T, eds. *Physical activity, fitness, and health.* Champaign, Illinois: Human Kinetics, 1994:551–68.

14 Rejeski WJ. Dose-Response issues from a psychosocial perspective. In: Bouchard C, Shephard RJ, Stephens T, eds. *Physical activity, fitness, and health.* Champaign, Illinois: Human Kinetics, 1994:1040–55.

15 Shephard R. *Aerobic fitness and health.* Champaign, Illinois: Human Kinetics, 1994.

16 Moses J, Steptoe A, Matthews A, *et al.* The effects of exercise training on mental well-being in the normal population: a controlled trial. *J Psychosom Res* 1989;**33**: 47–61.

17 Sexton H, Maere A, Dahl NH. Exercise intensity and reduction in neurotic symptoms. *Acta Psychiatr Scand* 1989;**80**:231–5.

18 International Society of Sport Psychology. Physical activity and psychological benefits: a position statement. *Sport Psychol* 1992;**6**:199–204.

19 Morgan WP, Goldston SE, eds. *Exercise and mental health.* New York: Hemisphere, 1987.

20 Berger BG, Owen DR. Stress reduction and mood enhancement in four exercise modes: Swimming, body conditioning, Hatha yoga and fencing. *Res Q Exerc Sport* 1988;**59**:148–59.

21 Biddle S, Mutrie N. *Psychology of physical activity and exercise.* London: Springer Verlag, 1991.

22 Martinson EW. Benefits of exercise for the treatment of depression. *Sports Med* 1990;**9**:380–9.

23 LaFontaine TP, DiLorenzo TM, Frensch PA, *et al. Aerobic exercise and mood. Sports Med* 1992;**13**:160–70.

24 North TC, McCullagh P, Vu Tran, Z. Effect of exercise on depression. *Exerc Sports Sci Rev* 1990;**18**:379–415.

25 Folkins CH, Sime WE. Physical fitness training and mental health. *Am Psychol* 1981;**36**:373–89.

26 Sachs ML. Exercise and running: effects on anxiety, depression and psychology. *Humanistic Educ Dev* 1982;**21**:51–7.

27 Morgan WP. Physical activity, fitness and depression. In: Bouchard C, Shephard RJ, Stephens T, eds. *Physical activity, fitness, and health*. Champaign, Illinois: Human Kinetics, 1994:851–67.

28 McDonald DG, Hodgdon JA. *The psychological effects of aerobic fitness training: research and theory*. New York: Springer-Verlag, 1991.

29 Nicoloff G, Schwenk TL. Using exercise to ward off depression. *Physician and Sportsmedicine* 1995;23:44–58.

30 Hill JW. Exercise prescription. *Prim Care* 1987;14:817–25.

31 Landers DM, Petruzzello SJ. Physical activity, fitness and anxiety. In: Bouchard C, Shephard RJ, Stephens T, eds. *Physical activity, fitness, and health*. Champaign, Illinios: Human Kinetics, 1994:868–82.

32 Long BC, Stavel RV. Effects of exercise training on anxiety: a meta-analysis. *J Appl Sport Psych* 1995;7:167–89.

33 Lambert MJ, Shapiro DA, Bergin AE. The effectiveness of psychotherapy. In: Garfield SL, Bergin AE, eds. *Handbook of psychotherapy and behavior change*. New York: Wiley, 1986:157–211.

34 Petruzzello SJ. Anxiety reduction following exercise: methodological artifact 'real' phenomenon? *J Sport Exerc Psychol* 1995;17:105–11.

35 McAuley E, Mihalko SL, Bane SM. Acute exercise and anxiety reduction: Does the environment matter? *J Sport Exerc Psychol* 1996;18:408–19.

36 Gauvin L, Brawley LR. Alternative psychological models and methodologies for the study of exercise and effect. In: Seraganian P, ed. *Exercise psychology: the influence of physical exercise on psychological processes*. New York: Wiley, 1993:146–71.

37 Tate AK, Petruzzello SJ. Varying the intensity of acute exercise: implications for changes in effect. *J Sports Med Phys Fitness* 1995;35:1–8.

38 Franks BD, Jette M. Manifest anxiety and physical fitness. *National College Physical Education Association for Men. Annual Proceedings*. Chicago, 1970.

39 Fillingim RB, Blumenthal JA. The use of aerobic exercise as a method of stress management. In: Lehrer PM, Woolfolk RL, eds. *Principles and practice of stress management*. London: Guilford, 1993: 443–62.

40 Blumenthal JA, Maddem DJ. Effects of aerobic exercise training, age and physical fitness on memory search performance. *Psychology Aging* 1988;3:230–85.

41 Sherwood A, Light KC, Blumenthal JA. Effects of aerobic exercise training on hemodynamic responses during psychosocial stress in normotensive and borderline hypertensive type A men: a preliminary report. *Psychosom Med* 1989;51:124–36.

42 Blumenthal JA, Fredrikson M, Kuhn CM, *et al*. Aerobic exercise reduces levels of cardiovascular and sympathoadrenal responses to mental stress in subjects without prior evidence of myocardial ischemia. *Am J Cardiol* 1990;65:93–8.

43 Roskies E, Seraganian P, Oseasohn R, *et al*. The Montreal type A intervention project: Major findings. *Health Psychol* 1986;5: 45–69.

44 Sinyor D, Golden M, Steiner Y, *et al*. Experimental manipulation of aerobic fitness and the response to psychosocial stress: heart rate and self-report measures. *Psychosom Med* 1986;48:324–37.

45 Sothmann M, Hart B, Horn T. Plasma catecholamine response to acute psychological stress in humans: relation to aerobic fitness and exercise training. *Med Sci Sports Exerc* 1991; 23:860–7.

46 Dishman R. Mental health. In: Seefeldt V, ed. *Physical activity and well-being*. Reston, Vancouver: AAPHERD, 1986:303–41.

47 Frazier SE, Nagy S. Mood state changes of women as a function of regular aerobic exercise. *Percept Mot Skills* 1989;68:283–7.

48 Madden DJ, Blumenthal JA, Allen PA, *et al*. Improving aerobic capacity in older adults does not necessarily lead to improved cognitive performance. *Psychology Aging* 1989;4:307–20.

49 McNair DM, Lorr M, Droppleman LF. Psychological effects of acute physical activity. *Arch Phys Med Rehabil* 1971;**52**:422–5.
50 Lennox SS, Bedell JR, Stone AA. The effect of exercise on normal mood. *J Psychosom Med* 1990;**34**:629–36.
51 Agaroff JA, Boyle GJ. Aerobic exercise, mood states and menstrual cycle symptoms. *J Psychosom Res* 1994;**38**:183–92.
52 Cramer SR, Nieman DC, Lee JW. The effects of moderate exercise training on psychological well-being and mood state in women. *J Psychosom Res* 1991;**35**:437–49.
53 Maroulakis M, Zervas Y. Effects of aerobic exercise on mood of adult women. *Percept Mot Skills* 1993;**76**:795–801.
54 Steinberg H, Sykes EA, LeBoutillier N. Exercise addiction: indirect measures of "endorphins"? In: Annett J, Cripps B, Steinberg H, eds. *Exercise addiction: motivation for participation in sport and exercise.* Leeds: British Psychological Society, 1997:6–14
55 Head A, Kendall MJ, Ferner R. Eagles C. Acute effects of β blockade and exercise on mood and anxiety. *Br J Sports Med* 1996;**30**:238–42.
56 McAuley E, Mihalko SL, Bane, SM. Exercise and self-esteem in middle-aged adults: multidimensional relationships and physical fitness and self-efficacy influences. *J Behav Med* 1997;**20**:67–83.
57 Sonstroem RJ. Exercise and self-esteem. *Exerc Sports Sci Rev* 1984;**12**:123–55.
58 Gruber JJ. Physical activity and self-esteem development in children: a meta-analysis. In: Stull G, Eckert H, eds. *Effects of physical activity on children: the Academy Papers No. 19.* Champaign, Illinois: Human Kinetics,1986:30–48.
59 Fox KR. *Physical self-perception profile manual.* Northern Illinois University: Office for Health Promotion, Dekalb, 1990.
60 Sonstroem RJ, Harlow LL, Gemma LM, *et al.* Test of structural relationships within a proposed exercise and self-esteem model. *J Pers Assess* 1991;**56**:348–64.
61 Sonstroem RJ, Speliotis ED, Fava JL. Perceived physical competence in adults: an examination of the physical self-perception profile. *J Sport Exerc Psychol* 1992;**14**:207–21.
62 Sonstroem RJ, Harlow LL, Josephs, L. Exercise and self-esteem: validity of model expansion and exercise association. *J Sport Exerc Psychol* 1994; **16**:29–42.
63 Israel RG, Sutton M, O'Brien KF. Effects of aerobic training on primary dysmenorrhea symptomatology in college females. *J Am Coll Health* 1985;**33**:241–44.
64 Timmonen S, Procope B. Premenstrual syndrome and physical exercise. *Acta Obstet Gynecol Scand* 1971;**50**:331–7.
65 Prior JC. Exercise-related adaptive changes to the menstrual cycle. In: Macleod D, Maughan R, Nimmo M, Reilly T, Williams C, eds. *Exercise: benefits, limits and adaptations.* London: Spon, 1987:239–54.
66 Choi PYL, Salmon P. Symptom changes across the menstrual cycle in competitive sportswomen, exercisers and sedentary women. *Br J Clin Psychol* 1995;**34**:447–60.
67 Shangold J. How I manage exercise amenorrhea. *Physician and Sportsmedicine* 1986;**14**:118–20.
68 Steptoe A, Cox S. Acute effects of aerobic exercise on mood. *Health Psychol* 1988;7:329–40.
69 Steptoe A, Bolton J. The short-term influence of high and low physical exercise on mood. *Psychological Health* 1988;2:91–106.
70 Cockerill IM, Lawson SL, Nevill AM. Mood states, menstrual cycle and exercise-to-music. In: Annett B, Cripps B, Steinberg H, eds. *Exercise addiction.* Leeds: British Psychological Society, 1995:61–9.
71 Steege JF, Blumenthal JA. The effects of aerobic exercise on PMS in middle-

aged women: a preliminary study. *J Psychosom Res* 1993;**37**:127–33.

72 Doyne EJ, Ossip-Klien DJ, Bowman ED, *et al.* Running vs weight lifting in the treatment of depression. *J Consult Clin Psychol* 1987;**55**:748–54.

73 Bonen A, Ling WY, MacIntyre KP, *et al.* Effects of exercise on the serum concentrations of FSH, LH, progesterone and estradiol. *Eur J Appl Physiol* 1979;**42**:15–23.

74 Baker ER, Mathur RS, Kirk RF, *et al.* Plasma gonadotropins, prolactin and steroid hormone concentrations in female runners immediately after a long-distance run. *Fertil Steril* 1982;**38**:38–41.

75 Cumming DC, Vickovic MM, Wall SR, *et al.* The effect of acute exercise on pulsatile release of luteinizing hormone in women runners. *Am J Obstet Gynecol* 1985;**153**:482–5.

76 Wells CL. *Women, sport and performance: a physiological perspective.* Champaign, Illinois: Human Kinetics, 1985.

77 Rauramaa R. Relationship of physical activity, glucose tolerance and weight management. *Prev Med* 1984;**13**:37–46.

78 Reid RL, Yen SSC. The premenstrual syndrome. *Clin Obstet Gynecol* 1983;**26**:710–8.

79 Johnson E, Gannon LR. *The endorphin theory of premenstrual syndrome: a synthesis of interdisciplinary research.* Paper presented at the Association of Women's Psychology, New York, 1985.

80 Tomlinson A. Introduction. In: Tomlinson A, ed. *Gender, sport and leisure.* Brighton: Chelsea School Research Centre, 1995:1–20.

81 Ryckman R, Hamel J. Male and female adolescents' motives related to involvement in organized team sports. *Int J Sport Psychol* 1995;**26**:383–97.

82 Scully DM, Clarke J. Gender issues. In: Kremer J, Trew K, Ogle S eds. *Young people's involvement in sport.* London: Routledge, 1997:25–56.

83 Scully DM, Reilly J, Clarke J. Perspectives on gender in sport and exercise. *Irish J Psychol* (special issue) 1999;**17**.

84 Franzoi SL. The body-as-object versus the body-as-process: gender differences and gender considerations. *Sex Roles* 1995;**33**:417–37.

85 Frederick CJ, Shaw SM. Body image as a leisure constraint: examining the experience of aerobic exercise classes for young women. *Leisure Science* 1995;**17**:57.

86 McAuley E, Bane SM, Rudolph DL, *et al.* Physique anxiety and exercise in middle-aged adults. *J Gerontol B Psychol Sci* 1995;**50**:229–35.

87 Frederick CM, Morrison CS. Social physique anxiety: personality constructs, motivations, exercise attitudes and behaviours. *Percept Mot Skills* 1996;**82**:963–72.

88 Sonstroem RJ, Potts SA. Life adjustment correlates of physical self-concepts. *Med Sci Sports Exerc* 1996;**28**:619–25.

89 Van Wersch A. Individual differences and intrinsic motivations for sport participation. In: Kremer J, Trew K, Ogle S, eds. *Young people's involvement in sport.* London: Routledge, 1997:57–77.

90 Biddle S, Goudas BA, Page BA. Social-psychological predictors of self report actual and intended physical activity in a university workforce sample. *Br J Sports Med* 1997;**28**:160–3.

91 Koff E, Bauman C. Effects of wellness, fitness and sport skills programs on body image and lifestyle behaviours. *Percept Mot Skills* 1997;**84**:555–62.

92 Furnham A, Greaves N. Gender and locus of control correlates of body image dissatisfaction. *Eur J Personality* 1994;**8**:183–200.

93 Cash TF, Henry PE. Women's body images: the results of a national survey in the USA. *Sex Roles* 1995;**33**:19–28.

94 Cash TF, Deagle EA. The nature and extent of body-image disturbances in anorexia nervosa and bulimia nervosa: a meta-analysis. *Int J Eating Dis* 1997;**22**:107–25.

95 Koenig LJ, Wasserman EL. Body image and dieting failure in college men and women: examining links between depression and eating problems. *Sex Roles* 1995;**32**:225–249.

96 Arena B. Hormonal problems in young female athletes. *Sports Exerc Inj* 1996;**2**:122–125.

97 Benson JE, Engelbert-Fenton KA, Eisenman PA. Nutritional aspects of amenorrhea in the female athlete triad. *Int J Sports Nutr* 1996;**6**:134–45.

98 Otis CL, Drinkwater B, Loucks A, *et al.* ACSM position stand: the female athlete triad. *Med Sci Sports Exerc* 1977;**29**:1–4.

99 Nattiv A. The female athlete triad: managing acute risk to long-term health. *Physician and Sportsmedicine* 1995;**22**:60–68.

100 Davis C, Kennedy SH, Ravelski E, Dionne M. The role of physical activity in the development and maintenance of eating disorders. *Psychol Med* 1994;**24**: 957–67.

101 Davis C. Eating disorders and hyperactivity: a psychobiological perspective. *Can J Psychiatry* 1997;**42**:168–75.

102 Troop NA, Holbrey A, Trowler R, *et al.* Ways of coping in women with eating disorders. *J Nerv Ment Dis* 1994;**182**:353–40.

103 Willcox M, Sattler DN. The relationship between eating disorders and depression. *J Soc Psychol* 1996;**136**:269–271.

104 Annett J, Cripps B, Steinberg H. *Exercise addiction.* Leeds: British Psychological Society, 1995.

105 Morgan WP, ed. *Physical activity and mental health.* Washington, DC: Taylor and Francis, 1996.

106 Grossman A, Bouloux P, Price P. The role of opioid peptides in the hormonal responses to acute exercise in man. *Clin Sci* 1984;**67**: 483–491.

107 Grant E. The exercise fix. *Psychol Today* 1992;**22**:24–8.

108 Sachs ML, Pargman D. Running addiction: a depth interview examination. *J Sport Behav* 1979;**2**:143–55.

109 Veale DMW. Exercise dependence. *Br J Addict* 1987;**82**:735–40.

110 Davis C, Kennedy SH, Ralevske E, *et al.* Obsessive compulsiveness and physical activity in anorexia nervosa and high-level exercising. *J Psychosom Res* 1995;**39**:967–76.

111 Veale DMW. Does primary exercise dependence really exist? In: Annett J, Cripps B, Steinberg H. *Exercise addiction.* Leeds: British Psychological Society, 1995:1–5.

112 Little JC. The athlete's neurosis: a deprivation crisis. *Acta Psychiatr Scand* 1969;**45**:187–97.

113 Mondin GW, Morgan WP, Piering PN, *et al.* Psychological consequences of exercise deprivation in habitual exercisers. *Med Sci Sports Exerc* 1996;**28**:1199–203.

114 Chan CS, Grossman HY. Psychological effects of running loss on consistent runners. *Percept Mot Skills* 1988;**66**:875–88.

115 Morris M, Steinberg H, Sykes EA, *et al.* Effects of temporary withdrawal from regular running. *J Psychosom Res* 1990;**34**:493–500.

116 Robbins JM, Joseph P. Experiencing exercise withdrawal: possible consequences of therapeutic and mastery running. *J Sport Psychol* 1985;**7**:25–39.

117 Annett J. Summing up. In: Annett J, Cripps B, Steinberg H. *Exercise addiction.* Leeds: British Psychological Society, 1995: 70–1.

118 Steinberg H, Sykes EA, LeBoutillier N. Exercise addiction: indirect measures of "endorphins". In: Annett J, Cripps B, Steinberg H. *Exercise addiction.* Leeds: British Psychological Society, 1995:6–14.

119 Berger BG, McInman A. Exercise and the quality of life. In: Singer RN, Murphy M, Tennant LK, eds. *Handbook of research on sport psychology.* New York: Macmillan, 1993:729–60.

120 McGeorge S, Harris J, Clark F. *Physical activity protocols for primary care.*

Loughborough: Department of Physical Education, Loughborough University, 1994.

121 Marcus BH, Simkin LR. The stages of exercise behaviour. *J Sports Med Phys Fitness* 1993;**33**:83–8.

122 British Heart Foundation. GP advice on exercise is worth more than £1000. *General Practitioner* 1996;July 12:24.

123 Health Education Authority. *Active for life*. London: HEA, 1996.

124 Hammond JM, Brodie DA, Bundred PE. Exercise on prescription: guidelines for health professionals. *Health Prom Int* 1997;**12**:33–41.

125 Iliffe S, Tai SS, Gould M, *et al.* Prescribing exercise in general practice. *BMJ* 1994;**309**:494–5.

126 Doctor in the gym, Sunday Times, Style Supplement. 1997; Sept 14:30–1.

127 Etnier JL, Salazar W, Landers DM, *et al.* The influence of physical fitness and exercise upon cognitive functioning: a meta-analysis. *J Sport Exerc Psychol* 1997;**19**:249–77.

Multiple choice questions

1 Which of the following does available evidence suggest that an effective physical exercise regimen for treating clinical depression should involve?
  (a) Short bursts of high intensity, anaerobic activity
  (b) Repetitive aerobic exercise extending over several months
  (c) Intensive aerobic exercise, compressed into a short period, for example a week
  (d) Non-aerobic exercise interspersed with group therapy
  (e) All of the above

2 According to Rejeski (1994) and other contemporary authors, which of the following best explains the effects of exercise on psychological wellbeing?
  (a) Cardiac-related cortical activity
  (b) Changes in neurochemical activity
  (c) The "time out" hypothesis
  (d) Physiological and/or psychosocial factors
  (e) The endorphin hypothesis

3 The profile of mood states (POMS) measures:
  (a) Mood state
  (b) Clinical depression
  (c) Symptoms of the premenstrual syndrome
  (d) Stress
  (e) Self esteem

4 Which of the following has NOT been associated with the positive effect of exercise on the premenstrual syndrome (PMS):
   (a) Oestrogen:progesterone ratio
   (b) Reduction in body fat
   (c) Glucose tolerance
   (d) Endorphin levels
   (e) Social-physique-anxiety (SPA)

5 The female athlete triad (FAT) refers to:
   (a) Depression, anxiety, and mood state
   (b) Depression, body image, and disordered eating
   (c) Disordered eating, amenorrhoea, and osteoporosis
   (d) Amenorrhoea, anorexia, and bulimia
   (e) Disordered eating, body image, and depression

Answers are on p. 364.

12   The athlete's heart

R J Shephard

Introduction

Osler commented "no man becomes a great runner or oarsmen who has not naturally a capable if not a large heart".[1] Nevertheless, for many years a substantial proportion of sports physicians were worried that the large heart of the endurance athlete, far from being advantageous, was actually a risk factor for sudden death on the sports field "because it indicates undue strain or because of the danger of eventual degeneration".[2]

In the early days of the Olympian movement, Henschen was able to demonstrate enlargement of the heart in cross country skiers by careful percussion of the chest.[3] He wrote "an enlarged heart is a good thing if it can perform more work over an extended period of time". Other features that can be detected on simple clinical examination include a prominent, displaced apical impulse and a right ventricular lift.[4] However, recognition of the large heart of endurance competitors became more widespread with the advent of radiography, as examination of the cardiac shadow began to supplement the very crude percussion techniques of clinicians such as Henschen.

At first, PA radiographs were used simply to measure cardiothoracic ratios.[2] Investigators quickly found that the cardiothoracic ratios of many athletes approached or exceeded the anticipated normal limit of 0.50.[5-7] Soon, German cardiologists with an interest in sports medicine had added a lateral view to the PA radiograph,[8] and, by taking three linear measurements from the radiographs, an estimate of cardiac volume was obtained. The measurement necessarily remained imprecise, for unless the x ray machine was ECG triggered, the radiographs might have been obtained either in systole or in diastole! In an average young man, the reported volume was about 700 ml, but in an endurance athlete the figure could rise as high as 1000–1100 ml, apparently without adverse consequences for health.

Later, the radiograph information was combined with an examination of ECG voltages.[9] Left ventricular hypertrophy was diagnosed if the sum of SV1 and RV5 exceeded 35 mm (3.5 mV), and right ventricular hypertrophy if the sum of RV1 and SV5 exceeded 10.5 mm (1.05 mV).[10,11] By using such criteria, the data of various authors suggest that 14–85% of Olympic athletes and marathon runners had developed left ventricular hypertrophy.[12] Other investigators developed more complicated evaluations of the ECG, based on voltage and non-voltage criteria,[13,14] but correlations with radiographic, echocardiographic, or ultimate necropsy evaluations remained poor,[15] in part because the hypertrophy of the chest muscles typical of many athletes attenuated electrocardiographic voltages.[4]

At this period in medical history, many of the population suffered from cardiac enlargement due to after effects of rheumatic heart disease such as mitral regurgitation. In such individuals, the size of the heart increased with the severity of the disease process, and it is thus not surprising that many physicians, particularly in the United States, also regarded the cardiac enlargement of an endurance athlete as an adverse sign. It is not easy to distinguish physiological from pathological hypertrophy on PA chest radiographs. In principle, there are important differences of appearance between the rheumatic heart and the heart of the endurance athlete. In a person with the end results of rheumatic valvar disease, the enlarged cardiac shadow is due mainly to a poor ejection fraction, so that the end systolic volume of the left ventricular chamber is generally increased. In contrast, much of the increase in end systolic cardiac dimensions of the endurance athlete is due to a hypertrophy of the ventricular wall. The firm, rounded contours of the hypertrophied heart should thus stand in marked contrast with the sagging, distended form of a failing myocardium.[16] However, in practice the PA cardiac silhouette is formed by variable contributions from the two ventricles and the atria, and it proved very difficult to distinguish the left ventricle from the other chambers. Many physicians were also slow to admit that they had erred in fulminating against competitors with a supposed pathological enlargement of the heart. Thus warnings against "athlete's heart" continued until quite recently.[17–20]

Echocardiographic and magnetic resonance imaging data

As is commonly the case in medical science, technological developments – the introduction of wide angle, two dimensional echocardiography[21–23] and magnetic resonance imaging[24,25] – led to new interest in the "athlete's heart" and hypertrophic cardiomyopathy as possible causes of sudden, exercise related death in athletes. Rost and Hollmann went so far as to describe hypertrophic myocardiopathy as an "ultrasound-specific" disease.[26]

The new techniques allowed cardiologists to make relatively accurate measurements of both wall thicknesses and the dimensions of the ventricular chambers.[27] A much clearer distinction could now be drawn between the distended heart of the person with cardiac failure and the strong hypertrophied heart of the person who was in good physical condition. Echocardiography also suggested differences between the heart of the endurance athlete, where the thicker ventricular walls seemed an adaptation to an increase in volume loading of the heart, and the heart of the competitor in sports with an isometric demand, where there was a thickening of both septal and free walls of the ventricle without any increase in left ventricular end diastolic diameter.[12,23, 28–30] Nevertheless, the limits of resolution for echocardiography, approximately 2 mm for an individual measurement,[31] remain of a similar order to many of the differences that have been discussed, both between athletes and sedentary individuals, and between the healthy and those with supposedly pathological enlargement of the heart. As with many laboratory procedures, the methodology allows the detection of group differences but provides limited information on the status of the individual patient.

Echocardiographic studies have shown as many as 60% of endurance athletes have a posterior wall diastolic thickness that exceeds the supposed normal values of 11 mm.[6,7,32,33] In consequence, normal limits for diastolic wall thickness have been revised upward, to 16 mm,[34–36] 18 mm,[37] or even 19 mm.[38] The new standards have left little margin of distinction between physiological hypertrophy and the 17–18 mm wall thickness typical of pathological forms of pressure overload (aortic stenosis, hypertension) or volume overload (aortic or mitral regurgitation).[15] Moreover, it is hard to believe that the hypertrophy seen in the athlete has any pathological significance, since even very high values regress towards normality over several months of inactivity, and the regression of moderate hypertrophy can be even more rapid.[39]

Part of the apparent problem is dimensional. Many athletes have a body mass that is much above the population average, and, if the cardiac dimensions of endurance athletes are expressed per unit of lean body mass, only the septal thickness is usually greater than in control subjects.[40] In resistance athletes, the body mass is usually very high, but the heart weight per kg of body mass remains normal.[28–30,41]

Diagnoses based on septal thickness and ventricular cavity ratios

In recent years, the diagnosis of pathological enlargement has been based on the thickness of the interventricular septum and the calculation of various ratios. There is substantial hypertrophy of the intraventricular septum in both endurance and resistance athletes, but again it is hard to accept this as a pathological finding, given its wide prevalence. Some 60% of basketball players[7] and 83% of child swimmers[42] have septal thicknesses that exceed accepted norms for sedentary populations.

Many cardiologists have been concerned if the ratio of interventricular septum to left posterior ventricular wall thickness exceeded some arbitrary limit (commonly 1.3:1).[12] But in fact septum to wall thickness ratios can rise as high as 2.0 in athletes, much higher than the values that are encountered in patients with pathological pressure or volume overload,[7,43,44] and it has yet to be shown convincingly that the high ratios observed in athletes are either dangerous or pathological.[12] Oakley and Oakley instanced an athlete who had a ratio of 1.5.[45] Four years after ceasing training, both the electrocardiogram and the echocardiogram of this individual were interpreted as normal.

Perhaps the most useful diagnostic measurement is the ratio of septal thickness to left ventricular end systolic or end diastolic diameter.[29,43,46–48] Currently, the upper limit of normality for the septal thickness to end systolic diameter ratio has been set at 0.48 (3 SD above normal values).[12] Other potential indicators of pathological enlargement include a discrepancy between cardiac dimensions and ergometric performance[29] and associated abnormalities of cardiac rhythm.

Cardiac hypertrophy and myocardial ischaemia

Many physicians have found it hard to believe that it is acceptable for the thickness of the heart wall to increase to the extent that is observed in top athletes. Although a little hypertrophy might help competitive performance, if a thickness or a thickness ratio increased beyond some figure (which it has been necessary to revise repeatedly in an upward direction), then they have maintained that the condition should be regarded as pathological, particularly if there are associated ECG abnormalities, limited ventricular compliance, or poor diastolic filling.[49]

It has been argued that as the cross section of the ventricular wall is increased, the diffusion pathway from the myocardial capillaries to the cardiac mitochondria is increased, leaving the heart more vulnerable to ischaemia and such fatal complications as cardiac arrest or ventricular fibrillation. Further, it has been recognised that in some instances, the situation of the enlarged heart is aggravated by a congenitally determined myocardial dystrophy,[50–54] with consequent disturbance of the electrical pathway,[55] mitral regurgitation,[34] or hypotension.[56]

There are several fallacies in the argument that an increase in heart size necessarily predisposes the individual to myocardial ischaemia. Firstly, when the heart hypertrophies, there is generally a parallel development of the myocardial capillaries, as in hypertrophied skeletal muscle. Thus the blood supply to a hypertrophied heart remains at least as good as that to a hypotrophic heart. More importantly, the main determinants of myocardial hypoxia are firstly, the relation of myocardial work rate to myocardial oxygen supply, secondly, the tension developed in the ventricular wall, and thirdly, the relative duration of the systolic phase of the cardiac cycle.

Relation of myocardial work rate to myocardial oxygen supply

The myocardial work rate during a bout of exercise is approximated by the product of heart rate and systolic blood pressure. Because of myocardial hypertrophy, the endurance athlete has a large ejection fraction and can sustain a larger stroke volume than a less well trained person during vigorous exercise. From this, it follows that a given external task can be performed at a lower heart rate and a lower cardiac work rate than would be the case in a sedentary individual (although of course the athlete will usually exercise to a much higher peak work rate than an untrained person). The myocardial oxygen consumption at a given external work rate is correspondingly reduced in the athlete, so that during ordinary daily life the risk of myocardial ischaemia is much less than in a sedentary person.

Tension developed in the ventricular wall

According to the Law of LaPlace (as modified for a thick walled structure), the total tension exerted by the ventricular wall is approximately proportional to the product of intraventricular pressure and the average ventricular radius.[57] In the endurance athlete, the large average radius of the ventricle may cause some increase of tension for a given arterial pressure. But because the gross section of the ventricular wall is also much greater in the athlete than in a sedentary individual, the force exerted per unit of wall cross section at any given level of intraventricular pressure is actually lower in the athlete than in the untrained person.[55]

Relative duration of the systolic phase of the cardiac cycle

The tension in the ventricular wall is high during systole, irrespective of the individual's training status. The high intramural pressure occludes perforating coronary vessels, and myocardial perfusion thus occurs mainly during diastole. Because ventricular hypertrophy is associated with a large stroke volume, the heart rate is slower and the relative length of the diastolic phase of the cardiac cycle is much longer for an athlete than for a sedentary person, both at rest and at a given submaximal work rate. This in turn allows greater myocardial perfusion in an athlete than in a sedentary person for much of the day, although training has little influence on the heart rate during maximal effort.

Box 12.1   Reputed dangers of myocardial hypertrophy

- Ventricular enlargement long considered as increasing risk of exercise-induced cardiac death
- Endurance training increases wall thickness without increase of risk
- Isometric training increases wall and septal thickness without increase of left ventricular end-diastolic diameter without increase of risk
- Rare inherited hypertrophic cardiomyopathy may increase risk of exercise-induced cardiac death
- Pathological hypertrophy not readily distinguished by measurements of wall thicknesses

---

Box 12.2 Benefits of myocardial hypertrophy

- Increase of myocardial capillarisation maintains local oxygen supply
- Increase of stroke volume allows lower heart rate at given cardiac work rate
- Lower heart rate decreases cardiac work rate and thus myocardial oxygen demand
- Lower heart rate allows longer diastolic phase, facilitating coronary perfusion
- Thicker ventricular wall reduces intramural tension for any given intraventricular pressure

---

Risk of sudden death during exercise

One of the main reasons for fear of hypertrophic cardiomyopathy is that occasionally a young endurance athlete dies on the sports field.[51,58] It is reasoned that cardiac hypertrophy provides an explanation of such deaths, and that the condition should have been detected by a careful preparticipation examination,[59-62] despite growing evidence that attempts at preparticipation screening are not cost-effective.[63]

The causes of sudden, exercise related death in the young athlete are varied.[50,64-67] Sometimes there is an undetected congenital anomaly – for instance, an abnormal origin of the coronary vessels – so that the chances of myocardial ischaemia during intensive exercise are increased. Sometimes there is an aneurysm of the circle of Willis, which ruptures, causing death from cerebral bleeding. Sometimes there is an infection of the myocardium due to recent influenza or some other viral disorder. But where no other cause can be assigned, blame is attached to myocardial hypertrophy, particularly a hypertrophy of the interventricular septum. Details of the hypothesis have changed a little in recent years – in place of fears regarding myocardial ischaemia, many cardiologists now argue that myocardial hypertrophy affects the electrical conducting system and that this predisposes to abnormalities of heart rhythm. Others maintain that the underlying problem is almost always an inherited dystrophy of cardiac muscle with a disarray of the myocardial fibres and that there is little relation between ventricular hypertrophy and sudden death in the absence of this anomaly.[56]

Many investigators have attached blame to an excessive interventricular septal thickness, a finding commonly established only at necropsy examination. However, the dice seem heavily loaded in favour of proving that septal hypertrophy is associated with athletic deaths, since training thickens both the ventricular wall and the interventricular septum and the necropsy examination is being performed on a person who has died on the sports field.

To establish the postulated pathological significance of septal thickening, it would be necessary to make either a prospective comparison of outcomes between athletes with supposedly normal septa and those with thickened septa or, alternatively, to carry out a blinded necropsy comparison between athletes who died on the sports field and others at a similar level of training who were killed in traffic accidents. The practical problem in arranging a prospective trial of this type is that the sudden death of young athletes on the sports field is an extremely rare event. Most physicians who are interested in studying the question have difficulty in accumulating more than 10 or 20 personal cases over a lifetime of practice, and in only a small proportion of the 10 or 20 cases is myocardial hypertrophy even a potential explanation of the incident. The costs of organising a prospective trial that would have a reasonable statistical probability of demonstrating a difference of septal thickness between athletes who die and those who survive would thus seem prohibitively large. Possibly, such a trial could be arranged on a cooperative, multicentre basis, by having each of a group of investigators identify and follow athletes in whom the septum appeared to be extremely thick, following also two or three control subjects with normal septa but matched for their involvement in endurance sport.

An alternative approach would be to focus retrospectively on those who have died during athletic competition. The distribution of septal thicknesses in this population could then be compared with that of a second group of endurance athletes who were killed in traffic accidents. To obtain adequate numbers, the trial would have to be organised on a multicentre basis, and one immediate obstacle would be that whereas details of the athletic involvement of a person dying on the sports field would be readily available at the inquest, it would be difficult to obtain adequate detail on the sports histories of those involved in traffic accidents, or indeed to ensure that other aspects of personal lifestyle were well matched between the two groups of cases.

We may conclude that, firstly, the case against cardiac enlargement is currently far from established, and secondly, experimental obstacles are such that it will be difficult to obtain conclusive proof from either prospective trials or retrospective necropsy examinations in the foreseeable future.

Box 12.3 Possible causes of sudden, exercise-induced death in young athletes

- Abnormal origin of coronary vessels
- Aneurysm of Circle of Willis
- Viral myocarditis
- Familial hypertrophic cardiomyopathy
- Marfan's syndrome
- Other undetected congenital cardiovascular abnormalities
- Conduction abnormalities (especially Wolff-Parkinson-White syndrome)
- Abuse of alcohol, cocaine or solvents

Sudden death from hypertrophic cardiomyopathy

Some investigators have boldly claimed that hypertrophic cardiomyopathy is the commonest cause of death in young athletes.[17–19,37,68] In fact, extreme forms of "athlete's heart" are quite uncommon, even in highly conditioned athletes, and the total number of exercise related deaths is very low (for example, around 100 per year in the United States).[67] Most incidents occur in the coronary-prone age range and are probably due to coronary atherosclerosis rather than ventricular hypertrophy. A computerised search of the literature covering a 50 year period unearthed a total of *four* likely cases of hypertrophic cardiomyopathy in athletes who were under the age of 40 years![64]

The conclusion that hypertrophic cardiomyopathy is a common cause of exercise related death seems to have stemmed from a paper by Maron *et al.*[18] These investigators collected case histories on 29 athletes between the ages of 13 and 30 who had died in the United States over a period of several years; 19 of the 29 were said to have hypertrophic cardiomyopathy, although only in eight of the 19 did the septum to free wall ratio meet the minimum diagnostic criterion of 1.3/1.0. At best, the whole hypothesis seems to have been built up on fewer than two deaths per year across the United States! Others have used extremely loose criteria, classifying as "probable hypertrophic cardiomyopathy" all deaths where the cardiac mass exceeded 400 g in the absence of other systemic, valvar, or cardiac disorders.[37] Even when this simplistic approach was adopted, the total incidence across the United States was apparently only about five cases a year. Spirito *et al.* have further pointed out that almost all reports of the condition around the world have come from two laboratories.[68] The view that the condition is widely prevalent is due, at least in part, to a repeated description of the supposed 19 cases of Maron *et al.*[18] in a minimum of 25 independent publications.

There remains the possibility that the individual who dies while exercising is affected by an extremely rare inherited malformation of the β myosin heavy chain,[69] but there is no particular reason for this disorder to affect endurance athletes. Moreover, the overall frequency of the anomaly is hardly high enough to form a basis for health policy.

Epidemiological evidence

In deciding on the health significance of cardiac hypertrophy, we are left with a final epidemiological option. We know that on average endurance athletes have a larger heart than sedentary individuals or competitors in other types of sport. What is the longevity of the endurance athlete relative to that of the general population?

A recent study by Sarna and associates looked at a sample of 2613 athletes who had represented Finland in either the Olympic Games, the World championships, or the European championships between 1920 and 1965.[70] Endurance athletes survived to an average age of 75.6 years, compared with 69.9 in a sample of 1712 sedentary adults and 71.5 years for those who had been Finnish champions in power sports. Thus there was no evidence that participation in endurance activity had led to any shortening of lifespan – rather, survival seemed to be enhanced by such competition. Sarna *et al.* adjusted their data for a number of covariates, but the comparison remains incomplete, as there are likely to have been differences of personal lifestyle, particularly cigarette consumption, between the endurance athletes and the general population. The effect of cigarette smoking is sufficiently powerful to have masked any small disadvantage from exercise precipitated sudden death. Moreover, it is uncertain how far either endurance athletes or the participants in power sports continued their exercise involvement in the long interval between competition and the average age at death.

Given that any risk of death during exercise is extremely small, and we cannot design a satisfactory experiment to see whether cardiac enlargement contributes to this phenomenon, the best advice for the moment is probably to avoid costly and ineffective preparticipation medical examinations that could precipitate costly invasive procedures, cardiac phobias, and premature cessation of sports involvement in those successful athletes who have large hearts.[63]

Benefits of cardiac hypertrophy

To this point, we have not considered possible benefits of cardiac hypertrophy. It is well established that cardiac hypertrophy is associated with a large stroke volume and thus a large maximum cardiac output. Peak oxygen transport in turn is closely associated with peak cardiac output. Thus the person with a large heart is likely to have a large maximum oxygen intake. In consequence, they are able to undertake any given physical task at a correspondingly smaller fraction of their maximum oxygen intake. Many aspects of exercise related strain, from the increase of blood pressure to the sense of personal fatigue, are less for the person who has developed a large maximum oxygen intake.

If cardiac hypertrophy is advantageous for a young person, it becomes even more important for an older individual. Peak oxygen intake decreases progressively with each year of survival beyond early adult life. In a sedentary person, the loss averages about 500 μl/[kg.min] per year.[71] Thus, by the age of 75–80 years, a sedentary person lacks a sufficient margin of aerobic power to climb even a slight slope without becoming excessively breathless. Soon, even the minor chores of daily life become very fatiguing, and the last 10 years of life are spent in growing institutional dependency.

The rate of ageing in an endurance athlete is difficult to ascertain because the volume of training is often reduced as a competitor becomes older. But tests on those who have maintained their training programmes suggest that the absolute rate of deterioration may be a little slower than in a sedentary person – a number of estimates for active individuals lie in the range 400–450 μl/[kg.min] per year.[72] Given a much higher initial aerobic power and possibly a slightly slower ageing effect the endurance athlete has a much greater maximum oxygen intake than a sedentary person at any given age during their retirement years. Equating subjects in terms of oxygen transport rather than chronological age, the advantage to the endurance competitor may be as much as a 10–20 year reduction of biological age.[71] Thus such a person does not need institutional support until an age of 90 or even 100 years. Given that regular exercise has a much smaller influence on the survival prospects of an elderly person,[73,74] the probability is that an endurance athlete will die before physical condition has deteriorated to the point that extensive institutional support is required.

This seems an important argument in favour of developing and maintaining a large heart. Physicians have for too long worried about the one in 10 million chance that athletic participation might cause sudden death, while neglecting the growing problem of sedentary senior citizens who require full time care in geriatric wards. Survival prospects are probably increased somewhat by endurance exercise.[73] But survival alone is not the most important goal of treatment. The true assessment of medical advice is its impact on quality adjusted life expectancy.[75] And in such terms a large heart is indeed beautiful.

Conclusions

Although ventricular hypertrophy is sometimes suggested to be the commonest cause of sudden exercise related death in the young adult, the total number of exercise induced deaths is very small and their relation to ventricular hypertrophy is far from established. There is a rare inherited form of myocardial dystrophy that predisposes to sudden death, but this is not peculiar to athletes. Detailed preparticipation studies of an athlete's heart are unwarranted unless there is a family history of early cardiac death. In general, the "athlete's heart" is a beneficial adaptation to training, enhancing work capacity and reducing the likelihood of dependency in old age.

1 Osler W. *The principles and practice of medicine*. New York: Appleton, 1892:635.
2 Keys A, Friedell HL. Size and stroke of the heart in young men in relation to physical activity. *Science* 1938;**88**:456–8.
3 Henschen S. Skilanglauf und Skiwettlauf. Eine medizinische Sport Studie. Jena: Mitt med Klin Uppsala, 1899. (Cited by Rost and Hollmann, ref. 26.)
4 Park RC, Crawford MH. Heart of the athlete. *Curr Probl Cardiol* 1985;**10**:1–73.
5 Gott PH, Roselle HA, Crampton RS. The athletic heart syndrome. *Arch Intern Med* 1968;**122**:340–4.

6 Raskoff WJ, Goldman S, Cohn K. The athletic heart. *JAMA* 1976;**236**:158–62.
7 Roeske WR, O'Rourke RA, Klein H, Leopold G, Karliner JS. Noninvasive evaluation of ventricular hypertrophy in professional athletes. *Circulation* 1976;**53**:286–92.
8 Reindell H, König K, Roskamm H. *Functionsdiagnostik des gesunden und kranken Herzens*. Stuttgart: Thieme, 1966.
9 Bramwell C, Ellis R. Some observations on the circulatory mechanism in marathon runners. *Q J Med* 1931;**24**:329–46.
10 Sokolow M, Lyon TP. The ventricular complex in left ventricular hypertrophy as obtained by unipolar precordial and limb leads. *Am Heart J* 1949;**37**:161–86.
11 Sokolow M, Lyon TP. The ventricular complex in right ventricular hypertrophy as obtained by unipolar precordial and limb leads. *Am Heart J* 1949;**38**:273–94.
12 Huston TP, Puffer JC, Rodney WM. The athletic heart syndrome. *N Engl J Med* 1985;**313**:24–32.
13 Romhilt DW, Estes EH. Point score system for the ECG diagnosis of left ventricular hypertrophy. *Am Heart J* 1968;**75**:752–8.
14 Scott RC. Ventricular hypertrophy. *Cardiovasc Clin* 1973;**5**:219–54.
15 George KP, Wolfe LA, Burggraf GW. The "athletic heart syndrome". A critical review. *Sports Med* 1991;**11**:300–31.
16 Shephard RJ. *Endurance fitness*. 1st ed. Toronto: University of Toronto Press, 1969.
17 Brandenburg RO. Syncope and sudden death in hypertrophic cardiomyopathy. *J Am Coll Cardiol* 1990;**15**:962–4.
18 Maron BJ, Roberts WC, McAllister HA, Rosing DR, Epstein SE. Sudden death in young athletes. *Circulation* 1980;**62**:218–29.
19 Nienhaber CA, Hiller S, Spielmann RP, Geiger M, Kuck H. Syncope in hypertrophic cardiomyopathy: multivariate analysis of prognostic determinants. *J Am Coll Cardiol* 1990;**15**:948–55.
20 Sandric S. Echocardiography in sports medicine: clinical diagnostic possibilities and limitations. In: Lubich T, Venerando A, eds. *Sports cardiology*. Bologna: Aulo Gaggi, 1980:707–16.
21 Dickhuth HH, Jakob E, Staiger L, Keul J. Two dimensional echocardiographic measurements of left ventricular volume and stroke volume of endurance athletes and untrained subjects. *Int J Sports Med* 1983;**4**:21–6.
22 Maron BJ, Gottdiener J, Bonow RO, Epstein SE. Hypertrophic cardiomyopathy: cardiomyopathy with unusual localizations of left ventricular hypertrophy undetectable by M-mode echocardiography. *Circulation* 1981;**63**:409–18.
23 Morganroth J, Maron BJ, Henry WL, Epstein SE. Comparative left ventricular dimensions in athletes. *Ann Intern Med* 1975;**82**:521–4.
24 Fleck SJ, Henke C, Wilson C. Cardiac MRI of elite junior Olympic weightlifters. *Int J Sports Med* 1989;**10**:329–33.
25 Milliken MC, Stray-Gundersen J, Pesjock RM, Katz J, Mitchell JH. Left ventricular mass as determined by magnetic resonance imaging in male endurance athletes. *Am J Cardiol* 1998;**62**:301–5.
26 Rost R, Hollmann W. Cardiac problems in endurance sports. In: Shephard RJ, Åstrand PO, eds. *Endurance in sport*. Oxford: Blackwell Scientific Publications, 1992:438–51.
27 Reichek N, Devereaux RB. Left ventricular hypertrophy: relationship of anatomic, echocardiographic and electrocardiographic findings. *Circulation* 1981;**63**:1391–8.
28 Snoeckx LHEH, Abeling HFM, Lambregts JAC, Schmitz JJF, Verstappen FTJ, Reneman RS. Echocardiographic dimensions in athletes in relation to their training programs. *Med Sci Sports Exerc* 1982;**14**:428–34.
29 Urhausen A, Kindermann W. Echocardiographic findings in strength- and endurance-trained athletes. *Sports Med* 1992;**13**:270–84.

30 Zeppilli S, Sandric S. Cecchiti F, Spataro A, Fanelli R. Echocardiographic measurements of cardiac arrangements in different sports activities. In: Lubich T, Venerando A, eds. *Sports cardiology.* Bologna: Aulo Gaggi, 1980:723–34.

31 Perreault H, Turcotte RA. Exercise-induced cardiac hypertrophy. Fact or fallacy? *Sports Med* 1994;**17**:288–308.

32 Ikåheimo MJ, Palatsi IJ, Takkunen JT. Noninvasive evaluation of the athletic heart: sprinters versus endurance runners. *Am J Cardiol* 1979;**44**:24–30.

33 Parker BM, Londeree BR, Cupp GV, Dubiel JP. The noninvasive cardiac evaluation of long-distance runners. *Chest* 1978;**73**:376–81.

34 Shapiro LM. Left ventricular hypertrophy in athletes in relation to the type of sport. *Sports Med* 1987;**4**:239–44.

35 Spirito P, Pelliccia A, Proschan MA *et al.* Morphology of the "athlete's heart" assessed by echocardiography in 9476 elite athletes representing 27 sports. *Am J Cardiol* 1994;**74**:802–6.

36 Williams CC, Bernhardt DT. Syncope in athletes. *Sports Med* 1995;**19**:223–34.

37 Van Camp SP, Bloor CM, Mueller FO, Cantu R, Olson HG. Nontraumatic sports death in high school and college athletes. *Med Sci Sports Exerc* 1995;**27**:641–7.

38 Reguero JJR, Cubero GI, de la Iglesia JL, *et al.* Prevalence and upper limit of cardiac hypertrophy in professional cyclists. *Eur J Appl Physiol* 1995;**70**:375–8.

39 Ehsani AA, Hagberg JM, Hickson RC. Rapid changes in left ventricular dimensions and mass in response to physical conditioning and deconditioning. *Am J Cardiol* 1978;**42**:52–6.

40 Hagan RD, Laird WP, Gettman LR. The problems of per-surface areas and per-weight standardization indices in the determination of cardic hypertrophy in endurance-trained athletes. *J Cardiopulm Rehab* 1985;**5**:554–60.

41 Longhurst JC, Kelly AR, Gonyea WJ, Mitchell JH. Echo-cardiographic left ventricular masses in distance runners and weight lifters. *J Appl Physiol* 1980;**48**:154–62.

42 Allen HD, Goldberg SJ, Sahn D, Schy N, Wojcik R. A quantitative echocardiographic study of champion childhood swimmers. *Circulation* 1976;**55**:142–55.

43 Menapace FJ, Hammer WJ, Ritzer TF, *et al.* Left ventricular size in competitive weight lifters: an echocardiographic study. *Med Sci Sports Exerc* 1982;**14**:72–5.

44 Shapiro LM. Physiological left ventricular hypertrophy. *Br Heart J* 1984;**52**:130–5.

45 Oakley DG, Oakley CM. Significance of abnormal electrocardiograms in highly trained athletes. *Am J Cardiol* 1982;**50**:985–9.

46 Colan SD, Sanders SP, Borrow KM. Physiological hypertrophy: effects on left ventricular systolic mechanics in athletes. *J Am Coll Cardiol* 1987;**9**:776–83.

47 Dickhuth HH, Röcker K, Hipp A, Heitkamp HC, Keul J. Echocardiographische Befunde beim Sportherz. In: Rost R, Webering F, eds. *Kardiologie im Sport.* Cologne: Deutscher Artze Verlag, 1987:132–45.

48 Pearson AC, Schiff M, Mrosek D, Labovitz AJ, Williams GA. Left ventricular diastolic function in weight lifters. *Am J Cardiol* 1986;**58**:1254–9.

49 Hillis WS, McIntyre PD, Maclean J, Goodwin JF, McKenna WJ. Sudden death in sport. *BMJ* 1994;**309**:657–60.

50 Rosenzweig A, Watkins H, Hwang D-S, *et al.* Preclinical diagnosis of familial hypertrophic cardiomyopathy by genetic analysis of blood lymphocytes. *N Engl J Med* 1991;**325**:1753–60.

51 Sadaniantz A, Thompson PD. The problem of sudden death in athletes as illustrated by case studies. *Sports Med* 1990;**9**:199–204.

52 Solomon SD, Jarcho JA, McKenna W, *et al.* Familial hypertrophic cardiomyopathy is a genetically heterogeneous disease. *J Clin Invest* 1990;**86**:993–9.

53 Thierfelder L, Watkins H, MacRae C, *et al.* Alpha tropomyosin and cardiac troponin T mutations cause familial hypertrophic cardiomyopathy: a disease of the sarcoma. *Cell* 1994;**77**:701–12.

239

54 Wigle ED, Sasson Z, Henderson MA, *et al.* Hypertrophic cardiomyopathy. The importance of the site and the extent of hypertrophy. A review. *Prog Cardiovasc Dis* 1985;**28**:1–83.

55 Maron BJ, Isner JM, McKenna WJ. Hypertrophic cardiomyopathy, myocarditis and other myopericardial diseases and mitral valve prolapse. *Med Sci Sports Exerc* 1994;**26**:S261–7.

56 McKenna WJ, Camm AJ. Sudden death in hypertrophic cardiomyopathy. Assessment of patients at high risk. *Circulation* 1989;**80**:1489–92.

57 Shephard RJ. *Physiology and biochemistry of exercise.* New York: Praeger Publishing, 1982.

58 Kohl HW, Powell KE. What is exertion-related sudden cardiac death? *Sports Med* 1994;**17**:209–12.

59 Dickhuth HH, Röcker K, Hipp A, Heitkamp HC, Keul J. Echocardiographic findings in endurance athletes with hypertrophic non-obstructive cardiomyopathy (HNCM) compared to non-athletes with HNCM and to physiological hypertrophy (athlete's heart). *Int J Sports Med* 1994;**15**:273–7.

60 Mitten MJ, Maron BJ. Legal considerations that affect medical liability for competitive athletes with cardiovascular abnormalities and acceptance of Bethesda Conference recommendations. *Med Sci Sports Exerc* 1994;**26**:S238–41.

61 Smith DM. Pre-participation physical evaluations. Development of uniform guidelines. *Sports Med* 1994;**18**:293–300.

62 Weidenbener EJ, Krauss MD, Waller BF, Talierco CP. Incorporation of screening echocardiography in the preparticipation exam. *Clin J Sports Med* 1995;**5**:86–9.

63 Franklin B, Kahn JK. Detecting the individual prone to exercise-related sudden cardiac death. *Sports Sci Rev* 1995;**4**(2):85–105.

64 Chillag S, Bates M, Voltin R, Jones D. Sudden death: myocardial infarction in a runner with normal coronary arteries. *Physician and Sportsmedicine* 1980; **18**(3):89–94.

65 Goodman JM. Exercise and sudden cardiac death. Etiology in apparently healthy individuals. *Sports Sci Rev* 1995;**4**:14–30.

66 Torg J. Sudden cardiac death in the athlete. In: Torg J, Shephard RJ, eds. *Current therapy in sports medicine.* Philadelphia: Mosby, 1995:8–10.

67 Winget JP, Capeless MA, Ades PA. Sudden death in athletes. *Sports Med* 1994;**18**:375–83.

68 Spirito P, Chiarella F, Carratino L, Berisso MZ, Bellotti P, Vecchio C. Clinical course and prognosis of hypertrophic cardiomyopathy in an outpatient population. *N Engl J Med* 1989;**320**:749–55.

69 Marian AJ, Kelly D, Mares A, *et al.* A missense mutation in the beta-myosin heavy chain gene is a predictor of premature sudden death in patients with hypertrophic cardiomyopathy. *J Sports Med Phys Fitness* 1994;**34**:1–10.

70 Sarna S, Sahi T, Koskwenvuo M, Kaprio J. Increased life expectancy of world class male athletes. *Med Sci Sports Exerc* 1993;**25**:237–44.

71 Shephard RJ. *Physical activity and aging.* 2nd ed. London: Croom Helm, 1987.

72 Kavanagh T, Mertens DJ, Matosevic V, Shephard RJ, Evans B. Health and aging of Masters athletes. *Clin J Sports Med* 1989;**1**:72–88.

73 Paffenbarger RS, Hyde RT, Wing AL, Lee I-M, Kampert JB. Some interrelations of physical activity, physiological fitness, health and longevity. In: Bouchard C, Shephard RJ, Stephens T, eds. *Physical activity, fitness and health.* Champaign, Illinois: Human Kinetics, 1994:119–33.

74 Pekkanen J, Marti B, Nissinen A, Tuomilehto J, Punsar S, Karvonen MJ. Reduction of premature mortality by high physical activity: a 20-year follow-up of middle-aged Finnish men. *Lancet* 1987;**i**:1473–7.

75 Shephard RJ. Physical activity and quality-adjusted life-expectancy. *Quest* 1996;**48**:354–65.

Multiple choice questions

1 When examining the heart of a young athlete, which of the following statements are true?
(a) The cardiothoracic ratio on a PA radiograph should not exceed 0.50
(b) A pathological hypertrophy should be diagnosed if the sum of the ECG voltages SV1 and RV5 exceeds 3.5 mV
(c) The upper limit of normality for the posterior wall diastolic thickness at echocardiography is 11 mm
(d) An abnormality should be diagnosed if the ratio of inter-ventricular septum to left posterior ventricular wall thickness exceeds 1.3
(e) The usual limits of resolution of echocardiography do not allow a reliable distinction between physiological and pathological increases in thickness of the ventricular wall

2 At any given intensity of exercise, which of the following statements about the possible benefits of myocardial hypertrophy is false?
(a) A lengthening of the capillary diffusion path for oxygen reduces the oxygen supply of the myocardium
(b) An increase of stroke volume reduces the heart rate
(c) A relative lengthening of the diastolic phase facilitates perfusion of the perforating coronary vessels
(d) A reduction of wall tension facilitates coronary perfusion
(e) Myocardial work rate is reduced

3 Which of the following is *not* an underlying cause of exercise-induced death in an 18-year old athlete?
(a) An undetected congenital cardiac anomaly
(b) Myocardial hypertrophy
(c) A viral myocarditis
(d) Solvent abuse
(e) A familial cardiomyopathy based on abnormality of the β myosin heavy chain

4 Which of the following statements about the aetiology of sudden, exercise-induced death in young athletes is incorrect?
(a) Hypertrophic cardiomyopathy is not a frequent cause of such deaths
(b) A careful 50-year literature search suggested that hypertrophic cardiomyopathy was causing several hundred such deaths in the US every year

(c) Loose diagnostic criteria have contributed to the apparent prevalence of hypertrophic cardiomyopathy as a cause of such deaths

(d) Even when using very loose diagnostic criteria, the apparent incidence of sudden exercise-related deaths from hypertrophic cardiomyopathy in the US is only about 5 cases per year.

(e) Repeated reporting of a short case series from one laboratory has increased the apparent prevalence of hypertrophic cardiomyopathy as a cause of sudden, exercise-related death

5 When examining for evidence of a pathological enlargement of the heart in a young athlete, which of the following is incorrect?

(a) Allowance must be made for the large lean body mass of many competitors

(b) Ergometric performance may fail to match cardiac dimensions

(c) A family history of premature sudden death is not a useful diagnostic criterion

(d) Some authors find a septal thickness/end-diastolic diameter ratio of more than 0.48 to be a pointer of pathology

(e) There are often associated abnormalities of cardiac rhythm

Answers are on p. 365.

13   The effect of altered reproductive function and lowered testosterone concentrations on bone density in male endurance athletes

K L Bennell, P D Brukner, S A Malcolm

Introduction

The effect of intense physical activity on female reproductive hormones is well recognised,[1-3] and there is evidence that menstrual disturbances associated with hypo-oestrogenism adversely affect bone density especially at the lumbar spine.[4,5] Physical activity can also have a range of effects on male reproductive function, depending on the intensity and duration of the activity and the fitness of the individual.[6] In particular, endurance training may be associated with reductions in circulating testosterone concentrations. As testosterone has important anabolic roles, alterations in reproductive hormone profiles may have detrimental skeletal consequences similar to those seen in women with menstrual disturbances. The aim of this chapter is to present the limited literature on the relation between bone density and testosterone concentrations in male endurance athletes.

An overview of male hypogonadal-pituitary-gonadal (HPG) axis regulation

The main functions of the testes are steroid biosynthesis and spermatogenesis. These are controlled by higher structures of the hypogonadal-pituitary-gonadal (HPG) axis operating under a negative feedback system, the major gonadal regulatory hormone being testosterone.[7] Gonadotropin-releasing hormone (GnRH), secreted in pulses by the hypothalamus, stimulates the pituitary gland to secrete the two gonadotropic hormones: luteinising hormone (LH) and follicle-stimulating hormone (FSH). LH stimulates the testis to secrete testosterone which is produced from cholesterol in the smooth endoplasmic reticulum. FSH, together with a small proportion of testosterone, facilitates sperm production with the seminiferous tubules. Prolactin, a stress hormone produced in the pituitary gland, may also be involved in regulation of testicular sex steroid production.[8]

Metabolic roles of testosterone

About 95% of circulating serum testosterone comes from production in the testis with the remainder produced in the adrenal glands. Testosterone is found in plasma primarily bound to proteins, albumin and sex-hormone binding globulin (SHBG), with a small portion (3%) circulating unbound and referred to as free testosterone.[6] The biologically active form of testosterone is that bound to albumin and the small unbound or free portion.[9] Half of the testosterone produced is cleared through the liver and the remainder is cleared through extrahepatic metabolism.

Testosterone serves as a circulating precursor for the formation of active metabolites which in turn mediate many of the physiological phenomena that are involved in androgen action.[10] One of these, dihydrotestosterone has a more pronounced anabolic effect than testosterone.

Testosterone and its active metabolites have important reproductive functions, being responsible for the development and maintenance of secondary sexual characteristics and for spermatogenesis. In addition, testosterone is a powerful anabolic hormone that stimulates tissue growth and development. Testosterone has important effects on bone mass as demonstrated by the finding that hypogonadism in males is a risk factor for osteoporosis.[11–13] Testosterone may have direct effects on bone formation given that androgen receptors have been identified on osteoblasts.[14] It may also act indirectly through augmented nocturnal secretion of growth hormone and subsequently insulin-like growth factor 1 (IGF-1), particularly during puberty, and by increased muscular

---

Box 13.1   The effects of testosterone

- Testosterone production by the testes is under the control of the hypothalamic-pituitary-gonadal axis
- Testosterone and its active metabolites, including dihydrotestosterone, are responsible for the development and maintenance of secondary sexual characteristics and for spermatogenesis. They also have anabolic functions stimulating tissue growth and development
- Testosterone may have direct effects on bone formation or it may act indirectly through augmented nocturnal secretion of growth hormone and subsequently insulin-like growth factor. This may be important during puberty and may be related to increasing muscularity

---

activity and stresses on the skeleton promoting bone mass at local sites.

Effects of exercise on testosterone concentrations

Relatively short duration exercise bouts at maximum or near maximum intensity seem to increase serum testosterone concentrations[15-21] with measurable changes evident within minutes. However, with prolonged acute submaximal exercise bouts of about 2 hours or longer [16,22] suppression of circulating testosterone is noted which may remain for several days.

There is controversy about the effects of chronic intense exercise on basal testosterone concentrations. Some cross-sectional studies have found reductions of total testosterone and measures of biologically available testosterone concentrations[15,22-28] in athletes compared with non-athletes, while others have reported no difference.[29-34] Similar conflict is apparent in the findings of prospective studies. In these, previously sedentary men were placed on a strenuous exercise programme or conditioned athletes significantly increased their normal training volume. While some noted a reduction in testosterone concentrations[35-40] others observed no changes[41-44] or an increase.[45,46] These results suggest that some male athletes who train intensively may experience reductions in testosterone concentrations although this is not a consistent phenomenon. Even where decreases have been noted, however, in general the testosterone levels are still within the normal range.

Discrepancies in the results of both cross-sectional and prospective studies may be attributable to differences in subject characteristics in terms of age, race and previous activity level, type of exercise programme and measurement procedures including sampling and analysing techniques. Since testosterone concentrations show fluctuations and a circadian pattern, the time of day when samples are obtained and the use of serial hormone determinations may influence study results. A further important point is that not all studies included assessment of free testosterone concentrations. These may be altered after exercise despite non-significant changes in total testosterone.

Possible mechanisms for suppression of testosterone concentrations with long term exercise

Long term suppression of serum testosterone associated with exercise may result from decreased production rates, decreased protein binding or increased clearance.[47] Of these, the most likely mechanism is decreased testosterone production arising from

---

Box 13.2   The effects of exercise on testosterone concentrations

- There is controversy in the literature about the effects of exercise on testosterone concentrations. Conflicting results may be explained by differences in the intensity and duration of the activity and physical characteristics of the individual including age and fitness level. Methodology issues including the study design and sampling, and analysing techniques for testosterone concentrations may also influence the results
- Relatively short duration intense activity may lead to transient increases in testosterone concentrations
- Prolonged acute submaximal exercise bouts may lead to a suppression of testosterone levels possibly lasting up to several days
- Male athletes who train intensively may experience reductions in basal testosterone concentrations, although this is not necessarily a consistent phenomena. Furthermore, concentrations still tend to be within normal clinical range
- Possible mechanisms for suppression of testosterone concentrations with long term exercise include decreased production rates due to intrinsic failure of the testis or to central dysfunction in the hypothalamic-pituitary-gonadal axis, decreased protein binding, or increased clearance

---

either intrinsic failure of the testis to maintain adequate steroid biosynthesis perhaps due to testicular microtrauma and temperature increase[48] or from central dysfunction in the HPG axis. The latter is supported by reports of decreases in LH pulse amplitude[15] and frequency[32] as well as changes in pituitary responses to hypothalamic stimulation by exogenous GnRH[26,32] in male athletes. In addition, factors may interact with the HPG axis including dietary intake[40,49] and raised concentrations of stress related hormones.[33]

Skeletal effects of lowered testosterone concentrations in male athletes

In female athletes menstrual disturbances have been found in association with lower bone density particularly at trabecular sites.[4,5] Furthermore, stress fractures seem to be more common in women with amenorrhoea or oligomenorrhoea with a relative risk that is between two to four times greater than that of their eumenorrhoeic counterparts.[50,52] There are few studies investigating the relation of testosterone levels to bone density and stress fracture risk in young male athletes. A recent case report described the clinical features of a 29-year-old male distance runner who presented with a pelvic stress fracture, greatly decreased bone density and symptomatic hypogonadotropic hypogonadism.[53] Using this case as an index, the authors hypothesised that exercise-induced hypogonadotropic hypogonadism could be identified in male athletes by the presence of one or more specific risk factors which included the presence of sexual dysfunction, a history of fracture, and the initiation of endurance exercise before age 18 years.[54] They compared concentrations of free testosterone and luteinising hormone in 15 male runners with one or more of the above risk factors and 13 runners with none of the risk factors. Only one of the runners in the first group was identified as having primary hypogonadism and there was no significant difference between groups for hormone concentrations. Bone density, however, was not measured in these runners and correlated with testosterone concentrations. From a clinical perspective, it is important to clarify that although some male athletes do present with reduced testosterone concentrations, these concentrations are generally still within the normal range for adult men. Therefore, detrimental effects on bone density may not be as dramatic as those described for women with athletic amenorrhoea in whom oestradiol concentrations are well below normal.

Several studies have reported lower bone density in male runners than in non-runners or those running shorter distances.[34,55,56] Male distance runners, averaging 92 km/week, were found to have 9.7% lower bone density at the lumbar spine compared with a group of non-runners. No differences in bone density were found at the radial or tibial shafts.[56] Although hormonal status was not measured, the authors speculated that lowered testosterone concentrations may have played a part in explaining their results. Another study also reported negative correlations between running distance and lumbar spine, proximal femur and total body bone density in male runners.[55] However, it was unable to show correlations between running distance and either serum total testosterone concentration or the free testosterone index (ratio between total testosterone and SHBG). The authors therefore suggested that the observed osteopenia—associated with increased running distance—was independent of male sex hormones.

MacDougall *et al.* compared 22 sedentary men with 53 male runners divided into five groups on the basis of their weekly running distance.[34] They showed that bone density of the trunk tended to be lower in those who ran more than 64 km (40 miles) per week while tibial bone density was greater in those who ran 24 to 32 km (15 to 20 miles) per week and tended to be lower in those who ran further than this. Nevertheless, total testosterone concen-

---

Box 13.3   The relationship between lowered testosterone concentrations and bone density in male athletes

- Some studies have reported lower bone density in male athletes compared with those training less intensely or with non-athletes
- However, no study has established a relation between lowered circulating testosterone concentrations and lowered bone density in male athletes
- There is no research investigating the effects of intense training on pubertal progression in men
- The effects of exercise on the male reproductive system do not seem to have the same skeletal consequences compared with female athletes, in whom menstrual disturbances can lead to a loss of bone, particularly at axial sites

trations were within the normal range for the runners and did not differ from the controls.

Male triathletes were found to have similar bone density at the spine as a group of sedentary men, whereas male rowers had significantly higher spinal bone density.[29] Although total serum testosterone concentrations of all groups fell within the normal range, triathletes had significantly lower concentrations than the controls. The authors claimed that the lower testosterone in the triathletes may have negated any positive skeletal effects arising from their higher levels of exercise. However, this cannot be stated conclusively without comparing the bone density of groups of triathletes with high and low testosterone concentrations. It is possible that some other factor common to triathlete training is affecting bone density independently of testosterone concentrations.

The results of these limited studies have failed to establish a relation between lowered circulating testosterone levels and osteopenia in male athletes. However, there are several methodological issues which should be considered. Only one study[55] included assessment of SHBG in addition to total serum testosterone to give an indication of the amount of free testosterone. As SHBG is the biologically active portion, levels of this fraction may be more relevant to skeletal health. Furthermore, none measured dihydrotestosterone, an active metabolite of testosterone which has a greater anabolic effect.[10] Most studies used single sampling procedures at differing times of the day which may not necessarily provide a true representation of the hormonal concentrations. Radioimmunoassays were used to measure testosterone and while these indicate the immunological activity of the hormone they do not necessarily reflect the biological activity. This depends not only on hormonal concentrations but also on receptor availability and sensitivity within the subject.[7] It is possible that some male athletes have reduced biological activity of testosterone despite normal circulating concentrations and this may lead to bone loss.

Delayed puberty

Pubertal development, as assessed by age of menarche, appears to be delayed in female athletes.[57-58] It has been suggested that intense training in the premenarcheal years may contribute to this phenomenon.[59] There is some evidence that women with a later menarcheal age have lower bone density.[60-64] This may result from failure to maximise peak bone mass during the pubertal years. An association has also been found between a later age of menarche and an increased risk of stress fracture in female track and field athletes.[52] For every 1 year increase in age at menarche, the risk of stress fracture increased four fold.

While there is no physiological index comparable with age of menarche in men, longitudinal data indicate that sporting participation has little effect on attained stature, the timing of peak height velocity, rate of statural growth or sexual maturation in men.[65,66] Whether these results necessarily apply to intense endurance exercise is less clear as most studies do not focus on such extreme forms of exercise. Although men with delayed puberty have been found to exhibit significant osteopenia,[12-13] the pubertal delay in these reports is not attributed to sporting pursuits but is part of some other disease process or disorder. Research investigating the effects of intense training on pubertal progression, testosterone concentrations, bone accrual and stress fracture risk in male athletes is warranted.

Summary

It is apparent that bone density in male athletes can be reduced without a concomitant decrease in testosterone, suggesting that bone density and testosterone concentrations in the normal range are not closely related in male athletes. Further research is necessary to monitor concurrent changes in bone density and testosterone over a period of time in exercising men. In any case, the effect of exercise on the male reproductive system does not appear as extreme as that which can occur in female athletes and any impact on bone density is not nearly as evident.

These results imply that factors apart from testosterone concentrations must be responsible for the observed osteopenia in some male athletes. Many factors have the potential to affect bone density adversely, independently of alterations in reproductive function. These include low calcium intake, energy deficit, weight loss, psychological stress and low body fat, all of which may be associated with intense endurance training. Future research investigating skeletal health in male athletes should include a thorough assessment of reproductive function in addition to these other factors.

1 Bonen A, Belcastro AN, Ling WY, Simpson AA. Profiles of selected hormones during menstrual cycles of teenage athletes. *J Appl Physiol* 1981;**50**:551.

2 Boyden TW, Pamenter RW, Stanforth P, Rotkis T, Wilmore JH. Sex steroids and endurance running in women. *Fertil Steril* 1983;**39**:629–32.

3 Ellison PT, Lager C. Moderate recreational running is associated with lowered salivary progesterone levels in women. *Am J Obstet Gynecol* 1986;**154**:1000–3.

4 Drinkwater BL, Nilson K, Chesnut CH, *et al*. Bone mineral content of amenorrheic and eumenorrheic athletes. *N Engl J Med* 1984;**311**:277–81.

5 Myburgh KH, Bachrach LK, Lewis B, Kent K, Marcus R. Low bone mineral density at axial and appendicular sites in amenorrheic athletes. *Med Sci Sports Exerc* 1993;**25**:1197–202.

6 Arce JC, de Souza M. Exercise and male factor infertility. *Sports Med* 1993;**15**:146–69.

7 Hackney AC. Endurance training and testosterone levels. *Sports Med* 1989;**8**:117–27.

8 Rubin RT, Poland RE, Sobel I, Tower BB, Odell WD. Effects of prolactin and prolactin plus luteinizing hormone on plasma testosterone levels in normal adult men. *J Clin Endocrinol Metab* 1978;**47**:447–52.

9 Pardridge WM. Serum bioavailability of sex steroid hormones. *Clin Endocrinol Metab* 1986;**15**:259–78.

10 Griffin JE, Wilson JD. Disorders of the testes and the male reproductive tract. In: Wilson JD, Foster DW, eds. *Williams textbook of endocrinology*. 8th ed. Philadelphia: WB Saunders Company, 1992: 799–852.

11 Seeman E, Melton LJ, O'Fallon WM, Riggs BL. Risk factors for spinal osteoporosis in men. *Am J Med* 1983;**75**:977–83.

12 Krabbe S, Christiansen C, Rodbro P, Transbol I. Effect of puberty on rates of bone growth and mineralisation with observations in male delayed puberty. *Arch Dis Child* 1979;**54**:950–3.

13 Finkelstein JS, Neer RM, Biller BMK, Crawford JD, Klibanski A. Osteopenia in men with a history of delayed puberty. *N Engl J Med* 1992;**326**:600–4.

14 Colvard DS, Eriksen EF, Keeting PE, *et al*. Identification of androgen receptors in normal human osteoblast-like cells. *Proc Natl Acad Sci USA* 1989;**86**:854–7.

15 McColl EM, Wheeler GD, Gomes P, Bhambhani Y, Cumming DC. The effects of acute exercise on pulsatile LH release in high-mileage male runners. *Clin Endocrinol* 1989;**31**:617–21.

16 Guglielmini C, Paolini AR, Conconi F. Variations of serum testosterone concentrations after physical exercise of different duration. *Int J Sports Med* 1984;**5**:246–9.

17 Kraemer RR, Kilgore JL, Kraemer GR, Castracane VD. Growth hormone, IGF-1, and testosterone responses to resistive exercises. *Med Sports Exerc* 1992;**24**:1346–52.

18 Gray AB, Telford RD, Weidemann MJ. Endocrine response to intense interval exercise. *Eur J Appl Physiol* 1993;**66**:366–71.

19 Hakkinen K, Pakarinen A, Alen M, Kauhanen H, Komi PV. Neuromuscular and hormonal adaptations in athletes to strength training in two years. *J Appl Physiol* 1988;**65**:2406–12.

20 Cadoux-Hudson TA, Few JD, Imms FJ. The effect of exercise on the production and clearance of testosterone in well trained young men. *Eur J Appl Physiol* 1985;**54**:321–5.

21 Kraemer WJ, Hakkinen K, Newton RU, *et al*. Acute hormonal responses to heavy resistance exercise in younger and older men. *Eur J Appl Physiol Occupat Physiol* 1998;**77**:206–11.

22 Tanaka H, Cleroux J, de Champlain J, Ducharme JR, Collu R. Persistent effects of a marathon run on the pituitary-testicular axis. *J Endocrinol Invest* 1986;**9**:97–101.

23 Arce JC, de Souza MJ, Pescatello LS, Luciano AA. Subclinical alterations in

hormone and semen profile in athletes. *Fertil Steril* 1993;**59**:398–404.

24 Ayers JWT, Komesu Y, Romani T, Ansbacher R. Anthropomorphic, hormonal, and psychologic correlates of semen quality in endurance-trained male athletes. *Fertil Steril* 1985;**43**:917–21.

25 Hackney AC, Sinning WE, Bruot BC. Reproductive hormonal profiles of endurance-trained and untrained males. *Med Sci Sports Exerc* 1988;**20**: 60–5.

26 Hackney AC, Sinning WE, Bruot BC. Hypothalamic-pituitary-testicular axis function in endurance-trained males. *Int J Sports Med* 1990;**11**:298–303.

27 Wheeler GD, Wall SR, Belcastro AN, Cumming DC. Reduced serum testosterone and prolactin levels in male distance runners. *JAMA* 1984;**252**:514–7.

28 Hackney AC, Fahrner CL, Gulledge TP. Basal reproductive hormonal profiles are altered in endurance trained men. *J Sports Med Phys Fitness* 1998;**38**:138–41.

29 Smith R, Rutherford OM. Spine and total body bone mineral density and serum testosterone levels in male athletes. *Eur J Appl Physiol* 1993;**67**:330–4.

30 Bagatell CJ, Bremner WJ. Sperm counts and reproductive hormones in male marathoners and lean controls. *Fertil Steril* 1990;**53**:688–92.

31 Gutin B, Alejandro D, Duni T, Segal K, Phillips GB. Levels of serum sex hormones and risk factors for coronary heart disease in exercise-trained men. *Am J Med* 1985;**79**:79–84.

32 MacConnie SE, Barkan A, Lampman RM, Schork MA, Beitins IZ. Decreased hypothalamic gonadotrophin-releasing hormone secretion in male marathon runners. *N Engl J Med* 1986;**315**:411–7.

33 Mathur DN, Toriola AL, Dada OA. Serum cortisol and testosterone levels in conditioned male distance runners and non-athletes after maximal exercise. *J Sports Med* 1986;**26**:245–50.

34 MacDougall JD, Webber CE, Martin J, *et al.* Relationship among running mileage, bone density, and serum testosterone in male runners. *J Appl Physiol* 1992;**73**:1165–70.

35 Griffiths RO, Dressendorfer RH, Fullbright CD, Wade CE. Testicular function during exhaustive endurance training. *Physician and Sportsmedicine* 1990;**18**:54–64.

36 Urhausen A, Kullmer T, Kindermann W. A 7-week follow-up study of the behaviour of testosterone and cortisol during the competition period in rowers. *Eur J Appl Physiol* 1987;**56**:528–33.

37 Wheeler GD, Singh M, Pierce WD, Epling WF, Cumming DC. Endurance training decreases serum testosterone levels in men without changes in luteinizing hormone pulsatile release. *J Clin Endocrinol Metabol* 1991;**72**:422–5.

38 Roberts AC, McClure RD, Weiner RI, Brooks GA. Overtraining affects male reproductive status. *Fertil Steril* 1993;**60**:686–92.

39 Hackney AC, Sharp RL, Runyan WS, Ness RJ. Relationship of resting prolactin and testosterone in males during intensive training. *Br J Sports Med* 1989;**23**:194.

40 Opstad PK. Androgenic hormones during prolonged physical stress, sleep, and energy deficiency. *J Clin Endocrinol Metabol* 1992;**74**:1176–83.

41 Fellman N, Coudert J, Jarrige JF, *et al.* Effects of endurance training on the androgenic response to exercise in man. *Int J Sports Med* 1985;**6**:215–9.

42 Peltonen P, Marniemi J, Hietanen E, Vuori I, Ehnholm C. Changes in serum lipids, lipoproteins, and heparin releasable lipolytic enzymes during moderate physical training in man: a longitudinal study. *Metabolism* 1981;**30**:518–26.

43 Seidman DS, Lolev E, Deuster PA, *et al.* Androgenic response to long-term physical training in male subjects. *Int J Sports Med* 1990; **11**:421–4.

44 Klausen T, Breum L, Fogh-Andersen N, Bennett P, Hippe E. The effect of short and long duration exercise on serum erythropoietin concentrations. *Eur J Appl Physiol* 1993;**67**:213–7.

45 Keizer H, Janssen GME, Menheere P, Kranenburg G. Changes in basal plasma testosterone, cortisol, and dehydroepiandrosterone sulfate in previously untrained males and females preparing for a marathon. *Int J Sports Med* 1989;**10**:S139–45.

46 Remes K, Kuoppasalmi K, Adlercreutz H. Effects of long-term physical training on plasma testosterone, androstenedione, luteinizing hormone and sex-hormone-binding globulin capacity. *Scan J Clin Lab Invest* 1979;**39**:743–9.

47 Cumming DC, Wheeler GD, McColl EM. The effects of exercise on reproductive function in men. *Sports Med* 1989;**7**:1–17.

48 Kandeel FR, Swerdloff RS. Role of temperature in regulation of spermatogenesis and use of heating as a method of contraception. *Fertil Steril* 1988;**49**:1–23.

49 Hamalainen EK, Adlercreutz H, Puska P, Pietinen P. Decrease of serum total and free testosterone during a low-fat high-fibre diet. *J Steroid Biochem* 1983;**18**:369–70.

50 Carbon R, Sambrook PN, Deakin V, *et al.* Bone density of elite female athletes with stress fractures. *Med J Aust* 1990;**153**:373–6.

51 Myburgh KH, Hutchins J, Fataar AB, Hough SF, Noakes TD. Low bone density is an etiologic factor for stress fractures in athletes. *Ann Intern Med* 1990;**113**:754–9.

52 Bennell KL, Malcolm SA, Thomas SA, *et al.* Risk factors for stress fractures in track and field athletes. A twelve-month prospective study. *Am J Sports Med* 1996;**24**:211–7.

53 Burge MR, Lanzi RA, Skarda ST, Eaton RP. Idiopathic hypogonadotropic hypogonadism in a male runner is reversed by clomiphene citrate. *Fertil Steril* 1997;**67**:783–5.

54 Skarda ST, Burge MR. Prospective evaluation of risk factors for exercise-induced hypogonadism in male runners. *West J Med* 1998;**169**:9–12.

55 Hetland ML, Haarbo J, Christiansen C. Low bone mass and high bone turnover in male long distance runners. *J Clin Endocrinol Metabol* 1993;**77**:770–5.

56 Bilanin JE, Blanchard MS, Russek-Cohen E. Lower vertebral bone density in male long distance runners. *Med Sci Sports Exerc* 1989;**21**:66–70.

57 Guler F, Hascelik Z. Menstrual dysfunction rate and delayed menarche in top athletes of team games. *Sports Med Training Rehabil* 1993;**4**:99–106.

58 Robinson TL, Snow-Harter C, Taaffe DR, *et al.* Gymnasts exhibited higher bone mass than runners despite similar prevalence of amenorrhea and oligomenorrhea. *J Bone Miner Res* 1995;**10**:26–35.

59 Frisch RE, Gotz-Welbergen AV, McArthur JW, *et al.* Delayed menarche and amenorrhea of college athletes in relation to age of onset of training. *JAMA* 1981;**246**:1559–63.

60 Katzman DK, Bachrach LK, Carter DR, Marcus R. Clinical and anthropometric correlates of bone mineral acquisition in healthy adolescent girls. *J Clin Endocrinol Metab* 1991;**73**:1332–9.

61 Armamento-Villareal R, Villareal DT, Avioli LV, Civtelli R. Estrogen status and heredity are major determinants of premenopausal bone loss. *J Clin Invest* 1992;**90**:2464–71.

62 Elliot JR, Gilchrist NL, Wells JE, *et al.* Historical assessment of risk factors in screening for osteopenia in a normal Caucasian population. *Aust N Z J Med* 1993;**23**:458–62.

63 Fox KM, Magaziner J, Sherwin R, *et al.* Reproductive correlates of bone mass in elderly women. *J Bone Miner Res* 1993;**8**:901–8.

64 Lu PW, Briody JN, Ogle GD, Morley K, Humphries IRJ. Bone mineral density of total body, spine, and femoral neck in children and young adults: a cross-sectional and longitudinal study. *J Bone Miner Res* 1994;**9**:1451–8.

65 Malina RM. Physical activity and training: effects on stature and the adolescent growth spurt. *Med Sci Sports Exerc* 1994;**26**:759–66.
66 Malina RM. Physical growth and biological maturation of young athletes. *Exerc Sports Sci Rev* 1994;**221**:389–433.

Multiple choice questions

1 Regarding the male hypogonadal-pituitary-gonadal axis (HPG), which of the following is true?
(a) Gonadotropic releasing hormone is secreted in pulses by the pituitary gland to stimulate the testes
(b) Follicle stimulating hormone stimulates the testes to secrete testosterone
(c) The male HPG works under a positive feedback system
(d) The hypothalamus secretes the two gonadotropic hormones: luteinising hormone and follicle stimulating hormone

2 Circulating testosterone:
(a) Is mainly found bound to proteins
(b) Is mainly found circulating unbound and referred to as free testosterone
(c) Has as its biologically active form that bound to sex hormone binding globulin
(d) Has a more pronounced anabolic effect than dihydro-testosterone

3 With regards to the effects of testosterone, which of the following are true?
(a) It is responsible for the development of secondary sexual characteristics
(b) It may have direct effects on bone resorption
(c) Hypogonadism in men is a risk factor for osteoporosis
(d) It may have indirect effects on bone via growth hormone and insulin-like growth factor

4 In general, what are the effects of exercise on testosterone concentrations?
(a) An initial decrease in concentrations with intense exercise bouts of short duration
(b) An increase with prolonged acute submaximal exercise bouts
(c) Always decreased concentrations with strenuous long term exercise
(d) Variable depending on a number of factors including type of exercise, fitness of the individual, and study methods

254

5 Which of the following are true for the relation between sex hormones and bone density in athletes?

(a) Lower bone density has been reported in some male athletes compared with those training less intensely and with non-athletes

(b) Female athletes with menstrual disturbances may have lower bone density particularly at axial sites

(c) A relation has been identified between lowered testosterone concentrations and bone density in male athletes

(d) Lower testosterone concentrations measured in some male athletes are still generally within clinically normal ranges

Answers are on p. 365.

14 Factors influencing the restoration of fluid and electrolyte balance after exercise in the heat

R J Maughan, J B Leiper, S M Shirreffs

Introduction

Sustained hard exercise in a hot environment presents a greater challenge to the body's homeostatic mechanisms than any other circumstance. The combination of a high rate of metabolic heat production and a restricted capacity for heat dissipation leads to hyperthermia, which may progress to heat illness; this will inevitably impair exercise performance, and may in extreme cases be fatal.[1]

The 1998 Commonwealth games held in Kuala Lumpur in September were but one example of a major sporting event held in unfavourable climatic conditions. The combination of high temperature and high humidity has major implications for everyone attending; this includes spectators, officials, and team management as well as competitors. Performance in all outdoor endurance events, which we can define as those lasting longer than a total time of about 20–30 minutes, is generally reduced, and there seems to be no way of avoiding some impairment of performance. A recent study under laboratory conditions has shown that endurance time on a bicycle ergometer at an exercise intensity that could be sustained for 92 minutes at a temperature of 11°C was reduced to 83 minutes when the temperature was increased to 21°C and to 51 minutes when the temperature was increased to 30°C;[2] in conditions experienced in Kuala Lumpur, the reduction would be even greater. If the athlete is dehydrated before exercise begins, the

256

reductions in performance observed in the heat are greatly magnified.

For those unaccustomed to living in the heat, the stress will be no different from that experienced by those who are accustomed to the heat, but the way in which the athletes deal with the conditions may be the largest factor influencing the impact of the climatic stress on their performance. The successful competitor will have prepared a coping strategy that includes acclimatisation, rehydration, and behavioural and psychological components. Aside from behavioural mechanisms to minimise or prevent overheating—such as moving indoors to an air conditioned cool environment—the physiological mechanisms activated by the acclimation process include an earlier onset of sweating and an increased sweating rate. Sweating can be very effective in removing heat from the body, and substantial amounts of fluid are likely to be lost in this way by many individuals. The acclimation process results in an increased sweat loss and therefore increases, rather than decreases, the need for fluid replacement. The water lost must be replaced to maintain body water balance and allow the best possible athletic performance to be achieved. In addition, it is well established that dehydration removes the thermoregulatory advantage and improved exercise tolerance that result from acclimatisation.[3]

Although the physician and physiologist disapprove, it seems to be beneficial, at least in terms of performance, for athletes in weight category sports, including wrestlers, boxers, and weightlifters, to perform while in a dehydrated state; the disadvantage arising from competing with a body water deficit has been found by trial, error, and the experience of coach and athlete to be outweighed by the advantages of competing in a weight category below the athlete's natural weight.[4] The advantage probably arises from biomechanical factors, including limb leverage advantages. However, the optimisation of rehydration after sweat loss induced to make weight at the time of the weigh-in may be of particular importance to performers in these sports. There are also many other athletes, including those who have to compete in more than one round of a competition on the same day or on successive days, for whom recovery and rehydration between events is of crucial importance.

The difficulty of achieving effective rehydration after thermal dehydration has long been recognised. Ingestion of water causes a prompt diuresis even when the individual is still hypohydrated, effectively preventing a return to euhydration.[5] More recent studies have confirmed that plain water is not the best solution to be consumed after exercise to replace the water lost as sweat.[6,7] These studies have highlighted the need for replacement of electrolytes as well as water, but have generally been non-systematic, with a number of variables changing simultaneously, leading to some difficulties in the interpretation of the results and in the formulation of recommendations for athletes. These reports have, however, also repeated earlier observations that voluntary fluid consumption generally stops short of the amount necessary to replace losses, leading to an involuntary dehydration. Levels of hypohydration equivalent to about 1% of body mass are sufficient to affect thermoregulatory responses to exercise; deficits of 2–3% of total body water, although sufficient to impair exercise performance, are not effective in initiating the drive to drink, and substantial fluid deficits (up to 5–10% of total body water) are well tolerated at rest by the healthy individual.[3] If physical work is to be sustained, however, the need for adequate hydration becomes critical at these levels of hypohydration.

This chapter will describe some of our recent work concerning issues which must be considered if optimisation of fluid replacement after sweating induced by exercising in the heat is to be achieved. The aim of this series of investigations has been to complete a systematic investigation of some of the factors that influence restoration of fluid balance after exercise-induced dehydration. The factors that govern fluid replacement during exercise have been extensively investigated and are the subject of a number of comprehensive reviews;[8–11] these issues will not be discussed further here. We have focused on replacement after exercise in preparation for the next bout of exercise, be it training or competition. Our concerns deal with the composition of the fluid consumed, with particular regard to its electrolyte content, the volume of fluid consumed, the effects of consuming food together with a drink, the effects of consuming alcohol on rehydration effectiveness, voluntary intake of fluid after exercise, and any special considerations for female athletes in view of possible menstrual cycle effects on the rehydration effectiveness of beverages. Finally, there has been an initial investigation of the possible implications of the restoration of fluid and electrolyte balance on the ability to perform an exhausting exercise task. These results are presented as a series of summaries of individual experiments, followed by a short discussion of the implications for the athlete in training or competition.

General outline of studies

In all of these individual experiments, a moderate level of dehydration was induced by intermittent exercise in a hot (about 34°C) humid (60–80% relative humidity) environment. Subjects exercised until body mass had decreased by about 2% of the initial value; for a 70 kg subject, this corresponded to a sweat loss of about 1.4 litres. Beginning 30 minutes after the end of this exercise period, drinks of varying volume or composition were provided over a fixed time (30 minutes in most of the studies), and thereafter no further intake was allowed until the end of the study period. Measurements of urine volume and composition and of a variety of plasma variables (electrolyte concentrations, hormone levels, osmolality, haemoglobin concentration, and haematocrit) were made throughout the study.

Electrolyte content of drinks

A study was undertaken to examine the effect of the sodium content of drinks on the rehydration process after exercise-induced dehydration equivalent to 1.9% of body mass of six fasted but euhydrated men.[12] After dehydration they consumed drinks with sodium concentrations of 1, 25, 50, and 102 mmol/l over a 60 minute period beginning 40 minutes after the end of exercise; the volume consumed was 1.5 times their mass loss by dehydration which amounted to about 2 litres in all trials. The entire volume of urine produced over the 6 hours after the end of the drinking period was collected and measured (no other food or drink was consumed after the rehydration period). The volume of urine produced was influenced by the quantity of sodium consumed, such that it was greatest when the 1 mmol/l drink was consumed and least when the 102 mmol/l drink was consumed (fig 14.1). The sweat secreted during the exercise was collected and the sodium content measured; the mean (SD) concentration was 49.2 (18.5) mmol/l. Calculations of whole body sodium balance can be made, taking the pre-exercise values as the zero point (fig 14.2); the results clearly show that there is a strong relation between the sodium content of the ingested fluid and its ability to restore water balance.

Blood samples were collected before and 40 minutes after the dehydration period (immediately before the test drink was consumed) and then at intervals until 6 hours after the end of the rehydration period. Plasma volume changes, calculated according

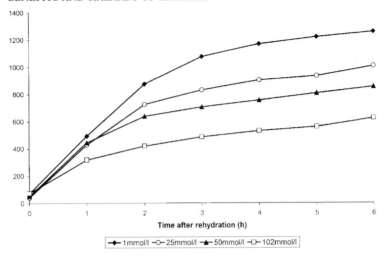

Fig 14.1 Cumulative urine output after rehydration over time after exercise-induced dehydration followed by ingestion of a fixed volume of electrolyte drinks with differing sodium content. Significant treatment effects were seen after the rehydration period (redrawn from Shirreffs and Maughan[12]).

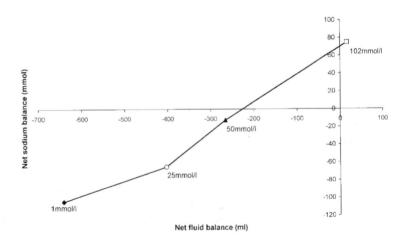

Fig 14.2 Relation between whole body water balance and sodium balance 6 hours after the end of exercise-induced dehydration followed by ingestion of a fixed volume of fluid with different sodium concentration (redrawn from Shirreffs and Maughan[12]).

to the formula of Dill and Costill,[13] decreased with dehydration in all trials and increased after rehydration in all trials. Restoration of plasma volume occurred less rapidly with the 1 mmol/l beverage, in that 1 hour after the end of the fluid ingestion period, the increase in plasma volume was 4.3% in this trial, with increases of 10.6% and 12.2%, with the 50 and 102 mmol/l drinks, respectively. Overall there was a tendency for the plasma volume recovery to be related to the quantity of sodium consumed, with the smallest increase with the 1 mmol/l beverage and the greatest increase with the 102 mmol/l beverage.

Sodium has an important function in assisting effective rehydration, largely as a consequence of its role as the major ion of the extracellular fluid. If sufficient sodium and water are ingested, some of the sodium remains in the vascular space, with the result that plasma osmolality and sodium concentration do not decline as may occur if plain water is ingested. As a result, the plasma levels of vasopressin and aldosterone are maintained, and an inappropriate diuresis—inappropriate because the body is still in net negative fluid balance—is prevented. Where ad libitum fluid intake is possible, maintaining the plasma osmolality and the circulating sodium concentration also plays a part in stimulating the drive to drink, and thus helps to ensure that an adequate volume is consumed.

Potassium is the major ion of the intracellular fluid, and it has been postulated that the inclusion of potassium in drinks consumed after sweat loss may aid rehydration by enhancing the retention of water in the intracellular space.[14] In a study designed to investigate this, eight male volunteers were dehydrated by 2.1% of body mass by intermittent cycle ergometer exercise in the heat.[15] Subjects ingested a glucose beverage (90 mmol/l), a sodium containing beverage (NaCl 60 mmol/l), a potassium containing beverage (KCl 25 mmol/l), and a beverage consisting of the addition of all three over a 30 minute period begining 45 minutes after the end of exercise. The drink volume consumed was equivalent to the volume of sweat lost and amounted to about 1.6 litres in all trials; no other food or drink was consumed during the study. The urine produced and excreted from the end of the rehydration period for the next 6 hours was again collected.

A smaller volume of urine was excreted after rehydration when the electrolyte containing beverages were ingested compared with the electrolyte free beverage (fig 14.3). An estimated plasma volume decrease of 4.4% was observed with dehydration over all

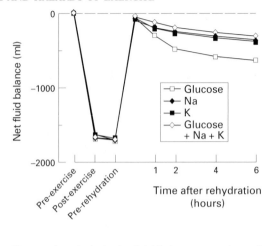

Fig 14.3 Changes in whole body fluid balance over time after exercise-induced dehydration followed by ingestion of drinks containing no electrolytes or containing sodium, potassium, or both sodium and potassium. Cumulative urine output was higher after ingestion of the electrolyte free drink than after ingestion of any of the other drinks causing a rapid return to a negative fluid balance (based on data from Maughan *et al.*[15]).

trials. After drink ingestion, plasma volume increased in all trials, but the rate of recovery was slower when the KCl beverage was consumed. However, by the end of the study period, 6 hours after the end of the rehydration period, the mean (SD) increase was not different between trials and amounted to 7.5 (5.1)% for the glucose-electrolyte beverage, 9.7 (6.2)% for NaCl, 7.8 (5.1)% for the KCl solution, and 7.9 (2.0)% for the beverage containing all three components. Although there were differences in the total amount of electrolytes present in the drinks, there was no difference in the fraction of ingested fluid retained 6 hours after the drinks that contained electrolytes had been finished. It could be postulated, however, that as the beverage volume consumed was equivalent to the volume of sweat lost, subjects were dehydrated throughout the entire study, even after the drinking period. The volumes of urine excreted were close to basal levels, and significant further reductions in output may not have been possible when both sodium and potassium were ingested, over and above the reductions already induced when the sodium and potassium were ingested separately. This highlights the need to ensure that the volume of fluid consumed is sufficient not only to meet the fluid deficit incurred by sweating, but also to provide for ongoing urine and other losses.

Effects of the volume of fluid consumed

As obligatory urine losses persist even in the dehydrated state, it is clear that any drink consumed after exercise-induced or thermal sweating must be consumed in a volume greater than the volume of sweat that has been lost. To investigate the influence of drink volume on rehydration effectiveness, 12 male volunteers performed intermittent exercise in the heat to induce a level of dehydration equivalent to a mean of 2.06% of their initial body mass.[16] Over a 60 minute period begining 30 minutes after the end of exercise, drink volumes equivalent to 50, 100, 150 and 200% of the sweat loss were consumed. In addition, to investigate the possible interaction between beverage volume and its sodium content, six of the subjects consumed a relatively low sodium concentration drink (23 mmol/l), and six a moderately high sodium concentration drink (61 mmol/l). For 6 hours after the end of the drinking period, subjects consumed no other food or drink, and the entire volume of urine produced and excreted was collected and measured. When either the low or high sodium beverage was consumed, the urine volume produced was, not surprisingly, related to the beverage volume consumed, such that the smallest volumes were produced when 50% of the loss was consumed and the greatest when 200% of the loss was consumed (table 14.1).

As different drink volumes were consumed in each of the trials, a calculation of fluid balance status relative to the situation before the dehydration allows easier comparisons than a simple measure of the urine volume produced (table 14.1). With dehydration, individuals move into negative fluid balance; by drinking they return towards a positive fluid balance status, and only if the volume consumed is greater than the sweat loss do they become positively hydrated. Urine output moves them towards and/or into a state of negative fluid balance status again. As shown in table 14.1, subjects were significantly hypohydrated when they consumed a volume equivalent to only half their sweat loss irrespective of the drink composition. With a drink volume equivalent to that of the sweat loss, subjects were also hypohydrated at this time, but significantly less so when the higher sodium beverage had been consumed, confirming the effectiveness of sodium at promoting rehydration. When a drink volume double the sweat loss was

Table 14.1 Volume of urine produced after ingestion of varying volumes (representing 50, 100, 150, or 200% of fluid loss) of drinks with low (23 mmol/l) or high (61 mmol/l) sodium content and calculated increase in plasma volume relative to the dehydrated value (0%). Values are mean (SD) or median (range) as appropriate. For net fluid balance: 0=euhydrated, +=hyperhydrated, −=hypohydrated

Drink volume as a percentage of fluid loss	Fluid intake			
Measure	50%	100%	150%	200%
Sodium concentration 23 mmol/l				
Sweat loss (ml)	1490 (73)	1450 (73)	1500 (135)	1460 (98)
Drink volume (ml)	746 (42)	1448 (73)	2255 (203)	2927 (198)
6 hour urine volume (ml)	135 (114 to 240)	493 (181 to 731)	867 (263 to 1191)	1361 (1014 to 1984)
6 hour net fluid balance (ml)	−909 (−1011 to −835)	−528 (−799 to −205)	−128 (−441 to 380)	−135 (−503 to 426)
Increase in plasma volume (%)	3.6 (2.9)	6.7 (5.1)	8.6 (4.7)	11.0 (4.4)
Sodium concentration 61 mmol/l				
Sweat loss (ml)	1530 (159)	1510 (140)	1500 (120)	1510 (164)
Drink volume (ml)	758 (81)	1522 (142)	2243 (176)	3180 (348)
6 hour urine volume (ml)	144 (124 to 162)	260 (137 to 376)	602 (350 to 994)	1001 (714 to 1425)
6 hour net fluid balance (ml)	−958 (−1018 to −826)	−286 (−415 to −159)	+111 (−379 to 394)	+427 (−139 to 828)
Increase in plasma volume (%)	7.9 (3.2)	10.9 (2.2)	12.4 (2.7)	13.9 (6.9)

consumed, subjects were still slightly hypohydrated 6 hours after drink ingestion when it had a low sodium concentration and indeed they were in a similar condition to when they drank the same beverage in a volume of only 150% of their sweat loss. With the high sodium drink, subjects had retained enough of the fluid to maintain them in a state of hyperhydration 6 hours after drink ingestion when they consumed either 150% or 200% of their sweat loss, and the excess retained would eventually be lost by urine production or by further sweat loss if the individual commenced exercise or moved to a warm environment. Calculated plasma volume changes indicated a decrease of about 5.3% with dehydration. At the end of the study period, the general pattern, irrespective of which drink had been consumed, was for the increases in plasma volume to be a direct function of the volume of fluid consumed; in addition, the increase tended to be greater for those individuals who ingested the high sodium drink.

Effects of solid food and fluid consumption

In many situations it is not uncommon to consume solid food between exercise bouts, and indeed in most situations it probably should be encouraged. We undertook a further study in which eight volunteers (five men, three women) dehydrated by 2.1% of their body mass by exercising in the heat and then, over a 60 minute period starting 30 minutes after the end of exercise, consumed either a solid meal plus virtually electrolyte free flavoured water or a commercially available sports drink;[17] the volume of fluid contained within the meal plus water was the same as the volume of sports drink consumed. For 6 hours after the end of the eating and/or drinking period, the entire volume of urine produced and excreted was collected. The volume of urine produced after food plus fluid ingestion was significantly less than that when the drink alone was consumed (table 14.2). It was calculated that plasma volume decreased by 5.4% with dehydration over all trials. The plasma volume increased after rehydration in all trials, and there was no difference in the mean (SD) increase between the food plus fluid trial (11.7 (2.0)%) and drink only trial (13.2 (4.2)%). The quantity of water consumed with both these rehydration methods was the same, but the meal had a greater electrolyte content (table 14.2), and it seems most likely that the greater efficacy of the meal plus water treatment in restoring whole body water balance was a consequence of the greater total cation content.

Table 14.2 Volume of urine produced following drink ingestion. Also shown is the fluid volume consumed and the quantities of major electrolytes ingested. Values are mean (SD) or median (range) as appropriate

Measure	Meal+water	Sports drink
Fluid volume (ml)	2076 (371)	2042 (373)
Electrolytes ingested (mmol)		
Na^+	63 (11)	43 (8)
K^+	21 (3)	7 (3)
6 hour urine volume (ml)	665 (396 to 1190)	934 (550 to 1403)

Alcohol consumption

Many people advise against the consumption of alcohol and caffeine containing beverages when fluid replacement is desired because they have been shown, at least in some circumstances, to act as diuretics. However, it is obvious that many people enjoy consuming these types of beverages in many circumstances. We therefore undertook a study to investigate the effect of consuming alcohol after exercise in the heat sufficient to induce dehydration equivalent to 2.01 (0.06)% of body mass.[18,19] Over a 60 minute period beginning 30 minutes after the end of exercise, subjects consumed a volume equivalent to 150% of their mass loss of drinks containing 0, 1, 2 or 4% alcohol; the drink composition was identical in all other respects. The volume of urine produced and excreted for the 6 hours after drink ingestion was measured and was found to be related to the quantity of alcohol consumed, with a larger volume the more alcohol that was consumed (table 14.3). However, despite the definite tendency for the urinary output to increase with increasing alcohol, only with the 4% beverage did the increased value approach significance. The calculated decrease in plasma volume with dehydration was about 7.6% across all trials. With rehydration the plasma volume increased, but the rate of increase seemed to be related to the quantity of alcohol consumed; at the end of the study period, the mean (SD) increase in plasma

Table 14.3 Volume of drink consumed and fraction of fluid retained 6 hours after ingestion of drink of various alcoholic strengths (0, 1, 2, or 4%). Values are mean (SD)

Measure	0%	1%	2%	4%
Drink volume (ml)	2178 (191)	2240 (147)	2275 (154)	2155 (125)
Fraction of fluid retained (%)	59.3 (15.7)	53.1 (11.0)	50.0 (16.2)	40.7 (13.7)

volume relative to the dehydrated value was 8.1 (3.2)% with 0% alcohol, 7.4 (2.7)% with 1%, 6.0 (3.4)% with 2%, and 5.3 (3.4)% with 4%.

Voluntary beverage consumption

We have already demonstrated and discussed the need for drinking more than the sweat volume lost to have a chance of rehydrating effectively. However, in practice it is left to the discretion of an individual how much they consume and what they choose to drink. In a study to examine the effect of palatability, together with the solute content of beverages, in promoting rehydration after sweat loss, eight men exercised in the heat to lose 2.1% of their mass.[20] Over a 2 hour period after exercise, subjects were allowed to drink ad libitum; the drinks they received, each on a separate occasion, were a glucose-electrolyte beverage, aerated water, a commercial sports drink, and an orange juice/lemonade mixture. Subjects drank a greater volume of the sports drink and orange juice/lemonade mixture, the taste of which was perceived as being more pleasant (table 14.4). As different volumes of drinks were consumed, a calculation of fluid balance status relative to the situation before the dehydration allows easiest comparisons; with dehydration, individuals move into a negative fluid balance status, and by drinking they move towards a positive fluid balance status, and, only if the volume consumed is greater than the sweat loss do they become positively hydrated, and urine production and excretion moves them towards and/or into the negative fluid balance status again. By consuming a greater volume, individuals give themselves a better chance of effectively rehydrating, and therefore the palatability of drinks, together with their composition, should be considered when free choice is given to individuals, as indeed occurs in most situations.

Menstrual cycle effects: concerns for female athletes

Almost all previous investigations into rehydration after exercise, as with so much human physiology, have been concerned exclusively with men. This is in part a consequence of the possibility that the steroid hormones, which are subject to cyclical variation in women, may have an influence on fluid balance, and the wish to avoid this confounding factor. We therefore undertook

267

Table 14.4 Volume of drink consumed and net fluid balance 4 hours after rehydration. Values are mean (SD). For net fluid balance: 0 = euhydrated, + = hyperhydrated, − = hypohydrated

Measure	Glucose 90 mmol/l + sodium 60 mmol/l + potassium 24 mmol/l	Aerated water	Sports drink (sodium 24 mmol/l + potassium 4 mmol/l)	Orange/lemonade (sodium 2 mmol/l + potassium 24 mmol/l)
Drink volume (ml)	1796 (758)	1750 (560)	2492 (661)	2488 (233)
4 hour net fluid balance (ml)	−123 (615)	−474 (333)	−135 (358)	45 (238)

Table 14.5   Volume of urine produced after drink ingestion at various stages of the menstrual cycle. Also shown is the volume of drink consumed. Values are mean (SD) or median (range) as appropriate

Measure	2 days before the onset of menses	5 days after the onset of menses	19 days after the onset of menses
Drink volume (ml)	1662 (195)	1550 (172)	1392 (241)
6 hour urine volume (ml)	714 (469 to 750)	476 (433 to 639)	534 (195 to 852)

a specific study to establish whether or not there is an acute effect of these hormones on fluid balance in the few hours after exercise-induced sweat loss.[21] Five women, each with a regular menstrual cycle, exercised in the heat to dehydrate themselves by 1.8% of their body mass. They did this at three different stages of their menstrual cycle (2 days before, and 5 and 19 days after the onset of menses), and, over a 60 minute period beginning 30 minutes after the end of exercise, they consumed the same quantity of the same beverage on each occasion; the volume consumed was 150% of the mass loss and the drink, a commercially available sports drink, was the same in all trials. For 6 hours after the end of the rehydration period, the entire volume of urine excreted was collected and measured. There was no difference in the volume of urine produced (table 14.5) and hence in the volume of the ingested fluid that was retained at the different stages of the menstrual cycle. These results suggest that the acute replacement of volume losses incurred by sweat loss due to exercising in the heat are not affected by the normal regular menstrual cycle. Therefore women seem not to be disadvantaged when rapid and complete restoration of exercise-induced sweat loss is required.

Performance effects

The studies described above have used restoration of fluid balance as an index of recovery after exercise-induced dehydration, but many other factors are involved in the restoration of exercise capacity. To investigate some of the factors that influence recovery of performance capacity, a further experiment was undertaken; the study design was similar to that used previously, but subjects performed a standardised exercise test 4 hours after the end of the rehydration period. Rehydration was achieved by administration of plain water, a flavoured placebo, or a drink containing carbo-hydrate (68 g/l) and electrolytes (25 mmol/l sodium, 4 mmol/l potassium) in a volume equal to 1.5 times the sweat loss of about

269

2% of body mass. The performance test consisted of an incremental cycling exercise test continued to the point of exhaustion.

The glucose-electrolyte test drink had an electrolyte content similar to that of most commercial sports drinks, and there was a tendency (P = 0.073) for the median (range) cumulative urine output over the 4 hour recovery period to be less in this trial (1162 (816–1429) ml) than in the placebo (1470 (1228–1667) ml) or water (1395 (954–1555) ml) trials. This is consistent with the results of the previous trials and confirms that this low level of electrolytes will give a small increase in the volume of fluid retained over this time scale.

All subjects recorded their best exercise performance, measured as the time to fatigue, on the carbohydrate-electrolyte trial, with a mean (SD) exercise time of 18.00 (2.43) minutes compared with 16.42 (2.15) minutes after consuming the plain water and 17.00 (1.76) minutes in the placebo trial. These results suggest that there is a benefit from the addition of electrolytes and glucose to drinks ingested after exercise but cannot distinguish between the various possible mechanisms that might be involved. It is, however, worth noting that there were no differences in the blood glucose concentration at any time between trials despite the ingestion of a substantial amount of carbohydrate on one of the trials. There is clearly a need for more systematic studies to resolve the outstanding questions.

Discussion and conclusions

Rapid and complete restoration of fluid balance after exercise is an important part of the recovery process and becomes even more important in hot humid conditions. The choice of drink to be consumed after exercise may and indeed should be different depending on the individual and their particular circumstances. Replacement of substrate in addition to water and electrolyte losses may be of concern in the period after exercise in preparation for a further bout of exercise. In terms of sustaining life, substrate (muscle and liver glycogen) depletion is unlikely to have an adverse effect in an otherwise healthy individual, but water depletion, if not reversed, may have serious consequences. Moderate levels of dehydration (2–3% reductions in body mass) will impair performance, and when an Olympic medal is at stake it might be wise to assume that even very low levels of dehydration may have a negative impact on performance; it is certainly the case that hypohydration of only 1% of body mass has a measurable effect on the thermoregulatory response to exercise.[3] Severe dehydration (losses of more than 6–7% of body mass) can result in a life threatening situation, and this scenario is rendered more likely when the ambient temperature is high.[1] Such extremes of water depletion should not occur in any athlete in the case of sports competition if a conscious effort is made to ensure adequate fluid replacement. However, even if the health concerns are ignored, the effects on performance of a fluid decrement should be enough to persuade all individuals to attempt to remain fully hydrated at all times, and particularly to ensure that they begin each bout of exercise in a water replete state.

Team doctors, coaches, and athletes must be aware of the factors

---

Box 14.1   Restoration of fluid and electrolyte balance after exercise

- Fluid balance can be effectively achieved only if a fluid volume greater than the sweat volume lost is consumed. This is necessary to surmount the obligatory urine losses
- Restoration of water losses as sweat will be achieved only if sodium is consumed in addition to water after exercise. The sodium should ideally be present in moderately high concentrations (for example, 50 mmol/l)
- Plain water may be sufficient to promote fluid balance recovery after exercise-induced dehydration if solid food is also consumed. The electrolytes necessary to promote fluid retention will be consumed as the food
- While not recommended to be the rehydration beverage of choice, in most situations, the diuretic effect of alcohol seems to be blunted when consumed by individuals dehydrated as a result of exercise-induced sweat production. To rehydrate effectively, however, a large volume must be consumed, and therefore the alcohol content must be low (not greater than 2%)
- In the field situation, when athletes chose when and how much to drink, a drink perceived as pleasant tasting is likely to be consumed in greater volumes than an unpleasant tasting drink and therefore is more likely to be effective at rehydrating the athlete
- While not essential for long term fluid balance restoration after exercise-induced dehydration, a source of carbohydrate may usefully be included in relatively low concentrations (up to 6%) in fluid replacement beverages to provide a substrate for muscle glycogen restoration or an energy source for exercise performance

271

that influence rehydration and of the electrolyte content of the available drinks. The amount of electrolytes lost in sweat is highly variable between individuals, and, although the optimum drink may be achieved by matching electrolyte loss with equal quantities from the drink, this is virtually impossible in a practical situation. Sweat composition varies considerably between individuals but also varies with time during exercise and will be further influenced by the state of acclimation.[22] However, a moderate excess of salt intake would appear to be beneficial as far as hydration status is concerned without any detrimental effects on health provided that fluid intake is in excess of sweat loss and that renal function is not impaired. Concerns over the possible adverse effects of a high salt intake have led some athletes to restrict dietary salt intake.[23] For the athletes with large sweat losses, sodium loss will be correspondingly high; loss of 5 litres of sweat with a sodium content of 50 mmol/l requires ingestion of almost 15 g of sodium chloride to restore balance. This amount of sweat can easily be lost in 2–3 hours of hard training or match practice in hot humid conditions. Although the diet will make a major contribution to replacement, normal daily salt intake from food is only about 6–8 g for the United Kingdom population, about half of whom rarely or never add salt to food at the table.[24] There is clearly a high risk of salt deficit when losses are high, unless a conscious effort is made to increase intake.

It is clear from the results described above, as well as those of many other studies, that rehydration after exercise can be achieved only if sweat electrolyte losses as well as water are replaced. The oral rehydration solution recommended by the World Health Organisation for the treatment of acute diarrhoea has a sodium content of 60–90 mmol/l, reflecting the high sodium losses that may occur in some types of diarrhoea.[25] In contrast, the sodium content of most of the major commercial sports drinks is in the range 10–25 mmol/l[22] and is even lower in some products that are marketed as sports drinks. Most commonly consumed soft drinks contain virtually no sodium, and these drinks are therefore unsuitable when the need for rehydration is crucial. The problem with a high sodium concentration in beverages is that it may exert a negative effect on taste, resulting in reduced consumption. It is equally clear, however, that drinks with a low sodium content are ineffective, and they will also reduce the stimulus to drink.[26]

It can generally be concluded that to achieve effective rehydration after exercise in the heat or heat exposure sufficient to cause sweat loss, the rehydration beverage should contain moderately high levels of sodium (at least 50 mmol/l), plus possibly some potassium; a source of substrate is not necessary for rehydration, although a small amount of carbohydrate (<2%) may improve the rate of intestinal uptake of sodium and water. The volume of beverage consumed should be greater than the volume of sweat lost to make provision for the ongoing obligatory urine losses. Therefore the palatability of the beverage is of importance; many individuals may lose substantial amounts of sweat and will therefore have to consume large amounts of fluid to replace them, and this is more likely to be achieved if the taste is perceived as being pleasant. Although we have shown that water alone is adequate for rehydration purposes when food that replaces the electrolytes lost in sweat is also consumed, there are many situations where intake of solid food is avoided. This is particularly true in weight category sports where the interval between the weigh-in and competition is short but is also the case in events where only a few hours intervene between succeeding rounds of the competition.

The above studies were carried out in a systematic way and did not attempt to replicate real life situations where many other factors will intervene. After the exercise in the heat, individuals were removed to a relatively cool indoor environment and undertook no further exercise. For athletes living in training camps or in the village at major championship events where the outside environment is hot for the majority of most days, it is highly likely that they will be unable to avoid some exposure to a thermally stressful environment. Team support staff, officials, and spectators will also be at risk. All must be aware of the need to maintain fluid balance and should consider rehydration after passive heat exposure as well as after exercise. Indicators such as a reduction in urine output and failure to maintain body mass are more reliable measures of dehydration than the feeling of thirst.

1 Sutton JR. Clinical implications of fluid imbalance. In: Gisolfi CV, Lamb DR, eds. *Perspectives in exercise science and sports science. Vol 3. Fluid homeostasis during exercise.* Carmel: Benchmark Press, 1990:425–56.
2 Galloway SDR, Shirreffs SM, Leiper JB, Maughan RJ. Exercise in the heat: factors limiting exercise capacity and methods for improving heat tolerance. *Sports Exerc Inj*, 1997;**3**:19–24.
3 Sawka MN, Pandolf KB. Effects of body water loss on physiological function

and exercise performance. In: Gisolfi CV, Lamb DR, eds. *Perspectives in exercise science and sports science. Vol 3. Fluid homeostasis during exercise.* Carmel: Benchmark Press, 1990:1–38.

4 Horswill CA. Physiology and nutrition for wrestling. In: Lamb DR, Knuttgen HG, Murray R, *et al.*, eds. *Perspectives in exercise science and sports science. Vol 7. Physiology and nutrition for competitive sport.* Carmel: Cooper, 1994:131–80.

5 Costill DL, Sparks KE. Rapid fluid replacement following thermal dehydration. *J Appl Physiol* 1973;**34**:299–303.

6 Gonzáles-Alonso J, Heaps CL, Coyle EF. Rehydration after exercise with common beverages and water. *Int J Sports Med* 1992;**13**:399–406.

7 Nielsen B, Sjogaard G, Uglevig J, Knudsen B, Dohlmann B. Fluid balance in exercise dehydration and rehydration with different glucose-electrolyte drinks. *Eur J Appl Physiol* 1986;**55**:318–25.

8 Coyle EF, Coggan AR. Effectiveness of carbohydrate feeding in delaying fatigue during prolonged exercise. *Sports Med* 1984;**1**:446–58.

9 Lamb DR, Brodowicz GR. Optimal use of fluids of varying formulations to minimise exercise-induced disturbances in homeostasis. *Sports Med* 1986;**3**:247–74.

10 Maughan RJ. Carbohydrate-electrolyte solutions during prolonged exercise. In: Lamb DR, Williams MH, eds. *Perspectives in exercise science and sports science. Ergogenics: the enhancement of sport performance.* Carmel: Benchmark Press, 1991:35–85.

11 Murray R. The effects of consuming carbohydrate-electrolyte beverages on gastric emptying and fluid absorption during and following exercise. *Sports Med* 1987;**4**:322–51.

12 Shirreffs SM, Maughan RJ. Volume repletion after exercise-induced volume depletion in humans: replacement of water and sodium losses. *Am J Physiol* 1999;**274**:868–75F.

13 Dill DB, Costill DL. Calculation of percentage changes in volumes of blood, plasma, and red cells in dehydration. *J Appl Physiol* 1974;**37**:247–8.

14 Nadel ER, Mack GW, Nose H. Influence of fluid replacement beverages on body fluid homeostasis during exercise and recovery. In: Gisolfi CV, Lamb DR, eds. *Perspectives in exercise science and sports medicine. Vol 3. Fluid homeostasis during exercise.* Carmel: Benchmark Press, 1990:181–205.

15 Maughan RJ, Owen JH, Shirreffs SM, Leiper JB. Post-exercise rehydration in man: effects of electrolyte addition to ingested fluids. *Eur J Appl Physiol* 1994;**69**:209–15.

16 Shirreffs SM, Taylor AJ, Leiper JB, Maughan RJ. Post-exercise rehydration in man: effects of volume consumed and sodium content of ingested fluids. *Med Sci Sports Exerc* 1996;**28**:1260–71.

17 Maughan RJ, Leiper JB, Shirreffs SM. Restoration of fluid balance after exercise-induced dehydration: effects of food and fluid intake. *Eur J Appl Physiol* 1996;**73**:317–25.

18 Shirreffs SM, Maughan RJ. The effect of alcohol consumption on fluid retention following exercise-induced dehydration in man. *J Physiol (Lond)* 1995;**489**:33–4P.

19 Shirreffs SM, Maughan RJ. The effect of alcohol consumption on the restoration of blood and plasma volume following exercise-induced dehydration in man. *J Physiol (Lond)* 1996;**491**:64–5P.

20 Maughan RJ, Leiper JB. Post-exercise rehydration in man: effects of voluntary intake of four different beverages. *Med Sci Sports Exerc* 1993;**25**:12S.

21 Maughan RJ, McArthur M, Shirreffs SM. Influence of menstrual status on fluid replacement after exercise-induced dehydration in healthy young women. *Br J Sports Med* 1996;**30**:41–7.

22 Maughan RJ. Fluid and electrolyte loss and replacement in exercise. In: Harries M, Williams C, Stanish WD, Micheli LJ, eds. *Oxford textbook of sports medicine.*

New York: Oxford University Press, 1994:82–93.

23 Bergeron MF. Heat cramps during tennis: a case report. *Int J Sport Nutr* 1996;**6**:62–8.

24 Gregory J, Foster K, Tyler H, Wiseman M. *The dietary and nutritional survey of British adults.* London: HMSO, 1990.

25 Walker-Smith JA. Recommendations for oral rehydration solutions for use in the treatment of diarrhoeal disease in European children. *J Pediatr Gastroenterol Nutr* 1992;**14**:113–15.

26 Nose H, Mack GW, Shi X, Nadel ER. Role of osmolality and plasma volume during rehydration in humans. *J Appl Physiol* 1988;**65**:325–31.

Multiple choice questions

1 Exercise in the heat is likely to cause which one of the following:
   (a) Dehydration as a result of sweat secretion and evaporation
   (b) A reduction in circulating blood volume
   (c) A reduction in exercise performance
   (d) All of the above

2 The purpose of sweat secretion during exercise is:
   (a) To induce exercise-induced dehydration
   (b) To provide a means for the body to regulate core temperature
   (c) To reduce blood volume
   (d) To induce thirst to stimulate beverage consumption

3 Consumption of which electrolyte is essential to the postexercise recovery of fluid balance status after exercise-induced dehydration?
   (a) Magnesium
   (b) Potassium
   (c) Sodium
   (d) Chloride

4 What volume of beverage should be consumed after exercise resulting in a fluid balance deficit to optimise the restoration of euhydration?
   (a) Any volume that the athlete can comfortably consume
   (b) Half of the sweat volume lost
   (c) A volume the same as the sweat volume lost
   (d) A volume greater than the sweat volume lost

275

5 Plain tap water is a sufficient rehydration beverage if:
   (a) It is consumed in a sufficiently large quantity
   (b) It is consumed in a sufficiently small quantity
   (c) It has flavouring added
   (d) It is consumed together with an electrolyte source

Answers are on p. 365.

15 Physiological adaptation to environmental hypoxia: implications for exercise performance

D M Bailey, B Davies

Introduction

Paul Bert was the first investigator to show that acclimatisation to a chronically reduced inspiratory partial pressure of oxygen (P_1O_2) invoked a series of central and peripheral adaptations that served to maintain adequate tissue oxygenation in healthy skeletal muscle,[1] physiological adaptations that have been subsequently implicated in the improvement in exercise performance during altitude acclimatisation. However, it was not until half a century later that scientists suggested that the additive stimulus of environmental hypoxia could potentially compound the normal physiological adaptations to endurance training and accelerate performance improvements after return to sea level. This has stimulated an exponential increase in scientific research, and, since 1984, 22 major reviews have summarised the physiological implications of altitude training for both aerobic and anaerobic performance at altitude and after return to sea level. Of these reviews, only eight have specifically focused on physical performance changes after return to sea level,[2-9] the most comprehensive of which was recently written by Wolski et al.[9]

Few reviews have considered the potentially less favourable physiological responses to moderate altitude exposure, which include decreases in absolute training intensity,[10] decreased plasma volume,[11] depression of haemopoiesis and increased haemolysis,[12] increases in sympathetically mediated glycogen depletion at altitude,[13] and increased respiratory muscle work after return to sea level.[14] In addition, there is a risk of developing more serious medical complications at altitude, which include acute mountain sickness, pulmonary oedema, cardiac arrhythmias, and cerebral hypoxia.[15] The possible implications of changes in immune function at altitude have also been largely ignored, despite accumulating evidence of hypoxia mediated immunodepression.[16]

In general, altitude training has been shown to improve performance at altitude, whereas no unequivocal evidence exists to support the claim that performance at sea level is improved. Table 15.1 summarises the theoretical advantages and disadvantages of altitude training for sea level performance.

This chapter summarises the physiological rationale for altitude training as a means of enhancing endurance performance after return to sea level. Factors that have been shown to affect the acclimatisation process and the subsequent implications for exercise performance at sea level will also be discussed.

Table 15.1 Physiological changes during altitude acclimatisation in native lowlanders; time course and theoretical implications for exercise performance at sea level

Physiological advantages	Response time	Physiological disadvantages	Response time
Increased free fatty acid mobilisation	Weeks	Increased ventilation	Immediate
Increased haemoglobin	Days	Decreased cardiac output	Days
Increased capillarity	Months/ years?	Decreased blood flow	Days
Increased oxidative enzyme activity	Weeks	Immunodepression	Immediate?/days
Increased mitochondrial volume	Weeks	Increased oxidative stress and tissue damage	Immediate
		Increased dehydration	Immediate
		Jet lag	Immediate
		Decreased training intensity	Immediate
		Acute mountain sickness	Days
		Sunburn due to increased ultraviolet B (290–320 nm)	Immediate
		Catecholamine mediated glycogen depletion	Days/weeks
		Increased haemolysis	Weeks

Method

Studies were located by using five major databases, which included Medline, Embase, Science Citation Index, Sports Discus, and Sport, in addition to extensive hand searching and cross referencing. All published English language studies, dating back from the present day to 1956, that included physiological measurements during exercise before and after hypoxic training were incorporated in the overall analysis. Ninety one investigations were selected, which included 772 hypoxically trained experimental and 209 normoxically trained control subjects.

The investigations were subdivided according to whether a normoxically trained control group was incorporated into the experimental design. Other classifications were made depending on the characteristics of the hypoxic stimulus, which included type (normobaric or hypobaric hypoxia; continuous or intermittent), duration, and magnitude (calculated ambient PO_2), and timing of physiological testing after the descent to sea level.

The continued popularity of altitude training has been influenced by two factors. Firstly, hypoxia in itself increases blood haemoglobin (Hb) concentration, which has been shown to improve endurance performance. Secondly, several of the best endurance runners in the world have originated from East African countries that are based at altitude (1500–2000 m). Is it possible that either living and/or training at altitude may contribute to their running success?

Physiological rationale for altitude training

Autologous blood reinfusion and endurance performance

One of the most documented physiological adaptations to a reduced P_IO_2 is the increased release of erythropoietin, which causes a transient increase in red blood cell mass.[17] The implications of secondary polycythaemia to both submaximal and maximal indices of endurance performance have been clearly shown by studies that have artificially induced erythrocythaemia after either autologous blood reinfusion[18] or subcutaneous injections of recombinant human erythropoietin.[19,20] Table 15.2 summarises the major research findings. It has been reported that absolute maximal oxygen uptake ($\dot{V}O_2MAX$) values are increased by about 200 ml/min per g/dl increase in Hb, irrespective of the methods by which polycythaemia is induced.[21]

Table 15.2   Effects of autologous blood reinfusion on $\dot{V}O_2$MAX

Author/reference	Volume of blood reinfused (ml)	Change in Hb after reinfusion (%)	Change in $\dot{V}O_2$MAX after reinfusion (%)
Ekblom[19]	1350	+9*	+8*
Celsing[21]	2250	+11	+7**
Buick[23]	900	+8**	+5**
Spriet[24]	1200	NR	+7*
Williams[25]	920	+7**	NR
Goforth[26]	760	+4*	+11**
Robertson[27]	750	+28*	+13*
Robertson[28]	475	+16*	+10*
Thompson[29]	1000	+12*	+11*
Sawka[30]	600	+10*	+11*
Robertson[31]	475	+16*	+10**

*Significantly different from before infusion (P<0.05).
**Significantly different from before reinfusion (P<0.01).
NR not reported.

However, the use of blood doping as an ergogenic aid is considered unethical and potentially dangerous and is banned by the International Olympic Committee.[22]

Physiological adaptations of the native highlander: a superior athlete?

Figure 15.1 illustrates the apparently disproportionate running success of the native highlander. This figure represents data obtained from athletes who were born and raised at a median altitude of 2000 m above sea level, which represents less than 1% of the world population. This phenomenon has prompted several comparative investigations into what, if any, physiological adaptations mediated by hypoxia could contribute to their superiority in distance running events. Much interest has focused on the four steps of the oxygen transport system—namely, alveolar ventilation, lung diffusion, circulatory oxygen transport, and tissue oxygen extraction. Studies have shown that the native highlander is characterised by a larger pulmonary diffusion capacity[32] and adaptations in the structural and metabolic organisation of skeletal muscle that result in a tighter coupling between ATP hydrolysis and oxidative phosphorylation.[33] These are the major factors that facilitate oxygen transport and utilisation. The significance of these adaptations has been elucidated in a series of investigations that have reported higher values for $\dot{V}O_2$MAX,[34] power output,[35] arterial

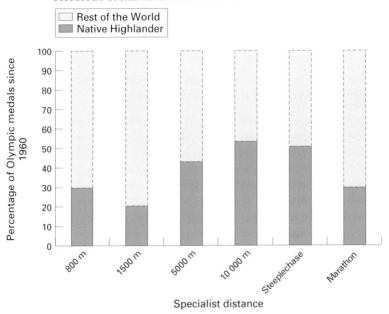

Fig 15.1   Percentage of Olympic medals for middle and long distance running events won by native highlanders since 1960.

oxygen saturation,[36] cerebral oxygen delivery[37] during maximal exercise and decreased blood lactate[33,35] and ammonia concentrations[38] for a given submaximal work rate.

To what extent these physiological adaptations are acquired as the result of inheritance or hypobaric hypoxia is not well defined. The influence of genetic factors on quantitative oxygen transport was recently investigated in a unique study by Beall et al.[39] They identified a major gene that enhances arterial oxygen saturation in sedentary Tibetan natives. The physiological significance of this was shown by Niermeyer et al. who concluded that genetic adaptations to hypobaric hypoxia resulted in improved oxygenation and conferred resistance to subacute infantile mountain sickness.[40] These adaptations were more pronounced in a cohort of Tibetan newborns whose ancestors have resided at altitude for 50 000 to 100 000 years, in comparison with Han newborns whose ancestors had resided at altitude for only 45 years.[41] In general, these findings would suggest that a lifetime or perhaps generations of altitude

281

exposure are responsible for the biological distinctiveness of the high altitude population.

Altitude training and sea level endurance performance in native lowlanders

Table 15.3 summarises the effects of altitude training on sea level endurance performance. The weight of scientific evidence does not support the potentiating effects of altitude training. However, it is becoming clearer that a number of methodological deficiencies may preclude the potential synergistic effects of hypoxia and physical exercise, the physiological implications of which will be discussed in the following sections.

Intensity and duration of the hypoxic stimulus and associated haematological adaptation

There is still much controversy about the optimal altitude and duration required for athletes to train in an attempt to optimise endurance performance at sea level. Much attention has focused on the erythropoietic response to hypoxia and subsequent haematological adaptation. Considering the inverse relation between PO_2 and resting Hb concentration,[78] it would seem logical that the higher the athlete can train the better. However, other factors that inhibit exercise performance are exacerbated with a reduction in PO_2. Acute mountain sickness presents at altitudes above 2000 to 3000 m,[79] with the possibility of the elite athlete suffering physiological symptoms at even lower altitudes.[15] Prolonged exposure to altitudes above 4500 m has been shown to result in a reduction in muscle mass, the underlying physiological mechanisms for which have been recently reviewed by Kayser.[80] Finally, the effects of training at a lower PO_2 may result in a reduction in work rate, so that detraining may override the potential benefits of altitude acclimatisation.[81]

Hypoxia and detraining

A recent study has shown that $\dot{V}O_2MAX$ is significantly reduced at an altitude as low as 610 m above sea level in elite endurance athletes.[82] This is a phenomenon peculiar to about 50% of trained subjects, with $\dot{V}O_2MAX$ values of above 65 ml/kg per min or 4 litres/

Table 15.3 Effects of hypoxic training on sea level endurance performance

Hypoxic stimulus	Altitude (m)	Exposure time (days)	Time tested after altitude (days)	Submaximal improvement	Change in $\dot{V}O_2$ MAX (%)	Control group
Potentiating effects						
IH[42]	2000	28	4	ND	+13†	Yes
IH[43]	4500	6	1/7	ND	+6†/+5†	No
CH[44]	1300–2500	28	1	Yes†	+4†	No
CH[45]	1900	21	1/14	Yes†	NS/NS	No
CH[46]	2100–2700	14	2	Yes†	NS	No
CH[47]	2300	23	3/21	Yes†	+8†/+10†	No
CH[48]	2500	28	7	ND	+6†	No
IH[49]	3049–4268	23	3–4	Yes†	NS	No
CH[50]	3800	35	14	ND	+14†	No
IH[51]	4020	21/28	1	Yes†	+8‡/+26‡	No
CH[52]	1250–2500	28	7	Yes†	+4†	Yes
IH[53]	2300	21–28	1	Yes†	NS	Yes
IH[54]	2300	28	1–2	Yes†	ND	Yes
IH[55]	4000	70	1	Yes†	NS	Yes
No potentiating effects						
CH[47]	2300	14	1	No	NS	No
CH[56]	1695–2700	7	4	ND	NS	No
CH[57]	2240	20	4/22	ND	+6/+9*	No
CH[58]	2300	42	4–5	No	NS	No
CH[59]	2300	70	5	ND	NS	No
CH[60]	2800	10	2–4	No	+7*	No
CH[61]	3090	17	1	ND	NS	No
CH[62]	3110	21	7	ND	-5*	No
CH[63]	4000	48–63	2–15	No	NS	No
IH[64]	4000	21	1	ND	NS	No
CH[38]	2000	14	6/12	ND	NS/NS	Yes
CH[65]	1600–1800	18–28	7	ND	NS	Yes
CH[66]	1640	28	20	No	NS	Yes
CH[67]	1700–2000	28	7	No	NS	Yes
CH[68]	2300	21	1	No	NS	Yes
IH[69]	2250	28	1	ND	+17.5*	Yes
IH[69]	3450	28	1	ND	+10.0*	Yes
IH[70]	2500	28	1	No	NS	Yes
IH[71]	2500	35	1	ND	NS	Yes
CH[72]	2600	11	1	ND	NS	Yes
IH[73]	3100	19	6	No	NS	Yes
IH[74]	3345	42	1	ND	NS	Yes
IH[75]	4020	15	1	ND	NS	Yes
IH[76]	4100–5700	21	1	ND	NS	Yes
CH[77]	4300	28	1–5	ND	NS	Yes

CH = chronic hypobaria; IH = intermittent hypobaria; ND = no data.
*Level of significance not reported.
†Significantly different from pre-altitude value (P < 0.05).
‡Significantly different from pre-altitude value (P < 0.01).
NS = not significantly different from pre-altitude value (P > 0.05).

Box 15.1 Altitude training guidelines

Strategy	Physiological rationale
Check iron stores 3 weeks before the altitude sojourn. If serum ferritin concentration is >40 μg/l start oral supplementation (200 to 300 mg daily); if <40 μg/l consider parenteral treatment (100 mg/w). Continue iron supplementation during the altitude sojourn. Beware of constipation	Optimise haematological adaptation
Supplement with vitamin C (0.5–1 g/day) and vitamin E (100–500 mg; 3 times daily) and ensure an adequate intake of polyunsaturated fatty acids	Increase gastrointestinal iron uptake/minimise haemolysis and free radical-mediated tissue damage
Avoid sunburn at altitude because of increased ultraviolet radiation intensity	Minimise free-radical mediated oxidative stress/maintain thermoregulatory function
Ensure adequate fluid intake and monitor hydration status regularly (for example, via body mass or urine volume/colour)	Prevent dehydration
Ensure adequate carbohydrate intake (>8 g/kg/day)	Maintain glycogen stores due to increased glycolytic flux mediated by increased β adrenergic activity (in particular during the first days)
Ensure adequate protein intake (1.2–1.8 g/kg/day)/administration of either BCAA (20 g/day) or L-glutamine (5 g/day)	Prevent loss of skeletal muscle mass. Minimise "central fatigue" phenomenon". "Boost" immunoreactivity
Avoid "communal living" training camp (ensure separate eating/living quarters)	Minimise the spread of infectious illness
Avoid maximal exercise during the first 5 days of altitude exposure. *Do not* attempt to train at the same absolute intensity as that performed at sea level	Prevent "overtraining" response
Decrease running distance if the altitude terrain is radically different to that at sea level	Minimise the risks of physical injury

min.[83] These elite athletes develop more severe levels of arterial hypoxaemia during maximal and submaximal exercise than sedentary controls both under normoxic and hypoxic conditions.[84,85] Several mechanisms have been proposed to explain these findings, which include hypoventilation, venoarterial shunting, ventilation-perfusion inequality, and an alveolar-capillary diffusion limitation.[86,87]

These observations led early investigators to hypothesise that altitude exposure may result in a detraining response.[81] Daniels and Oldridge[59] have shown the importance of training intensity at altitude and its effects on sea level performance. They suggested that intermittent exposures to altitudes of 2300 to 3300 m and sea level optimised the balance between hypoxic acclimatisation and training intensity. Despite the experimental limitations of a single group design, two world records and 12 personal best times were recorded by athletes on return to sea level, which presented a reasonable endorsement for such an approach. However, from our experience, it is equally possible to have expected similar improvements in a control group training at sea level.[66]

The detraining effect induced during chronic exposure to hypobaric hypoxia has been quantified in a sequence of studies by Levine et al.[52,70] In their recent study,[52] 39 competitive runners were randomly assigned to four weeks of living high (2500 m) and training low (1250 m), living high (2500 m) and training high (2500 m), or living low (150 m) and training low (150 m). They showed that, although $\dot{V}O_2$MAX values significantly improved 5 km race performance times by 4% in the two altitude trained groups, the running velocity that corresponded to $\dot{V}O_2$MAX and the ventilatory threshold at sea level were significantly improved only in the group that lived high and trained low. An unusual finding was that 5 km performance time was 31 seconds slower in the sea level control group, which would suggest that the training stimulus was not absolutely controlled during the experimental period. Nevertheless, it was concluded that the potentiating effects of altitude training were due to a high altitude acclimatisation effect (improved haematology) and a low altitude training effect (increased training intensity). Thus the authors advocated the practice of living high and training low as the optimal approach to altitude training. This has popularised the use of "altitude houses", recently developed in Finland, which are portable hypobaric chambers used by elite athletes, who alternate living and sleeping at simulated altitude with normobaric training.[88] However, the effectiveness of this procedure should at present be considered equivocal, and further scientific investigation is warranted to endorse this approach to altitude training.

Concept of a critical PO_2 and haematological adaptation

Few athletes can afford the costs inherent in a "live high, train low" approach to altitude training. Therefore is it possible that a "threshold" altitude exists that optimises the benefits of haemato-logical acclimatisation and minimises the negative effects of detraining? Weil et al.[89] have presented the most comprehensive evidence indicating the existence of such a threshold, albeit in sedentary highland natives (B Levine, personal communication). They identified a biphasic relation between the arterial partial pressure of oxygen (PaO_2) and red blood cell mass and shown a clear inflection point at a "critical" PaO_2 of 67 mm Hg, equivalent to an interpolated arterial oxygen saturation of 92%. This point corresponds to the steeper portion of the oxygen-Hb dissociation curve. The equivalent PO_2 would equate to about 135 mm Hg, which is comparable with an altitude of 2200–2500 m above sea level required to stimulate sufficient haemopoiesis at rest to influence endurance performance.[4] However, it has been shown that the decrement in $\dot{V}O_2MAX$ measured in hypobaric hypoxia is directly proportional to $\dot{V}O_2MAX$ measured in normoxia.[90] This would suggest that elite athletes are more prone to developing arterial hypoxaemia and may gain more benefit haematologically by training at lower altitudes in comparison with sedentary controls. This contention was supported by Ingjer et al. who showed that 3 weeks of altitude training at 1900 m in elite cross country skiers was sufficient to increase Hb concentration by 5% ($P < 0.02$) and decrease blood lactate concentration during a standardised submaximal test, despite no changes in $\dot{V}O_2MAX$.[45] However, it should be noted that these authors did not measure their subjects' plasma volumes, and their comments that the polycythaemia was independent of a haemoconcentration remains only speculative. The scarcity of training studies conducted at moderate altitudes of 1500 to 2000 m in elite athletes does not allow definitive conclusions to be made.

A retrospective investigation by Chapman et al.[91] based on an original study by Levine et al.[92] clearly showed the individuality of haematological adaptation at altitude. The authors characterised

286

two distinct cohorts of subjects, which they classified as responders and non-responders. Those who responded to altitude training with an improvement in 5 km run time after return to sea level (responders) exhibited more pronounced increases in erythropoietin concentration (EPO) and total red cell volume at altitude whereas no measurable haematological adaptations or performance improvements were observed in the group of non-responders. Individual differences in hypoxic ventilatory drive, P_{50} of Hb, and renal EPO response to hypoxia are possible explanations for their observations.

Optimal duration

Few data are available on the optimal time an athlete should spend training at altitude. On the basis of subjective coaching opinion as opposed to objective scientific evidence, it would seem that 3 weeks are sufficient to gain a performance advantage at sea level.[93] However, the longer the duration of the hypoxic stimulus the greater the erythropoietic response and associated haematological adaptation.[17] This was shown by Berglund,[94] who summarised the haematological changes during previous altitude training studies conducted between 1829 m and 3048 m.[94] He identified a "true" increase in Hb concentration of 1% per week, which was independent of a haemoconcentration. Thus, assuming that the detraining response could be minimised and polycythaemia did not approach pathological values, the longer the athlete spends at altitude, the greater the potential benefit for endurance performance.

Iron status during altitude training

Hypoxia in itself increases iron demand and mobilisation,[95,96] such that endurance athletes training at altitude may be prone to iron deficiency. Lack of this critical erythropoietic factor has been shown to inhibit complete haematological adaptation.[97] Despite its importance, few studies have actually reported iron status of athletes during their hypoxic exposure. Suboptimal iron stores may account for the vast majority of training studies that have failed to show increases in Hb concentration and endurance performance on return to sea level after the hypoxic exposure. The differences in iron status may also characterise the highly individualised haematological responses observed during altitude training.[45]

Interval between descent and event

There is some evidence to suggest that endurance performance is affected by the timing of the descent to sea level after a sojourn to altitude. The general consensus among top coaches would suggest that endurance performance is optimised following 14 days at sea level after a bout of altitude training,[93] yet there is no scientific evidence to support this claim. Suslov characterised the undulating nature of endurance performance after altitude training.[98] His research was based on over 1000 competitive track results obtained from middle and long distance runners after different periods of altitude training (1300–2500 m) and repeated sea level $\dot{V}O_2MAX$ tests conducted after training at 1800 m. He identified a decrease in competition performance during the first 2 days at sea level and the first phase of enhanced work capacity occurring between days 3 and 7, followed by a decrease between days 8 and 10. Performance was shown to continue to improve between days 12 and 13, with the best results achieved on days 18 to 20. He also identified an additional upsurge in performance between days 36 and 48 after altitude. He failed to identify the physiological mechanisms responsible for this phenomenon.

Few studies have tested subjects on more than one occasion after return to sea level. Asahina et al.[57] and Faulkner et al.[47] did not show any signficant changes in $\dot{V}O_2MAX$ values after either 3 or 22 days at sea level. Ingjer et al. showed that after a group of elite cross country skiers had trained for 3 weeks at an altitude of 1900 m, submaximal blood lactate values were lower than pre-altitude values on day 1 but not day 14 at sea level.[45] The authors concluded that a 0.8 g/d increase in Hb concentration measured on day 1 was responsible for the observed improvement in submaximal exercise. However, their failure to quantify plasma volume and blood flow changes weakens the validity of their haematological findings. Svedenhag et al. studied a group of Swedish middle distance runners who trained for a period of 2 weeks at altitude (2000 m) and were tested after 6 and 12 days on return to sea level.[38] They did not identify any significant changes in $\dot{V}O_2MAX$, maximal oxygen deficit, and submaximal blood lactate values compared with pre-altitude values or between days 6 and 12 at sea level. However, they showed a significant reduction in heart rate, Borg rating of perceived exertion, and plasma ammonia concentration during a standardised submaximal treadmill test, which was more apparent after 12 days at sea level.

The physiological mechanisms responsible for these subtle changes in performance at sea level remain elusive. Intermittent altitude training has been shown to increase the hypoxic ventilatory response in a group of sedentary subjects, whereas an equivalent training programme at sea level had no effect.[14,99] Acute exposure to altitude in the native lowlander may potentiate the hypoxic ventilatory response because of an increased peripheral chemoreceptor sensitivity, which would subsequently increase the work performed by the respiratory muscles. This has not been quantified in the elite athlete but may be implicated in the performance decrements shortly after return to sea level. Plasma volume has been shown to decrease by 25% during chronic exposure to hypobaric hypoxia[11] and may take as long as 2 months to normalise.[95] After return to sea level, this may remain depressed for 6 days,[100] which may also negatively affect performance. Altitude training may also involve considerable travelling time, and the negative impact of jet lag on exercise performance cannot be ignored[101] (see chapter 16).

Measurement of the altitude effect independent of training

Figure 15.2 shows that, since 1956, only 27 (30%) of the 91 hypoxic training studies reviewed have incorporated a normoxically trained control group. This makes it impossible to determine whether the physiological changes that occur after a bout of altitude training can be attributed to an improvement in physical conditioning or to the additive effects of hypoxia itself.

To our knowledge, the altitude training studies conducted by Asano et al.,[55] Terrados et al.,[53,54] Levine et al.,[92] and Bailey et al.[42] seem to be the only investigations to use a control group that have reported significant improvements in aerobic performance after return to normoxia. Asano et al.[55] studied 10 elite middle to long distance male runners, who trained for a 10 week period at the same relative exercise intensity at either sea level or a simulated altitude of 4000 m. After training, there were no improvements in $\dot{V}O_2MAX$ at sea level, yet 10 km personal best running times improved by about 6% ($P < 0.05$). By using a one legged training model, Terrados et al. attributed the potentiating effects of intermittent hypobaric training to increases in citrate synthase activity and myoglobin content.[53,54] The findings of Levine et al.[52] have already been described in this chapter.

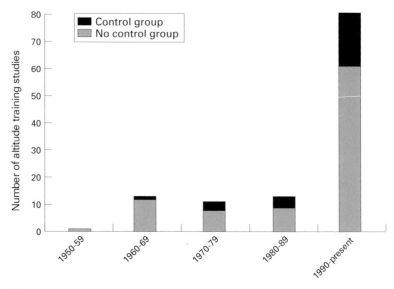

Fig 15.2   Number of hypoxic training studies conducted with or without a normoxically trained control group since 1950.

While previous investigations have dealt primarily with aerobic responses to altitude training, there is some evidence to suggest that anaerobic performance is improved on return to sea level.[46,102,103] Mizuno et al. showed that exercise time to exhaustion after altitude training improved by 17% ($P < 0.05$) when compared with pre-altitude values, which they attributed to a 6% increase ($P < 0.05$) in muscle buffer capacity.[46] However, the validity of these findings is questionable because of the lack of a normoxically trained control group. A well controlled investigation by Martino et al., which incorporated a performance matched control group based at sea level, investigated the effects of 3 weeks of altitude training at 2800 m on anaerobic measures of swimming performance.[102] Sea level sprint performance time over 100 m was 2.4 seconds quicker in the altitude trained group than the control group ($P < 0.05$). The largest improvements in the altitude trained group were noted in an upper body Wingate test. Peak power output increased by 27.9 W more than the control group ($P < 0.05$). In a recent investigation, Nummela et al. showed that 10 days of living high (~2200 m) and training low (sea level) resulted in greater improvements in 400 m running time ($P < 0.05$) and running velocity at a fixed concentration of blood lactate ($P < 0.05$) when compared with an equivalent programme of sea level training.[103]

However, the vast majority of altitude training studies have not identified performance improvements at sea level. While a decrease in absolute training intensity may be implicated,[10] a decrease in muscle perfusion may also have a contributory role; oxygen transport, determined as a product of blood flow and arterial oxygen concentration, is regulated during changes in PaO_2 possibly mediated by the release of endothelium-derived dilating/constricting factors. Reductions in blood flow during the inhalation of a hyperoxic gas mixture regulates oxygen delivery to the working muscles, such that total oxygen delivery is similar to that observed in normoxia.[104] Autoregulation of this mechanism has been investigated at altitude and after return to sea level.[105,106] While chronic exposure to hypobaric hypoxia increased arterial oxygen content as the result of an increase in Hb concentration, sympathetically mediated arterial vasoconstriction and a reduction in total cardiac output caused a reduction in blood flow, thus preventing an increase in oxygen transport.[105] This decrease in muscle perfusion has been shown to persist after return to sea level. By using Xenon-133 (^{133}Xe) blood flow to the vastus lateralis was shown to decrease by up to 39% ($P<0.001$) during submaximal exercise after a 3 month expedition to 8398 m.[106] The decrease in regional and systemic blood flow may serve to optimise pulmonary function at high altitude. Any increase in $\dot{Q}$ would effectively decrease pulmonary capillary transit time resulting in incomplete O_2 diffusion equilibration at the pulmonary and tissue level. This would ultimately limit O_2 flux to the mitochondrion, which has been identified in recent years as the major component of the integrative theory that sets $\dot{V}O_2MAX$. Research in our laboratory is currently focusing on the physiological role of the endothelium in this response. Are the changes in oxygen tension sensed by endothelial receptors and is the antagonistic vasoconstriction more pronounced because of a more severe erythropoiesis? Whatever the significance of these findings may be, it clearly highlights the complexity of the interactions between the components that constitute convective and diffusive O_2 transport to skeletal muscle.

Favier et al. suggested that the negative findings reported in the literature could, in part, be attributed to the fact that subjects were not fully acclimatised to hypobaric hypoxia.[74] In a unique experiment they used three groups of sedentary high altitude residents, who trained for 30 minutes a day at a constant work rate on a bicycle ergometer, during a 6 week period. Group 1 trained at a PO_2 that was equivalent to an interpolated altitude of 3345 m at 70% of $\dot{V}O_2MAX$ determined in hypoxia. The remaining two groups trained under normoxic conditions at either the same relative work rate (70% of the normoxic $\dot{V}O_2MAX$) or the same absolute work rate (70% of the hypoxic $\dot{V}O_2MAX$) as the hypoxically trained group. An incremental test to exhaustion was performed by all groups in normoxia and hypoxia immediately before and after training in an attempt to ascertain the physiological responses to submaximal and maximal exercise. The authors showed that $\dot{V}O_2MAX$ values improved similarly in all groups. However, they suggested that a lower reduction in base excess and bicarbonate stores observed in the hypoxically trained group could only potentially benefit anaerobic metabolism and, although time to exhaustion was not measured, facilitate exercise performance.

Hypoxia and immune function

Changes in total leucocyte, granulocyte, monocyte, lymphocyte, natural killer cell and T cell count, helper/suppression cell ratio, cell proliferation in response to mitogens, and serum immunoglobin levels have all been implicated in some form of immunodepression, which may subsequently cause underperformance in the athlete at sea level.[107] The additive stress of a reduction in the inspiratory PO_2, in conjunction with the extensive training loads used by athletes at altitude, may explain why some investigators have reported physiological evidence for a less favourable modulation of immune function in vivo during acute and chronic exposure to hypobaric hypoxia.[65,108–110]

Human studies have shown that chronic exposure to hypobaric hypoxia results in a depression of cell mediated immunity, whereas B cell function remains unimpaired.[16] Animal studies have further shown that murine host defences against bacterial pathogens are also impaired in hypoxia. The contributory immuno-modulatory role of endogenous glucocorticoids and neuropep-tides, which are increased at altitude, may contribute to the observed alterations in immune competence. In an experiment that used elite distance runners and matched controls, we showed that plasma glutamine concentrations decreased significantly in comparison with pre-altitude values after 20 days of endurance training at an altitude of 1640 m above sea level ($PO_2 = 135$ mm Hg).[112] A reduction in glutamine concentration has been identified in "overtrained" athletes and may be a contributory factor leading to

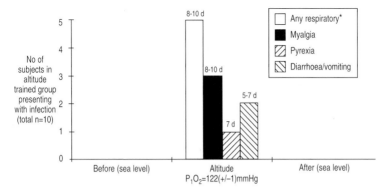

Fig 15.3 Frequency and duration (in days) of infectious illnesses encountered during intermittent normoxic and hypoxic training. (Any respiratory* indicates any one of the following symptoms: sore throat, cough, runny nose, sinusitis, earache.)

immunodepression and underperformance due to its importance as a substrate for key cells of the immune system in particular macrophages and lymphocytes.[111] These metabolic changes were associated with a marked increase in the frequency of upper respiratory tract and gastrointestinal infections (fig 15.3). While communal living may have contributed to the higher incidence of infectious illness at altitude, there were no reports of any physical symptoms for subjects in the sea level based group, despite identical living and training conditions.[112] In a separate study, again characterised by a high incidence of infectious illness during the altitude sojourn, two men who were particularly ill were subsequently diagnosed with infectious mononucleosis shortly after return to sea level.[113] The onset of physical symptoms that are characteristic of the first 3 to 5 days of the prodrome suggested that these subjects were exposed to the Epstein-Barr virus during the initial stages of altitude acclimatisation, presumably when the host is most hypoxaemic before complete haematological adaptation and potentially more susceptible to an antigenic challenge. It is difficult to comment on the physiological mechanisms responsible for these changes, but there is evidence that suggests that chronically increased concentrations of circulating catecholamines decrease the rate of glutamine transport out of muscle incubated in vitro (Parry-Billings M, unpublished data). In addition to this, Wagenmakers[114] has proposed an alternative mechanism, again related to increased catecholamine concentration observed at altitude.[11] He suggested that hypoxia induced glycogen depletion would result in a reduction in the availability of tricarboxylic acid cycle intermediates, in particular 2-oxoglutarate. This is required for the activation of the branched chain amino acid aminotransferase reaction, which ultimately produces glutamine. Alternatively, hypoxia may accelerate the hepatic uptake of glutamine which is a precursor for the production of the antioxidant glutathione.[115] Hypoxia is associated with an increased production of free radicals[116,117] and thus the production of effective free radical scavengers would prove beneficial. The implications of the immunodepressive influence of hypobaric hypoxia for endurance performance warrants further investigation to elucidate potential mechanisms that may modulate performance after return to sea level.

Research in our laboratory is currently focusing on the metabolic changes that predispose individuals to suffer from the debilitating symptoms associated with acute mountain sickness (AMS) during high altitude sojourns. A theoretical model is proposed which describes the relation between free radical activity, antioxidant status, glutamine metabolism, and the incidence of AMS at altitude (fig 15.4). It is hypothesised that free radical activity and free tryptophan concentrations increase whereas total antioxidant

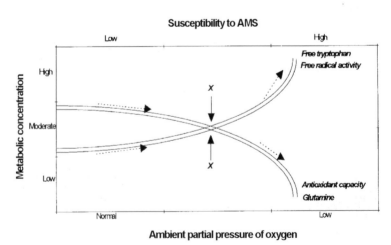

Fig 15.4 Theoretical relation between amino acid metabolism, free radical activity, total antioxidant capacity, and the incidence of AMS at altitude.

capacity and plasma glutamine concentrations decrease beyond a physiological and as yet unquantified concentration (denoted as X) mediated by a combination of physical exercise and a decreased P_IO_2 at altitude. The physical manifestation of these biochemical changes may be associated with some of the symptoms characteristic of AMS. While only speculative, it would also be interesting to investigate the effects of vitamin C, α tocopherol, and branched chain amino acid supplementation in the prevention or attenuation of AMS.

The catabolic effects of high altitude resulting in significant loss of skeletal muscle mass may be linked either directly or indirectly to glutamine metabolism; a theory that we investigated during the 1998 Mount Kanchenjunga medical expedition. While previously considered a maladaptive response, an increased net rate of protein degradation in skeletal muscle at altitude would provide a constant supply of branched chain amino acids (BCAA) which, via a series of transamination reactions, would donate their nitrogen for the subsequent synthesis of glutamine (fig 15.4). This metabolic pathway may be more active during chronic exposure to hypoxia to provide glutamine for the enhanced activity of lymphocytes and macrophages and thus enhance immunoreactivity. The proposed accelerated uptake and oxidation rate of BCAA by skeletal muscle at altitude may decrease the plasma concentration of BCAA resulting in an increase in the concentration of free tryptophan (that is, not bound to albumin) leading to an increase in 5-hydroxytryptamine (5-HT) in the brain, causing a general state of fatigue. This mechanism may be more pronounced in the subject who is more prone to or suffers from the physical symptoms associated with AMS. These hypotheses await investigation.

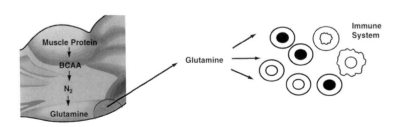

Fig 15.5   Cachexia theory at high altitude.

Reactive oxygen species at altitude

There is a limited body of evidence suggesting that oxidative injury mediated by free radicals is increased at altitude.[116,118,119] Simon-Schnass identified significant increases in indirect indices of free radical mediated lipid peroxidation at altitude, which included increased pentane excretion and thiobarbituric acid reactive substances, decreased erythrocyte filterability, and increased leucocyte and granulocyte counts.[116] Daily supplementation with an antioxidant such as tocopherol (vitamin E) equivalent to 300–400 mg has been shown to improve endurance performance, by theoretically limiting tissue damage.[116,118] Vasankari *et al.* most recently showed evidence for increased oxidative stress after 2 weeks at moderate altitude in nine elite skiers.[117] Relative to sea level values, serum diene conjugation, a marker of lipid peroxidation, was 20% higher at rest after a 20–30 km race ($P < 0.05$). Serum antioxidant potential increased during the race at altitude, whereas no changes were observed during the race at sea level. However, no studies have quantified free radical activity at altitude by using spin trapping techniques and electron spin resonance, which are the only direct methods for quantifying free radical activity *sine qua non*. An accelerated production of the highly toxic hydroxyl radical may occur as a consequence of an increased production of free iron derived from altitude induced and training induced destruction of red blood cells.[119] Thus it would seem that hypobaric hypoxia significantly increases oxidative stress, which has been shown to influence energy metabolism and membrane integrity negatively.

Recent research findings: clinical applications of intermittent normobaric hypoxic training

Recent research conducted in our laboratory has identified that the duration of the hypoxic stimulus seems to be an important determinant of physiological adaptation, which has implications for an individual's physical wellbeing and exercise capacity. We have shown in a randomised, placebo controlled, double blind study that 4 weeks of intermittent hypoxic training in healthy men induced significant increases in $\dot{V}O_2\text{MAX}$ and plasma glutamine concentration.[42] Rate pressure product during maximal exercise and plasma total homocysteine concentration decreased.[120] These changes were not observed in response to an identical programme of normoxic training. We are examining the physiochemical bases for the additive cardioprotective effects invoked by intermittent exposure to normobaric hypoxia, which may have important clinical implications.

Summary and future research

Physiological acclimatisation to a chronically reduced P_IO_2 is a prerequisite to achieve optimal physical performance in environmental hypoxia. However, scientific evidence to support the claim that either continuous or intermittent hypoxic training will enhance sea level performance remains at present equivocal. Future research should focus on methodological technicalities that optimise the balance between the favourable and less favourable responses to hypoxia and potential mediators of performance after return to sea level. Preliminary evidence showing that the additive stress of hypobaric hypoxia may provoke an adverse immune response and further potentiate free radical mediated oxidative injury has important implications which, if confirmed by scientific rigour, would present a threat to both the fitness and health of the elite competitor.

1 Bert P. *Barometric pressure: researches in experimental physiology.* Columbus: College Book, 1943. (Translated by MA Hitchcock and RA Hitchcock.)
2 Smith MH, Sharkey BJ. Altitude training: who benefits? *Physician and Sportsmedicine* 1984;**12**:48–62.
3 Terrados N. Altitude training and muscular metabolism. *Int J Sports Med* 1992;**13**:S206–9.
4 Levine BD, Stray-Gundersen J. A practical approach to altitude training: where to live and train for optimal performance enhancement. *Int J Sports Med* 1992; **13**:S209–12.
5 Levine BD, Roach RC, Houston CS. Work and training at altitude. In: Sutton JR, Coates G, Houston CS, eds. *Hypoxia and mountain medicine.* Texas: Queen City Printers, 1992:192–201.
6 Sutton JR. Exercise training at high altitude: does it improve endurance performance at sea-level? *Sports Science Exchange* 1993;**6**:4.
7 Hahn AG. The effect of altitude training on athletic performance at sea-level: a review. *Sports* 1993;**13**:1–7.
8 Saltin B. Exercise and the environment: focus on altitude. *Res Q Exerc Sport* 1996;**67**:1–10.
9 Wolski LA, McKenzie DC, Wenger HA. Altitude training for improvements in sea level performance. Is there scientific evidence of benefit? *Sports Med* 1996;**22**:251–63.
10 Stine TA, Levine BD, Taylor S, Schultz W, Stray-Gundersen J. Quantification of altitude training in the field [abstract]. *Med Sci Sports Exerc* 1992;**24**:S103.
11 Young AJ, Young PM. Human acclimatization to high terrestrial altitude. In: Pandolf KB, Sawka MN, Gonzalez PR, eds. *Human performance physiology and environmental medicine at terrestrial extremes.* Indianapolis: Benchmark Press, 1988:497–543.

12 Szygula Z. Erythrocytic system under the influence of physical training and exercise. *Sports Med* 1990;**10**:181–97.

13 Young A. Energy substrate utilization during exercise in extreme environments. *Exerc Sports Sci Rev* 1990;**18**:65–118.

14 Levine BD, Friedman DB, Engfred K, *et al.* The effect of normoxic or hypobaric hypoxic endurance training on the hypoxic ventilatory response. *Med Sci Sports Exerc* 1992;**24**:769–75.

15 Shephard RJ. Problems of high altitude. In: Shephard RJ, Astrand PO, eds. *Endurance in sport.* Oxford: Blackwell, 1992:471–8.

16 Meehan RT. Immune suppression at high altitude. *Ann Emerg Med* 1987;**16**:974–9.

17 Schmidt W, Spielvogel H, Eckardt KU, Quintela A, Penaloza R. Effects of chronic hypoxia and exercise on plasma erythropoietin in high-altitude residents. *J Appl Physiol* 1993;**74**:1874–8.

18 Gledhill N. The influence of altered blood volume and oxygen transport capacity on aerobic performance. *Exerc Sports Sci Rev* 1985;**13**:75–93.

19 Ekblom B, Berglund B. Effect of erythropoietin administration on maximal aerobic power. *Scand J Sports Med* 1991;**1**:88–93.

20 Metra M, Cannella G, La Canna G. Improvement in exercise capacity after correction of anaemia in patients with end stage renal failure. *Am J Cardiol* 1991;**68**:1060–6.

21 Celsing F, Svedenhag J, Pilhstedt P, Ekblom B. Effects of anaemia and stepwise-induced polycythaemia on maximal aerobic power in individuals with high and low haemoglobin concentrations. *Acta Physiol Scand* 1987;**31**:47–54.

22 American College of Sports Medicine. Position stand on the use of blood doping as an ergogenic aid. *Med Sci Sports Exerc* 1996;**28**:i–viii.

23 Buick FJ, Gledhill N, Froese AB, Spriet L, Meyers EC. Effect of induced erythrocythemia on aerobic work capacity. *J Appl Physiol* 1980;**48**:636–42.

24 Spriet LL, Gledhill N, Froses AB, Wilkes DL, Meyers EC. The effects of induced erythrocythemia on central circulation and oxygen transport during maximal exercise. *Med Sci Sports Exerc* 1980;**12**:122–3.

25 Williams MH, Wesseldine S, Somma T, Schuster R. The effect of induced erythrocythemia upon 5-mile treadmill run time. *Med Sci Sports Exerc* 1981;**13**:169–75.

26 Goforth HW, Campbell Jr NL, Hodgdon JA, Sucec AA. Hematologic parameters of trained distance runners following induced erythrocythemia. *Med Sci Sports Exerc* 1982;**14**:174.

27 Robertson RJ, Gilcher R, Metz KF, *et al.* Effect of induced erythrocythemia on hypoxia tolerance during physical exercise. *J Appl Physiol* 1982;**53**:490–5.

28 Robertson RJ, Gilcher R, Metz KF, *et al.* Hemoglobin concentration and aerobic work capacity in women following induced erythrocythemia. *J Appl Physiol* 1984;**57**:568–75.

29 Thompson JM, Stone JA, Ginsburg AD, Hamilton P. O_2 transport during exercise following blood reinfusion. *J Appl Physiol* 1982;**53**:1213–19.

30 Sawka MN, Dennis RC, Gonzalez RR, *et al.* Influence of polycythemia on blood volume and thermoregulation during exercise-heat stress. *J Appl Physiol* 1987;**62**:912–18.

31 Robertson RJ, Gilcher R, Metz KF, *et al.* Effect of simulated altitude erythrocythemia in women on hemoglobin flow rate during exercise. *J Appl Physiol* 1988;**64**:1644–9.

32 Dempsey JA, Reddan WG, Birnbaum ML. Effects of acute through life-long hypoxic exposure on exercise pulmonary gas exchange. *Respir Physiol* 1971;**13**:62–89.

33 Hochachka PW, Stanley C, Matheson GO, McKenzie DC, Allen PS, Parkhouse WS. Metabolic and work efficiencies during exercise in Andean natives. *J Appl Physiol* 1991;**70**:1720–30.

34 Sun SF, Droma TS, Zhang JG, *et al.* Greater maximal O_2 uptake and vital capacities in Tibetan than Han residents of Lhasa. *Respir Physiol* 1990;**79**:151–62.

35 Ge RL, Chen QH, Wang LH, Gen D, Yang P, Kubo K. Higher exercise performance and lower $\dot{V}O_2\text{MAX}$ in Tibetan than Han residents at 4700 m altitude. *J Appl Physiol* 1994;**77**:684–91.

36 Favier R, Spielvogel H, Desplanches D, Ferretti G, Kayser B, Hoppeler H. Maximal exercise performance in chronic hypoxia and acute normoxia in high-altitude natives. *J Appl Physiol* 1995;**78**:1868–74.

37 Huang SY, Sun S, Draoma T, *et al.* Internal carotid arterial flow velocity during exercise in Tibetan and Han residents of Lhasa (3658 m). *J Appl Pysiol* 1992;**73**:2638–42.

38 Svedenhag J, Saltin B, Johansson C, Kaijser L. Aerobic and anaerobic exercise capacities of elite middle-distance runners after two weeks of training at moderate altitude. *Scand J Med Sci Sports* 1991;**1**:205–14.

39 Beall CM, Blangero J, Williams-Blangero S, Goldstein MC. Major gene for percent of oxygen saturation of arterial hemoglobin in Tibetan highlanders. *Am J Phys Anthropol* 1994;**95**:271–6.

40 Niermeyer S, Yang P, Drolkar S, Zhuang J, Moore LG. Arterial oxygen saturation in Tibetan and Han infants born in Lhasa, Tibet. *N Engl J Med* 1995;**333**:1248–52.

41 Ward MP, Milledge JS, West JB. *High altitude medicine and physiology.* 2nd ed. London: Chapman Hall, 1995:344.

42 Bailey DM, Davies B, Castell LM, *et al.* Intermittent normobaric hypoxia: changes in plasma amino acids and implications for exercise performance. *J Physiol* 1998;**C17**:52.

43 Katayama K, Sato Y, Ishida K, Mori S, Miyamura M. The effects of intermittent exposure to hypoxia during endurance exercise on the ventilatory responses to hypoxia and hypercapnia in humans. *Eur J Appl Physiol* 1998;**78**:189–94.

44 Levine BD, Stray-Gundersen J, Duhaime G, Snell PG, Friedman DB. Living high-training low: the effect of altitude acclimatization/normoxic training in trained runners. *Med Sci Sports Exerc* 1991;**23**:[abstract 145].

45 Ingjer F, Myhre K. Physiological effects of altitude training on elite male cross-country skiers. *J Sports Sci* 1992;**10**:37–47.

46 Mizuno M, Juel C, Bro-Rasmussen T, *et al.* Limb skeletal muscle adaptation in athletes after training in altitude. *J Appl Physiol* 1990;**68**:496–502.

47 Faulkner JA, Daniels JT, Balke B. Effects of training at moderate altitude on physical performance capacity. *J Appl Physiol* 1967;**23**:85–9.

48 Stray-Gundersen J, Mordecai N, Levine BD. O_2 transport response to altitude training in runners. *Med Sci Sports Exerc* 1996;**27**(S5):[abstract 1131].

49 Loeppky JA, Bynum WA. Effects of periodic exposure to hypobaria and exercise on physical work capacity. *J Sports Med Phys Fitness* 1970;**10**:238–47.

50 Klausen K, Robinson S, Michael ED, Myhre LG. Effect of high altitude on maximal working capacity. *J Appl Physiol* 1966;**21**:1191–4.

51 Banister EW, Woo W. Effects of simulated altitude training on aerobic and anaerobic power. *Eur J Appl Physiol* 1978;**38**:55–69.

52 Levine BD, Friedman B, Stray-Gundersen J. Confirmation of the "high-low" hypothesis: living at altitude-training near sea level improves sea level performance. *Med Sci Sports Exerc* 1996;**28**:[abstract 742].

53 Terrados N, Melichna J, Sylven C, Jansson E, Kaijser L. Effects of training at simulated altitude on performance and muscle metabolic capacity in competitive road cyclists. *Eur J Appl Physiol* 1988;**57**:203–9.

54 Terrados N, Jansson E, Sylven C, Kaijser L. Is hypoxia a stimulus for synthesis of oxidative enzymes and myoglobin? *J Appl Physiol* 1990;**68**:2369–72.

55 Asano K, Sub S, Matsuzaka A, Hirakoba K, Nagai J, Kawaoka T. The

influences of simulated high altitude training on work capacity and performance in middle and long distance runners. *Bull Inst Health Sports Sci* 1986;**9**:195–202.

56 Klausen T, Mohr T, Ghisler U, Nielsen OJ. Maximal oxygen uptake and erythropoietic responses after training at moderate altitude. *Eur J Appl Physiol* 1991;**62**:376–9.

57 Asahina K, Ikai M, Agawas Y, Kuroda Y. A study on acclimatization to altitude in Japanese athletes. *Schweizerische Zeitschrift für Sportsmedizin* 1966;**14**:240–5.

58 Faulkner JA, Kollias J, Favour CB, Buskirk ER, Balke B. Maximum aerobic capacity and running performance at altitude. *J Appl Physiol* 1968;**24**:685–91.

59 Daniels J, Oldridge N. The effects of alternate exposure to altitude and sea-level on world-class middle-distance runners. *Med Sci Sports* 1970;**2**:107–12.

60 Balke B, Nagle FJ, Daniels J. Altitude and maximum performance in work and sports activity. *JAMA* 1965;**194**:176–9.

61 Dill DB, Adams WC. Maximal oxygen uptake at sea-level and at 3090 m altitude in high school champion runners. *J Appl Physiol* 1971;**30**:854–9.

62 Reeves JT, Grover RF, Cohn JE. Regulation of ventilation during exercise at 10,200 ft in athletes born at low altitude. *J Appl Physiol* 1967;**22**:546–54.

63 Buskirk ER, Kollias J, Akers RF, Prokop EK, Reategui EP. Maximal performance at altitude and on return from altitude in conditioned runners. *J Appl Physiol* 1967;**23**:259–66.

64 Vallier JM, Chateau P, Guezennec CY. Effects of physical training in a hypobaric chamber on the physical performance of competitive triathletes. *Eur J Appl Physiol* 1996;**73**:471–8.

65 Rusko HK, Kirvesniemi H, Paavolainen L, Vahasoyrinki P, Kyro KP. Effect of altitude training on sea level aerobic and anaerobic power of elite athletes. *Med Sci Sports Exerc* 1996;**28**(S5):[abstract 739].

66 Bailey DM, Davies B, Romer L, Gandy G. Physiological implications of moderate altitude training (1640 metres) on sea-level endurance performance in elite distance runners. *Br J Sports Med* 1996;**30**:370 [abstract].

67 Telford RD, Graham KS, Sutton JR, *et al.* Medium altitude training and sea-level performance. *Med Sci Sports Exerc* 1996;**28**(S5):[abstract 741].

68 Adams WC, Bernauer EM, Dill DB, Bomar Jr JB. Effects of equivalent sea-level and altitude training on $\dot{V}O_2$MAX and running performance. *J Appl Physiol* 1975;**39**:262–6.

69 Roskamm H, Landry F, Samek L, Schlager M, Weidemann H, Reindell H. Effects of a standardized ergometer training program at three different altitudes. *J Appl Physiol* 1969;**27**:840–7.

70 Levine BD, Engfred K, Friedman DB, *et al.* High altitude endurance training: effect of aerobic capacity and work performance. *Med Sci Sports Exerc* 1990;**22**:[abstract 209].

71 Friedman DB, Levine BD, Hanel B, Engfred K, Clifford PS, Secher NH. Endurance training and the hypoxic ventilatory response. *Med Sci Sports Exerc* 1990;**22**(S99):[abstract 592].

72 Rahkila P, Rusko H. Effects of high altitude training on muscle enzyme activities and physical performance characteristics of cross-country skiers. In: Komi P, ed. *Exercise and sport biology.* Champaign, Illinois: Human Kinetics, 1982:143–51.

73 Hahn AG, Telford RD, Tumilty DM, *et al.* Effect of supplementary hypoxic training on physiological characteristics and ergometer performance of elite rowers. *Excel* 1992;**8**:127–38.

74 Favier R, Spielvogel D, Desplanches D, *et al.* Training in hypoxia vs training in normoxia in high-altitude natives. *J Appl Physiol* 1995;**78**:2286–93.

75 Davies CT, Sargeant AJ. Effects of hypoxic training on normoxic maximal aerobic power output. *Eur J Appl Physiol* 1974;**33**:227–36.

76 Desplanches D, Hoppeler H, Linoissier MT, *et al.* Effects of training in

normoxia and normobaric hypoxia on human muscle ultrastructure. *Eur J Physiol* 1993;**425**:263–7.

77 Hansen JE, Vogel JA, Stelter GP, Consolazio CF. Oxygen uptake in man during exhaustive work at sea-level and high altitude. *J Appl Physiol* 1967;**23**:511–22.

78 Winslow RM, Monge CC. *Hypoxia, polycythemia and chronic mountain sickness.* Baltimore: Johns Hopkins University Press, 1987.

79 Milledge JS. High altitude. In: Harries M, Williams C, Stanish W, Micheli L, eds. *Oxford textbook of sports medicine.* London: Oxford University Press, 1994:217–30.

80 Kayser B. Nutrition and energetics of exercise at altitude. Theory and possible practical implications. *Sports Med* 1994;**17**:309–23.

81 Saltin B. Aerobic and anaerobic work capacity at 2,300 metres. *Medical Thoracics* 1967;**24**:205–10.

82 Gore CJ, Hahn AG, Watson DB, *et al.* V̇O$_2$MAX and arterial O$_2$ saturation at sea level and 610 m. *Med Sci Sports Exerc* 1996;**27**(S5):[abstract 42].

83 Anselme F, Caillaud C, Courret I, Prefaut C. Exercise induced hypoxemia and histamine excretion in extreme athletes. *Int J Sports Med* 1992;**13**:80–1.

84 Lawler J, Powers SK, Thompson D. Linear relationship between V̇O$_2$MAX and V̇O$_2$MAX decrement during exposure to acute hypoxia. *J Appl Physiol* 1988;**64**:146–9.

85 Koistinen P, Takala T, Martikkala V, Leppaluoto J. Aerobic fitness influences the response of maximal oxygen uptake and lactate threshold in acute hypobaric hypoxia. *Int J Sports Med* 1995;**26**:78–81.

86 Rowell LB, Taylor HL, Wang Y. Saturation of arterial blood with oxygen during maximal exercise. *J Appl Physiol* 1964;**19**:284–6.

87 Dempsey JA. JB Wolffe memorial lecture. Is the lung built for exercise? *Med Sci Sports Exerc* 1986;**18**:143–55.

88 Nummela A, Jouste P, Rusko H. Effect of living high and training low on sea level anaerobic performance in runners. *Med Sci Sports Exerc* 1996;**28**(S5):[abstract 740].

89 Weil JV, Jamieson G, Brown DW, Grover RF. The red cell mass-arterial oxygen relationship in normal man. *J Clin Invest* 1968;**47**:1627–39.

90 Shephard RJ, Bouhlel E, Vandewalle H, Monod H. Peak oxygen intake and hypoxia. *Int J Sports Med* 1988;**9**:279–83.

91 Chapman RF, Stray-Gundersen J, Levine BD. Individual variation in response to altitude training. *J Appl Physiol* 1998;**85**:1448–56.

92 Levine BD, Stray-Gundersen J. "Living high-training low": effect of moderate altitude acclimatization with low-altitude training on performance. *J Appl Physiol* 1997;**83**:102.

93 Dick FW. Training at altitude in practice. *Int J Sports Med* 1993;**13**:S203–5.

94 Berglund B. High-altitude training. Aspects of haematological adaptation. *Sports Med* 1992;**14**:289–303.

95 Rejnafarje C, Lozano R, Valdivieso J. The polycythemia of high altitudes: iron metabolism and related aspects. *Blood* 1959;**14**:433–55.

96 Hannon JP, Shields JL, Harris CW. Effects of altitude acclimatization on blood composition of women. *J Appl Physiol* 1969;**26**:540–7.

97 Stray-Gundersen J, Alexander C, Hochstein A, de Lomos D, Levine BD. Failure of red cell volume to increase to altitude exposure in iron deficient runners. *Med Sci Sports Exerc* 1992;**24**(suppl):S90.

98 Suslov FP. Basic principles of training at high altitude. In: *New studies in athletics, the IAAF quarterly magazine for NSA* 1994;**2**:45–9.

99 Benoit H, Costes F, Castells J, *et al.* Endurance training in normobaric hypoxia: ventilatory response and ability to exercise. *Int J Sports Med* 1992;**13**:90 [abstract].

100 Dill DB, Braithwaite K, Adams WC, Bernauer EM. Blood volume of middle distance runners: effect of 2300 m altitude and comparison with non-athletes.

Med Sci Sports Exerc 1974;**6**:1–7.

101 Reilly T. Circadian rhythms. In: Harries M, Stanish W, Micheli L, eds. *Oxford textbook of sports medicine*. London: Oxford University Press, 1994:238–54

102 Martino M, Myers K, Bishop P. Effect of 21 days training at altitude on sea-level anaerobic performance in competitive swimmers. *Med Sci Sports Exerc* 1996;**27**(S5):[abstract 37].

103 Nummela A, Jouste P, Rusko H. Effect of living high and training low on sea level anaerobic performance in runners. *Med Sci Sports Exerc* 1996;**38**(S5):[abstract 740].

104 Hogan MC, Welch HG. The effect of altered arterial oxygen tensions on muscle metabolism in dog skeletal muscle during fatiguing work. *Am J Physiol* 1986;**251**:C216–22.

105 Wolfel EE, Groves BM, Brooks GA, *et al.* Oxygen transport during steady-state submaximal exercise in chronic hypoxia. *J Appl Physiol* 1996;**70**:1129–36.

106 Boutellier U, Marconi C, diPrampero PE, Cerretelli P. Effects of chronic hypoxia on maximal performance. *Clin Respir Physiol* 1982;**18**(S4):39–44.

107 Shephard RJ, Pang NS. Potential impact of physical activity and sport on the immune system: a brief review. *Br J Sports Med* 1994;**84**:247–55.

108 Uchakin P. Immunological adaptations to altitude training [abstract]. In: *The third world congress for sport science* 1995:209–210.

109 Klokker M, Kharazmi A, Galbo H, Bygberg I, Pedersen BK. Influence of in vivo hypobaric hypoxia on function of lymphocytes, neutrocytes, natural killer cells and cytokines. *J Appl Physiol* 1993;**74**:1100–6.

110 Meehan RT, Duncan U, Neale LS, *et al.* Operation Everest II: alterations in the immune system at high altitudes. *J Clin Immunol* 1988;**8**:397–406.

111 Parry-Billings M, Blomstrand E, McAndrew N, Newsholme E. A communicational link between skeletal muscle, brain, and cells of the immune system. *Int J Sports Med* 1990;**11**(S2):S122–8.

112 Bailey DM, Davies B, Romer L, Castell L, Newsholme E, Gandy G. Implications of moderate altitude training for sea-level endurance in elite distance runners. *Eur J Appl Physiol* 1998;**78**:360–8.

113 Bailey DM, Davies B, Budgett R, Gandy G. Recovery from infectious mononucleosis following altitude training on elite middle distance runner. *Br J Sports Med* 1997;**31**:153–4.

114 Wagenmakers AJM. Amino acid metabolism, muscular fatigue and muscle wasting. Speculations on adaptations at high altitude. *Int J Sports Med* 1992;**13**:S110–13.

115 Hong RW, Rounds JD, Helton WS, Robinson MK, Wilmore DW. Glutamine preserves liver glutathione after lethal hepatic injury. *Ann Surg* 1992;**215**:114–19.

116 Simon-Schnass I. Risk of oxidative stress during exercise at high altitude. In: Sen CK, Packer L, Hanninen O, eds. *Exercise and oxygen toxicity*. Amsterdam: Elsevier, 1994:1:191–210.

117 Vasankari TJ, Kujala UM, Rusko H, Sama S, Ahotupa M. The effects of endurance exercise at moderate altitude on serum lipid peroxidation and antioxidative functions in humans. *Eur J Appl Physiol* 1997;**75**:396–9.

118 Nagawa T, Kita H, Aoki J, Maeshima T, Shiozawa K. *Asian Medicine* 1968;**11**:619–33.

119 Biselli R, Pecci G, Oliva C, Fattorossi A, D'Amelio R, Barsotti P. Effects of hypobaric hypoxia (HH) on polymorphonuclear granulocytes (PMNL) respiratory activity in HH-acclimatized and non-acclimatized rats [abstract]. *Int J Sports Med* 1992;**13**:94.

120 Bailey DM, Baker J, Richards M, *et al.* Coronary artery disease risk factor response following intermittent hypoxic training. *Med Sci Sports Exerc* 1999;**31**(5):S182(abstract 812).

Multiple choice questions

1 Convective O_2 transport is a product of:
   - (a) Blood flow and arterial oxygen content (caO_2)
   - (b) Blood flow only
   - (c) caO_2 only
   - (d) Haemoglobin (Hb) saturation

2 caO_2 is a product of:
   - (a) Hb only
   - (b) $Hb \times SaO_2 \times 1.34$
   - (c) SaO_2 only
   - (d) None of the above

3 The inspired partial pressure of oxygen (P_IO_2) is calculated by:
   - (a) Barometric pressure (BP) only
   - (b) Inspired fraction of oxygen (F_IO_2) only
   - (c) $(BP \times 0.2093) - 47$
   - (d) None of the above

4 What is the F_IO_2 on the summit of Mount Everest?
   - (a) 8%
   - (b) 10%
   - (c) 20.9%
   - (d) 0%

5 If the BP on Mount Everest is 240 mm Hg, what is the P_IO_2?
   - (a) 40 mm Hg
   - (b) 60 mm Hg
   - (c) 80 mm Hg
   - (d) 100 mm Hg

6 Chronic exposure to environmental hypoxia is associated with a decrease in plasma volume. What would happen to the plasma concentration of selected metabolites at rest and/or during physical exercise as a consequence of this haemoconcentration?
   - (a) Stay the same
   - (b) Be artificially raised
   - (c) Decrease
   - (d) Stay the same and then decrease

Answers are on p. 365.

16 Circadian rhythms, athletic performance, and jet lag

R Manfredini, F Manfredini, C Fersini, F Conconi

Introduction

Chronobiology can be defined as the study of rhythmic patterns in biological phenomena. Oscillatory fluctuations, called biological rhythms, occur in cells, tissues, organs, and more complex control systems. They are endogenous, arise within the organism, and persist under constant environmental conditions. Although they may show a wide range of periods, circadian rhythms (from the Latin *circa diem* meaning about 24 hours) are the most extensively investigated. Rhythms are not imposed by the environment but can be adjusted by exogenous synchronising cues—for example, alternation of light and dark. However, the night-day cycle has progressively lost some of its importance because of the invention of artificial light, which allows work by night. Together with shift work, the most important cause of internal desynchronisation is the rapid crossing of several time zones, called jet lag.[1] Travel across several time zones has become a necessity for international sports competitors, with possible impairments of performance until adjustment to the local time is achieved.

Both the 2000 and winter 2002 summer Olympic Games (scheduled, respectively, in Australia and the United States) will require the crossing of several time zones, especially for European teams, and chronobiology may be a useful tool for defining the optimal time for training and competing, thereby increasing personal performance and alleviating possible jet lag induced disturbances. In this chapter we will review briefly current knowledge on the possible effects of jet lag on physical performance in athletes and potentially alleviating strategies.

Jet lag

Rapid air travel across several time zones exposes the traveller to a shift in the internal biological clock. The result is a transient desynchronisation of rhythm, lasting until the biological rhythms adjust to the new environmental conditions. The subjective symptoms usually associated include sleep disorders, difficulties with concentrating, irritability, depression, disorientation, distorted estimation of time, space and distance, lightheadedness, loss of appetite, and gastrointestinal disturbances.[1,2] Air crews report sleep disturbances in about 60–70% of cases on the first night after crossing a time zone, which is reduced to 30% on the third day;[3] loss of sleep amounts to as much as 5 or 6 hours per night flight.[4] Moreover, female flight attendants experience more irregular

---

Box 16.1   Biological rhythms and exercise

- Chronobiology investigates the rhythmic patterns in biological phenomena. Biological rhythms are endogenous and inherited with the DNA, but can be adjusted (though not imposed) by environmental synchronising cues
- Biological rhythms may show a wide range of periods. The most extensively studied are circadian rhythms (from the Latin *circa diem* meaning about 24 hours), but both ultradian (< 24 hours) and infradian (> 24 hours, for example, circaseptan, circannual) also exist
- Many physiological mechanisms, each of them contributing to overall athletic performance, show a peculiar circadian pattern. Body temperature starts rising before waking, reaches a peak in the afternoon, then falls during sleep. An afternoon peak is also shown for heart rate, stroke volume, cardiac output, blood flow, and arterial blood pressure
- As a consequence, most components of sports performance show a rhythmic variation during the day, characterised by an afternoon-early evening peak. This is true for reaction time, isometric hand grip strength, elbow flexion and back strength, and long term memory recall. However, other aspects of performance, for example, mental arithmetic and short term memory peak in the early morning, so probably favouring sports demanding accuracy
- Circadian oscillation in biological parameters may condition one's personality "chronotype". In fact, both morning ("larks") and evening ("owls") type persons exist. The former get up and perform well early but must go to bed early. The latter wake up late and can retire late. All intermediate aspects, of course, are possible

menstrual cycles.[5] It is well known that westward flights (characterised by a phase delay) are followed by faster recovery and resynchronisation than eastward flights (phase advance), and sleep quality decreases particularly after eastward flights.[6] Klein and Wegmann calculated that 3 days were needed to resynchronise psychomotor performance rhythms after a westward flight from Germany to the United States, whereas 8 days were required for the reverse direction.[7] After a time zone crossing of several hours you can recover day by day. After a westward flight the mean re-entrainment shift rate is about 92/min/day, and only 57/min/day after eastward flights.[8] However, there is a considerable variation in the rate of readaptation between individuals for a given rhythm and between rhythms in a given individual. About 30% of transmeridian travellers have little or no difficulty adjusting to the temporary circadian desynchronisation and have no symptoms, but another 30% do not adjust well at all.[9] Symptoms are commonly reported during the 48 hours immediately after a flight, and the more time zones that have been traversed, the longer is the period of recovery, although the relation is not linear.[10] Individual factors associated with widely differing rates of rhythmic readaptation are direction of flight, synchroniser strength, rhythm stability, personality chronotype, rhythm amplitude, behavioural traits, and sleep habits.[9] Thus, for example, evening type people are less sensitive than morning types, people with low amplitudes in body temperature seem to be less resistant to phase shift than individuals with large circadian amplitudes,[1] and older travellers suffer more than younger ones.[11] It has also been reported that re-entrainment after transmeridian flights is more rapid in summer than in winter, possibly because the longer day permits greater exposure to natural daylight.[12]

Jet lag and athletic performance

Some aspects of chronobiology are important to physical performance—for example, the normal cyclic variation observed in the physiological mechanisms that contribute to overall athletic performance, the effect of abnormal rhythmicity or desynchronisation on athletic performance, and the alleviating countermeasures.

Human circadian rhythms at rest

Body temperature

Body temperature starts to rise before waking, reaches a peak at about 1800 hours, then falls during sleep with a nadir at around 0400 hours; an amplitude of 0.4–0.5°C is seen in young adults.[13] The circadian rhythm of body temperature is mainly the result of fluctuations in heat loss mechanisms rather than heat production,[13] maybe with the intervention of noradrenergic peaks.[14]

Heart rate, blood pressure, and ventilation

Heart rate oscillates during the day, with a peak at around 1500 hours and an amplitude of 5–15%.[15] An analogous pattern is demonstrable for stroke volume, cardiac output, blood flow, and blood pressure.[16] Both heart rate and blood pressure are greatly influenced by exogenous factors, such as sleep, posture, diet, and activity,[17] although it has been shown that the temporal organisation of blood pressure is mainly controlled by neuroendocrine mechanisms, coupled to either sleep or an endogenous pacemaker which is usually predominantly (although not solely) circadian.[18]

Gastrointestinal and urinary function

Circadian rhythms are associated with several gastrointestinal functions—for example, motility patterns, enzyme activity, and acid secretion.[19] Gastric emptying rates, for example, are over 50% slower for evening than morning meals.[20] As for urinary function, urinary electrolytes show an afternoon peak,[21] and urinary pH is lower during sleep and higher in the morning.[22]

Chronotype

An important factor is the personality "chronotype"—that is, whether one is a morning person ("lark") who gets up and goes to bed early, or an evening person ("owl"), who wakes up and retires late. There is a difference of about 65 minutes in the peaks of body temperature rhythm between morning and evening types, and morning types secrete significantly more adrenaline in the morning than do evening types. Furthermore, the timing of mood and activity rhythms differs by several hours between distinct morning and evening types.[23]

Circadian variations in sports performance

For more in depth information readers should read the excellent review by Atkinson and Reilly.[24] We will summarise the data from it. Although considerations such as environmental influences, temperature, meteorological conditions, and scheduled time of events make generalisation difficult, most components of sports

---

Box 16.2   Jeg lag and athletic performance

- The transient desynchronisation of a traveller's biological rhythms after a rapid air travel across several time zones, is called jet lag. Such disruption lasts until biological rhythms adjust to the new environmental conditions
- The most common subjective symptoms associated with jet lag include sleep disorders, difficulties with concentrating, disorientation, distorted estimation of time, space, and distances, mood disorders, and gastrointestinal disturbances. Westward flights (characterised by a phase delay) are usually tolerated more than eastward flights (phase advance)
- Selecting the best circadian time for exercise can result in an increase in athletic performance. On the other hand, an athletic task performed several hours before or after the optimal circadian window will potentially lead to less than optimal results
- Due to the shift in the circadian window jet lag may cause negative effects in competitive athletes required to travel rapidly all over the world. However, negative effects of jet lag are difficult to investigate because of the masking effects of stress, fatigue by the flight itself, motivation, etc. Thus, no final conclusions are at this time available

---

performance exhibit a rhythmic variation during the day, with a peak in the early evening. The time of day is characterised by peaks in reaction time,[25] isometric hand grip strength,[26] elbow flexion strength,[27] back strength,[28] total work performed in high-intensity constant work-rate exercise,[29] and lactate production[30] and lowest levels of joint stiffness[31] and pain perception.[32] When subjects are free to choose their submaximal work-rate during exercise of less than 40 minutes' duration, higher work rates are achieved in the early evening without any change in the perception of effort.[33] Moreover, in young adults the mean work rate over 80 minutes of exercise was found to be higher in the afternoon than in the morning.[34] Improvements in muscle strength after training sessions scheduled in the evening have been found to be 20% higher than those after training carried out in the morning.[35] In untrained male volunteers aerobic exercise performance did not show variations during the time frame within which exercise is normally conducted, although some physiological responses to exercise did.[36] In fact, resting plasma lactate concentrations and lactate responses to maximal exercise showed a circadian pattern, as well as absolute plasma noradrenaline concentrations after exercise, and noradrenaline responses to exercise. Long term memory recall, in which data must be retained for 1 week or longer, is 8% higher when the material is presented at 1500 hours than at 0900 hours.[37] The implications are important for the timing of coaching instructions and strategy as the 8% difference in memory retention is similar to the performance decrement induced when sleep is restricted to 3 hours. When individual differences in performances were controlled for, a significant early evening peak was found for length of jump,[38] and vertical jumping performance.[39] Swimming performance shows an evening peak too,[40] having rhythm amplitudes of 11 to 14% of the 24 hour mean values. The circadian variation in swimming performance is greater than the effect of obtaining only 3 hours of sleep for three successive nights.[41] It has to be stressed that there is an inverse relation between speed and accuracy in a simple repetitive test,[42] with accuracy being worse in the early evening. Remembering that other aspects of performance—for example, mental arithmetic and short term memory—peak in the early morning rather than evening hours,[43] it is possible that times of day other than the evening may be better for sports that demand accuracy, for competitive strategies, and for delivery and recall of coaching instructions.

Desynchronisation and athletic performance

A poor competitive performance may result when an athlete does not take into consideration his or her circadian performance profile, as an athletic task undertaken several hours before or after the circadian peak "window" will potentially be performed with less than optimal efficiency. Taking circadian rhythms into consideration can produce major benefits in tasks involving endurance, mental function, physical strength, and others. Selection of the best circadian time can result in as much as a 10% increase in athletic performance. A 10% decrement in peak performance can be compared with a performance after less than 3 hours of sleep, after drinking the legal limit of alcohol,[44] or after taking barbiturates.[45]

Jet lag may cause a shift in the circadian peak window. A recent study by Reilly *et al.* showed that, in British Olympic squad members, several performance measures—for example, leg and back strength, choice reaction time and subjective jet lag symptoms—were impaired for 5 days after a trip from the United Kingdom to Florida.[46] The first to be re-established was the sleep-wake cycle, then body temperature, and absence of jet lag symptoms before the complete normalisation of rhythms in performance measures. It has been reported that the performances of travelling American football teams depend on how closely the game time corresponds to the usual afternoon peaks in performance.[47] West coast teams, in fact, appear to be at an advantage over east and central teams for night games.

Although it is somewhat difficult to investigate the negative effects of jet lag in competitive athletes because of the masking of negative effects of stress, fatigue caused by the flight itself, and the forced situation of competing in a "different" environment a very interesting contribution has been recently provided by Recht and coworkers.[48] They analysed records for three complete seasons (1991–1993) of the 19 North American major league baseball teams based in cities of the Eastern and Pacific time zones. These teams had significantly more victories when they were playing at home than away (54% v 46%), and it was found that the probability of winning depended on whether the visiting team had just travelled eastward. The home team could, in fact, expect to score 1.24 more runs than usual when the visitors had just completed an eastward journey. The authors concluded that, although there are many factors, one critical component of the "home field" advantage involved previous transcontinental travel by the visiting team within the precedent 2 days but only in the case of an eastward direction. In accordance with such results, previous studies on a series of surveys on the scores of international games held in Japan and their relation to the length of stay of the visiting team,[49] showed an increase in performance level (as judged by the outcome of their matches) in parallel with adjusting to the new time zone. Again, Smith et al. tried to confirm the circadian time hypothesis by analysing the data from all Monday night football games between United States teams of both east and west coast.[50] As these games always start at 2100 hours in the east the authors hypothesised that the west coast teams would have an advantage. Thus, they analysed the data with respect to the Las Vegas point spread, which is designed to equalise several factors—for example, time zone, playing surface, home field advantage, etc. It was found that the west coast teams won significantly more games (63.5% v 36.5%), and outscored the east coast teams significantly more than predicted by the Las Vegas point spreads. On the other hand, another recent paper by Steenland and Deddens analysed the results of National Basketball Association (NBA) games over 8 years (1987–95).[51] As for the subanalysis of east versus west teams, when teams had equal rest and only the visitors had travelled, no significant differences in performance were found. From all these retrospective studies, however, no conclusive data on negative effects of jet lag performance can be drawn. A recent critical update of the literature by Youngstedt and O'Connor concluded that because of the serious flaws in previous research there is no compelling evidence that transmeridian air travel impairs athletic performance.[52] On the other hand, most of the above quoted retrospective studies were conducted in the United States, with a crossing of about three time zones, which may be insufficient to determine a clear shift in circadian biological rhythms. An international prospective field study designed to verify the negative effects of jeg lag on athletic performance is currently underway.

Measures to alleviate jet lag

Several measures have been suggested to reduce the negative effects of circadian rhythm desynchronisation, although treatment of shift workers, competitive athletes, and simple international travellers is quite different. The measures include preadaptation, meal timing and composition, phototherapy, and chronobiotic drugs.

Preadaptation

Theoretically, the negative effects of jet lag can be reduced by changing bedtime for several days before a transcontinental journey, remembering that sleep changes should correspond to the direction of travel (eastward or westward). Adaptation should be disturbed by behaviour that anchors the circadian rhythms to the previous phase—for example, taking prolonged naps at the new destination.[53] To lock the circadian rhythms to home time, at least 4 hours' sleep taken within the window of normal sleep in the home time zone are needed.[9] However, in practice, preadaptation is superfluous when people are travelling west, arriving late, and only a few hours phase advance can be recommended before travelling east.[54] Moreover, because of the difficulty of manipulating other synchronising factors (light, social constraints), preadjusting the sleep-wake cycles is largely ineffective.[55]

Timing and composition of meals

Certain food constituents seem to have effects on rhythm adjustment. A high carbohydrate low protein meal, facilitating brain uptake of tryptophan and its conversion to serotonin, may induce drowsiness and sleep. On the other hand, a high protein low carbohydrate meal, which enhances tyrosine uptake and conversion to noradrenaline, increases levels of arousal.[56] Moreover, programmed use of theophylline and caffeine can speed rhythm readaptation and help to raise arousal levels in the morning. However, although studies on military personnel consuming such diets reported reduced sleep disturbance and less subjective feelings of fatigue in the days immediately after a transmeridian flight compared with controls,[2] a clear link between diet and jet lag has not been formally established.

Phototherapy

When an individual's circadian phase is known, it is possible to act on the central clock mechanism, advancing or delaying the clock itself. Exposure to bright light, with specified intensity, duration, and timing, may advance or delay the phase of some human circadian rhythms.[57] Most available studies have used jet lag simulations, so the subjects are not exposed to the full complement of time cues normally encountered by transmeridian travellers; this has been reviewed by Boulos et al.[58] Two studies have investigated the effects of light treatment on sleep patterns after flights. In the former, 19 subjects returning to the United States from Oriental or South Pacific localities (advance shifts of 6.5 to 10 hours) were instructed to expose themselves to either bright white light (2000 lux) or dim red light (<100 lux) for 2 or 3 hours on awakening in the morning for 3 days.[59] No differences were found between the group means for any sleep measure, but exposure to bright light early in the morning appeared to facilitate the consolidation of sleep into a single night-time episode. In the latter, four subjects were polysomnographically recorded before and after a flight from Tokyo to San Francisco (8 hour advance).[60] In San Francisco, the subjects were requested to go bed at 2300 hours and wake up by 1000 hours and were exposed for 3 consecutive days to either bright (>3000 lux) or dim (<500 lux) light for 3 hours starting at 1100 hours (0300 hours Tokyo time). The bright light treatment seemed to be effective in accelerating circadian re-entrainment. However, the sparse number of field studies and the small sample population considered do not yet allow a clear judgment on the beneficial effect of bright light treatment for jet lag.[61] In fact, the Consensus Report for Light Treatment for Sleep Disorders[58] concluded that "much remains to be learned before procedures can be developed that are at once effective, reliable, and practical. For this to happen, optimal combinations of several light exposure parameters must be first defined and tailored to specific flight situations".

Chronobiotic drugs

Chronobiotic drugs are drugs that specifically affect some aspects of biological time structure, but they must be administered at the right time of the day. In the past few years, several putative chronobiotic drugs have been evaluated—for example, barbiturates,[62] short-acting benzodiazepines,[63] serotonin-depleting agents,[64] and corticosteroids,[65] with unsatisfactory or inconclusive results.[10]

The pineal hormone melatonin (*N*-acetyl-5-methoxytryptamine) is a very interesting chronomodulating substance. It is normally secreted at night and in animals serves to transmit information about the light-dark cycle to the body.[66] However, melatonin acts in a highly pleiotropic fashion, also eliciting secondary humoral immunological responses—for example, via interleukin-4 and other cytokines—or acting as a powerful radical scavenger.[67] The first reported administration of melatonin[68] induced a mild sedative effect, which was initially considered to be a pharmacological side effect. In fact, the hypnotic effect of melatonin is considered to be an integral part of its physiological action. In an early study with polysomnography,[69] intravenous infusion of melatonin before bedtime was associated with significantly increased sedation, reduced psychomotor activity, and shortened sleep-onset latency. A recent study on healthy volunteers provided further evidence that nocturnal melatonin secretion may be involved in sleep onset and that exogenous melatonin may be useful in treating insomnia.[70] Low oral doses of melatonin, just enough to increase serum melatonin concentrations to levels normally occurring at night,[71] produce hypnotic effects when given in the evening. Moreover, in humans, melatonin is likely to be an effective hypnotic agent to combat sleep disruption associated with increased temperature due to low circulating melatonin concentrations, and it may also improve sleep disruption caused by drugs that interfere with melatonin production—for example, β blockers and benzodiazepines.[72] Melatonin has been utilised for treatment of jet lag induced rhythm disturbances. In an early study reporting its use in transmeridian travellers, Arendt *et al.* administered melatonin to 17 subjects over a period of 14 days after a westward flight from London to San Francisco.[73] Compared with placebo, melatonin significantly reduced the negative feelings of jet lag and increased subjective alertness. Moreover, treated subjects also reported significantly reduced sleep onset latency and improved sleep quality, and endogenous melatonin and cortisol rhythms resynchronised more rapidly than in those consuming a placebo. In another study, 20 volunteers with experience in transcontinental flights were pretreated with melatonin (5 mg, orally) for three days before the flight, during the flight, and for 3 days after arrival at their destination.[74] The subjects pretreated with melatonin, compared with those taking placebo, reported significantly reduced feelings of jet lag and less time to establish a normal sleep pattern, reaching a "normal energy level" earlier than the controls and reporting lower levels of tiredness during the day. Nickelsen *et al.* administered 5 mg of melatonin or placebo at bedtime with no treatment before the flight in a cross over design. An accelerated adaptation of cortisol and a consistent, though non-significant, improvement of subjective jet lag with melatonin both westward and eastward were found.[75] A controlled double blind trial with melatonin was performed in healthy volunteers flying between North America and France selected for their sensitivity to eastward jet lag.[76] The protocol was simple, as one daily capsule of melatonin was administered on the day of return and the three consecutive evenings thereafter. A significant difference in self rating for global treatment efficacy, morning fatigue, and evening sleepiness was found in the melatonin compared with placebo group. Another study investigated the efficacy of oral melatonin in alleviating jet lag in flight crew after a series of international flights and the optimal time for consumption; it was shown that benefits are especially likely to occur when melatonin is consumed after arrival.[77] Subjects taking melatonin for 5 days at home after the return flight showed a more rapid recovery of energy and alertness than those taking melatonin from 1 day before departure. It has been reported that the amount and the direction of the phase shift depends on the time of melatonin ingestion: evening administration advances the body clock and morning administration delays it.[78]

Conclusions

Competitive athletes of many sport disciplines are nowadays, as never before, earning considerable sums of money by taking part in worldwide competitions. A growing series of events—tournaments, international meetings, world series, world cup challenges, and sponsored trophies—have greatly lengthened the competitive season. Only a few years ago, worldwide competitions were limited to the Olympic Games, World Championships, and a few other "top events". Thus, athletes are now required to travel quickly all over the world with no allowance for any "synchronisation" other than television network schedules. Both the next Winter and Summer Olympic Games (scheduled to take place in Australia and the United States respectively) will require the crossing of several time zones especially by European teams.

As for measures for alleviating jet lag in athletes, preadaptation (because of social and behavioural constraints) is hardly practicable and also ineffective, and adaptation at the place of competition requires time and money. Appropriate timing and composition of meals may be useful for accelerating the adaptation of circadian

---

Box 16.3   Management of jet lag

- Several measures to alleviate jet leg have been suggested, although treatment of simple international travellers or competitive athletes is quite different. They include preadaptation, meal time and composition, phototherapy, and chronobiotic drugs
- Theoretically, preadaptation is the most simple measure. Effects of jet lag can be reduced by changing bedtime for several days before a transcontinental flight, taking into consideration sleep changes and direction of travel (eastward or wesward). In practice, due to a series of practical and social difficulties, readaptation is largely ineffective
- It is possible that some food constituents may have effects on rhythm adjustment. Programmed use of theophylline and caffeine can speed up readaptation, and high carbohydrate-low protein or high protein-low carbohydrate meals can induce, respectively, drowsiness and sleep or increase of arousal. However, a clear link between diet and jet lag has not been formally established
- Exposure to bright light with specified intensity, duration, and timing may advance or delay the body central clock. However, though results of studies conducted on small sample populations are promising, definite conclusions cannot be drawn yet
- Several putative chronobiotic drugs, for example, benzodiazepines, barbiturates, corticosteroids, and serotonin-depleting agents have been evaluated with unsatisfactory or inconclusive results. The pineal hormone melatonin seems to be an interesting and promising chronomodulating substance, though results of exhaustive studies on athletes are not available yet

rhythms to the timing of environmental synchronisers at the athlete's destination, although limitations set by commercial airlines and/or restrictions of the training diet have to be considered. Phototherapy is undoubtedly of interest but still far too broad a practical standardisation. Probably, in the future, the combined use of bright light and melatonin will give satisfactory results, although further exhaustive studies specifically targeted for competitive athletes are needed. While short term studies indicate that melatonin has very low toxicity, there are no long term safety data. All the reported studies deal with healthy adult volunteers and the use of a preparation licensed for human experimental use and available on a named patient basis on prescription. There are no data on uncontrolled preparations available over the counter in some countries.[79]

The efficacy of melatonin in alleviating symptoms of jet lag is not in dispute but to what extent the beneficial effects of melatonin extend to promoting performance and mood in the new daytime is less clear.[80] Although melatonin is not licensed for use in Europe, it is freely available in the United States at varying grades of purity and most frequent flyers and/or top athletes regularly consume it. Unfortunately, the dosage and timing is not always correct, and it should be emphasised that the hypnotic action of melatonin may have disappointing consequences on athletic performance. The British Olympic Association has recently recommended caution in the use of melatonin and hypnotics, especially in subjects in whom beneficial effects without adverse side effects have not been shown.[81] In any case, however, the indiscriminate use of unlicensed preparations is not advisable. Specialists should always be consulted for personalised administration schedules.

1 Winget CM, DeRoshia CW, Markley CL, et al. A review of human physiology and performance changes associated with desynchronosis of biological rhythms. Aviat Space Environ Med 1984;551:1085–96.

2 Graeber RC. Alterations in performance following rapid transmeridian flight. In: Brown FM, Graeber RC, eds. Rhythmic aspects of behavior. Hillsdale, New Jersey: Lawrence Erlbaum Associates, 1982:173–212.

3 Lavernhe J, LaFontaine E, Pasquet J. Les réactions subjectives et objectives aux ruptures des rythmes circadiens lors des vols commerciaux long courriers est-ouest et vice-versa. Revue de Medecine Aeronautique Spatiale 1968;7:121–3.

4 Preston FS. Further sleep problems in airline pilots on worldwide schedules. Aerospace Medicine 1973;44:775–82.

5 Preston FS, Bateman SC, Short RV, et al. Effects of flying and of time changes on menstrual cycle length and performance in airline stewardesses. Aerospace Medicine 1973;44:438–43.

6 Suvanto S, Prtinen M, Harma M, *et al.* Flight attendents' desynchronosis after rapid time zone changes. *Aviat Space Environ Med* 1990;**61**:543–7.

7 Klein K, Wegmann H. The resynchronization of human circadian rhythms after transmeridian flights as a result of flight direction and mode of activity. In: Scheving LE, ed. *Chronobiology.* Tokyo: Igaku-Shoin, 1974:564–70.

8 Aschoff J, Hoffmann K, Pohl H, *et al.* Re-entrainment of circadian rhythms after phase-shifts to the zeitgeber. *Chronobiologia* 1975;**2**:23–78.

9 Winget CM, Soliman MRI, Holley DC, *et al.* Chronobiology of physical performance and sports medicine. In: Touitou Y, Haus E, eds. *Biologic rhythms in clinical and laboratory medicine.* Berlin and Heidelberg: Springer Verlag, 1992:230–42.

10 Redfern P, Minors D, Waterhouse J. Circadian rhythms, jet lag, and chron-obiotics: an overview. *Chronobiol Int* 1994;**11**:253–65.

11 Moline ML, Pollack CP, Monk TH, *et al.* Age-related differences in recovery from simulated jet-lag. *Sleep* 1992;**15**:28–40.

12 Suvanto S, Härma M. The prediction of the adaptation of circadian rhythms to rapid time zone changes. *Ergonomics* 1993;**36**:111–6.

13 Minors D, Waterhouse J. *Circadian rhythms and the human.* London: Wright PSG, 1981.

14 Akerstedt T. Altered sleep/wake patterns and circadian rhythms. *Acta Physiol Scand Suppl* 1979;**469**:1–48.

15 Reilly T. Human circadian rhythm and exercise. *Crit Rev Biomed Eng* 1990;**18**:165–80.

16 Smolensky MH, Tatar SE, Bergman SA, *et al.* Circadian rhythmic aspects of human cardiovascular function: a review by chronobiologic statistical methods. *Chronobiologia* 1976;**3**:337–71.

17 Pickering TG. The influence of daily activity on ambulatory blood pressure. *Am Heart J* 1988;**116**:1141–5.

18 Portaluppi F, Vergnani L, Manfredini R, *et al.* Endocrine mechanisms of blood pressure rhythms. *Ann NY Acad Sci* 1996;**783**:113–31.

19 Moore JG. Chronobiology of the gastrointestinal system. In: Touitou Y, Haus E, eds. *Biological rhythms in clinical and laboratory medicine.* Berlin: Springer-Verlag, 1992:410–7.

20 Goo RH, Moore JG, Greenberg E, *et al.* Circadian variation in gastric emptying of meals in man. *Gastroenterology* 1987;**93**:513–18.

21 Touitou Y, Touitou C, Bogdan A, *et al.* Circadian and seasonal variations of electrolytes in ageing humans. *Clin Chim Acta* 1989;**180**:245–54.

22 Robertson WG, Hodgkinson A, Marshall DH. Seasonal variations in the composition of urine from normal subjects: a longitudinal study. *Clin Chim Acta* 1977;**80**:347–53.

23 Winget CM, DeRoshia CW, Holley DC. Circadian rhythms and athletic performance. *Med Sci Sports Exerc* 1985;**17**:498–516.

24 Atkinson G, Reilly T. Circadian variation in sports performance. *Sports Med* 1996;**21**:292–312.

25 Kleitman N. *Sleep and wakefulness.* Chicago: University of Chicago Press, 1963.

26 Gifford LS. Circadian variation in human flexibility and grip strength. *Aust J Physiother* 1987;**33**:3–9.

27 Coldwells A, Atkinson G, Reilly T. Sources of variation in back and leg dynamometry. *Ergonomics* 1993;**37**:79–86.

28 Atkinson G, Greeves J, Cable T, *et al.* Day-to-day and circadian variability of leg strength measured with the LIDO isokinetic dynamometer. *J Sports Sci* 1995;**13**:18–9.

29 Hill DW, Borden DO, Darnaby KM, *et al.* Effect of time of day on aerobic and anaerobic responses to high intensity exercise. *Can J Sports Sci* 1992;**17**:316–9.

30 Reilly T, Baxter C. Influence of time of day on reactions to cycling at a fixed high

intensity. *Br J Sports Med* 1983;**17**:128–30.

31 Wright V, Dawson D, Longfield MD. Joint stiffness: its characterisation and significance. *Biol Med Eng* 1969;**4**:8–14.

32 Procacci P, della Corte M, Zoppi M, *et al.* Rhythmic changes of the cutaneous pain threshold in man. *Chronobiologia* 1974;**1**:77–96.

33 Coldwells A, Atkinson G, Reilly T, *et al.* Self-chosen work-rate determinates day-night differences in work capacity. *Ergonomics* 1993;**36**:313.

34 Atkinson G, Reilly T. Effects of age and time of day on preferred work rates during prolonged exercise. *Chronobiol Int* 1995;**12**:121–34.

35 Hildebrandt G, Gutenbrunner C, Reinhart C. Circadian variation of isometric strength training in man. In: Morgan E, ed. *Chronobiology and chronomedicine.* Frankfurt: Peter Lang, 1990:322–9 (vol 2).

36 Deschenes MR, Sharma JV, Brittingham KT, *et al.* Chronobiological effect on exercise performance and selected physiological responses. *Eur J Appl Physiol* 1998;**77**:249–56.

37 Folkard S, Monk TH, Bradbury R, *et al.* Time of day effects in school children's immediate and delayed recall of meaningful material. *Br J Psychol* 1977;**68**:45–50.

38 Reilly T, Down A. Circadian variation in the standing broad jump. *Percept Mot Skills* 1986;**62**:830.

39 Reilly T, Down A. Investigation of circadian rhythms in anaerobic power and capacity of the legs. *J Sports Med Phys Fitness* 1992;**33**:343–7.

40 Reilly T, Marshall S. Circadian rhythms in power output on a swim bench. *J Swim Res* 1991;**7**:11–3.

41 Sinnerton S, Reilly T. Effect of sleep loss and time of day in swimmers. In: Maclaren D, Reilly T, Lees A, eds. *Biomechanics and medicine in swimming: swimming science VI.* London: E and FN Spon, 1992:399–405.

42 Monk TH, Leng VC. Time of day effects in simple repetitive tasks: some possible mechanisms. *Acta Psychol (Amst)* 1982;**51**:207–21.

43 Monk TH. Chronobiology of mental performance. In: Touitou Y, Haus E, eds. *Biological rhythms in clinical and laboratory medicine.* Berlin: Springer-Verlag, 1992:208–13.

44 Folkard S, Monk TH. Chronopsychology: circadian rhythms and human performance. In: Gale A, Edwards JA, eds. *Attention and performance.* New York: Academic Press, 1983:55–78 (vol 2).

45 Klein KE, Bruner H, Wegmann HM, *et al.* Die Veränderung der psychomotorischen Leistungsbereitschaft als Folge pharmakodynamischer Einwirkung verschiedener Substanzen mit potentiell sedierenden Effekt. *Arzneimittelforschung* 1967;**17**:1048–51.

46 Reilly T, Atkinson G, Budgett R. Effects of temazepam on physiological and performance variables following a westerly flight across five time zones. *J Sports Sci* 1997;**15**:62.

47 Jehue R, Street D, Huizenga R. Effect of time zone and game time changes on team performance: National Football League. *Med Sci Sports Exerc* 1993;**25**:127–31.

48 Recht LD, Lew RA, Schwartz WJ. Baseball teams beaten by jet lag. (Letter). *Nature* 1995;**377**:583.

49 Sasaki T. Effect of jet lag on sports performance. In: Scheving LE, Halberg F, eds. *Chronobiology: principles and applications to shifts in schedules.* Rockville: Sijthoff and Noordhoff, 1980:417–34.

50 Smith RS, Guilleminault C, Efron B. Circadian rhythms and enhanced athletic performance in the National Football League. *Sleep* 1997;**20**:362–5.

51 Steenland K, Deddens JA. Effect of travel and rest on performance of professional basketball players. *Sleep* 1997;**20**:366–9.

52 Youngstedt SD, O'Connor PJ. The influence of air travel on athletic performance: an update. *Sports Med* (in press).

53 Minors DS, Waterhouse JM. Anchor sleep as a synchronizer of abnormal routine. *Int J Chronobiol* 1981;7:165–88.

54 Reilly T, Atkinson G, Waterhouse J. *Biological Rhythms and Exercise.* Oxford: Oxford University Press, 1997.

55 Reilly T, Atkinson G, Waterhouse J. Travel fatigue and jet-lag. *J Sports Sci* 1997;15:365–9.

56 Wurtman RJ. Nutrients that modify brain function. *Sci Am* 1982;246:50–9.

57 Czeisler CA, Allan JS, Strogatz SH, *et al.* Bright light resets the human circadian pacemaker independent of the timing of the sleep-wake cycle. *Science* 1986;233:667–71.

58 Boulos Z, Campbell SC, Lewy AJ, *et al.* Light treatment for sleep disorders: consensus report. VII. Jet lag. *J Biol Rhythms* 1995;10:167–76.

59 Cole RJ, Kripke DF. Amelioration of jet lag by bright light treatment: effects on sleep consolidation. *Sleep Res* 1989;18:411.

60 Sasaki M, Kurosaki Y, Onda M, *et al.* Effects of bright light on circadian rhythmicity and sleep after transmeridian flight. *Sleep Res* 1989;18:442.

61 Samuel A, Wegmann HA. Bright light: a countermeasure for jet lag? *Chronobiol Int* 1997;14:173–83.

62 Simpson HW. Chronobiotics: selected agents of potential value in jet lag and other dyschronisms. In: Scheving LE, Halberg F, eds. *Chronobiology: principles and applications to shift and schedules.* Rockville: Sijthoff and Noordhoff, 1980:433–46.

63 Wee BE, Turek FW. Midazolam, a short acting benzodiazepine, resets the circadian clock of the hamster. *Pharmacol Biochem Behav* 1989;32:901–6.

64 Simpson HW, Bellamy N, Halberg F. Double blind trial of a possible chronobiotic (quiadon): field studies in N.W. Greenland. *Int J Chronobiol* 1973;1:287–311.

65 Christie GA, Moore-Robinson M. Project Pegasus: circadian rhythms and new aspects of corticosteroids. *Clin Trials J* 1970;7:7–135.

66 Tamarkin L, Baird CJ, Almeida OFX. Melatonin: a co-ordinating signal for mammalian reproduction. *Science* 1985;227:714–20.

67 Hardeland R, Rodriguez C. Versatile melatonin: a pervasive molecule serves various functions in signaling and protection. *Chronobiol Int* 1995;12:157–65.

68 Lerner AB, Case JD. Melatonin. *Fed Proc* 1960;19:590–2.

69 Cramer H, Rudolph J, Consbruch U. On the effects of melatonin on sleep and behavior in man. *Adv Biochem Psychopharmacol* 1974;2:187–91.

70 Zhdanova IV, Wurtman RJ, Lynch HJ, *et al.* Sleep-inducing effects of low doses of melatonin ingested in the evening. *Clin Pharmacol Ther* 1995;57:552–8.

71 Dollins AB, Zhdanova IV, Wurtman RJ, *et al.* Effect of inducing nocturnal serum melatonin concentrations in daytime on sleep, mood, body temperature, and performance. *Proc Natl Acad Sci USA* 1994;91:1824–8.

72 Dawson D, Encel N. Melatonin and sleep in humans. *J Pineal Res* 1993;15:1–12.

73 Arendt J, Aldhous M, English J, *et al.* The effects of jet-lag and their alleviation by melatonin. *Ergonomics* 1987;30:1379–93.

74 Petrie K, Conaglen JV, Thompson L, *et al.* Effect of melatonin on jet lag after long haul flights. *BMJ* 1990;298:705–7.

75 Nickelsen T, Lang A, Bergan L. The effect of 6-, 9- and 11-hour time shifts on circadian rhythms: adaptation of sleep parameters and hormonal patterns following the intake of melatonin or placebo. In: Arendt J, Pevet P, eds. *Advances in pineal research* 1991;5:303–6.

76 Claustrat B, Brun J, David M, *et al.* Melatonin and jet-lag: confirmatory result using a simplified protocol. *Biol Psychiatry* 1992;32:705–11.

77 Petrie K, Dawson AG, Thompson L, *et al.* A double-blind trial of melatonin as a treatment for jet-lag in international cabin crew. *Biol Psychiatry* 1993;33:526–30.

78 Lewy AJ, Ahmed S, Jackson JM, *et al.* Melatonin shifts human circadian rhythms according to a phase response curve. *Chronobiol Int* 1992;**9**:380–93.
79 Arendt J, Deacon S. Treatment of circadian rhythm disorders—melatonin. *Chronobiol Int* 1997;**14**:185–204.
80 Waterhouse J, Reilly T, Atkinson G. Melatonin and jet lag. *Br J Sports Med* 1998;**32**:98–9.
81 Reilly T, Maughan R, Budgett R. Melatonin: a position statement of the British Olympic Association. *Br J Sports Med* 1998;**32**:99–100.

Multiple choice questions

1 Which of the following are true for biological rhythms?
  (a) They are endogenous, inherited with DNA
  (b) They are determined by environmental cues
  (c) They may be revealed and predicted on the basis of the date of birth
  (d) They may have a wide range of periods, from seconds to years

2 Which of the following are true for chronotype?
  (a) It is an important factor in personality
  (b) All people can be categorised into "morning" or "evening" types
  (c) Morning or evening types also exhibit different patterns in biological parameters
  (d) Different chronotypes may result in different results in athletic performance

3 Which of the following are true for jet lag?
  (a) It occurs after every flight
  (b) Its subjective associated symptoms include sleep and mood disorders and gastrointestinal disturbances
  (c) Westward flights are followed by a faster recovery than eastward flights
  (d) Jet lag symptoms are reported by all transcontinental travellers
  (e) The intensity of sleep disturbances usually decreases from the first night onwards

4 For rhythms of physiological variables which are true?
  (a) Body temperature shows a circadian pattern, with its peak in the evening
  (b) This rhythm is determined by metabolic processes leading to heat production
  (c) Main cardiovascular parameters—for example, heart rate and blood pressure—show an afternoon circadian peak

(d) Blood pressure rhythm is the result of both exogenous and endogenous factors

(e) Digestion is faster after lunch than after dinner

5 Which of the following are true for circadian variations in sports performance?

(a) Most components of sports performance show a rhythmic variation during the day, with a peak in afternoon–early evening hours

(b) Improvements in muscle strength after training sessions scheduled in the evening are higher than those in the morning

(c) Joint stiffness and pain perception have their lowest levels in the afternoon

(d) Though these circadian variations exist, no evidence is available in experimental controlled studies

6 Also regarding circadian variations in sports performance, which of the following show characteristic peaks in the afternoon?

(a) Isometric hand grip strength

(b) Elbow flexion strength

(c) Back strength

(d) Reaction time

(e) Long term memory recall

(f) Short term memory

(g) Speed in a single repetitive test

(h) Accuracy in a simple repetitive test

7 Which of the following are true regarding measures to alleviate jet lag?

(a) Though theoretically preadaptation is the most simple one, in practice it is largely ineffective

(b) Certain food constituents can speed up rhythm readaptation

(c) It is possible to advance or delay the central clock mechanism of an individual by means of exposure to a source of light

(d) The pineal hormone melatonin is only an hypnotic substance

(e) No double blind, controlled studies on melatonin administration have been carried out in athletes

(f) Amount and direction of the phase shift depend on the time of melatonin ingestion

Answers are on p. 365.

17 Intermittent exercise patterns

A E Hardman

Introduction

Physical activity is recognised as an important component of a healthy lifestyle, by the population at large as well as by scientists and clinicians. Nevertheless, most adult men and women in this country are physically inactive.[1] To alleviate the considerable public health burden of this level of inactivity requires nothing less than a major shift of behaviour to a more active style of living.[2] A start has been made with efforts to develop a physical activity strategy for England[3] and the Health Education Authority's campaign "Active Living". Both initiatives reflect a change of emphasis in making recommendations for physical activity. Traditionally, recommendations were for 20 to 60 minutes of moderate to high intensity endurance-type exercise performed three or more times a week. By contrast, recent consensus statements from expert bodies in the United States (on which the United Kingdom recommendations are modelled) encompass the notion that many health gains may be acquired through moderate intensity physical activities outside formal exercise programmes.[4-6] This chapter is concerned with one particular aspect of these recommendations—namely, that one effective pattern of physical activity is several short sessions during the day.

Methods

A search was made through Medline from 1970 to the present, with combinations of the following terms: "accumulation", "exercise", "training", "intermittent", "continuous", "short bout(s)", "long bout(s)", "session(s)", "physical activity recommendations" and "splitting distance/time". A large number of publications were found through use of the terms intermittent and continuous but, with one exception, these compared the effects of training through rather long bouts of exercise with those of "interval training"—that is, high intensity efforts separated by brief recovery periods but within the same session. As the key feature of accumulating exercise is performance of several short separate exercise sessions throughout the day, this literature was not pursued further. Only five original papers were found describing studies comparing the effects of increasing levels of physical activity through several short sessions of exercise a day with those from one longer session. Because of the paucity of literature covering this topic specifically, additional indirect evidence has been invoked (with a personal library) in evaluating the rationale for the proposition that physical activity accumulated through the day confers health benefits.

Observational studies

Guidelines for the amount of exercise needed to confer health gains were originally developed from two lines of evidence: first, epidemiological findings of a lower risk of coronary heart disease and premature mortality in men who engaged in considerable amounts of physical activity; and second, the literature describing the amount and type of exercise needed to increase endurance fitness (usually assessed as maximal oxygen uptake ($\dot{V}O_2MAX$)) in healthy adults. The common feature was planned exercise or training of a fairly vigorous nature. In fact, in one landmark study of English civil servants, only "vigorous" exercise was associated with a lower risk of heart attack. Thus the accepted view was that activities that increase fitness confer many, maybe most, health benefits. This view is probably sound as studies that have related physical fitness to all-cause mortality and cause specific mortality and morbidities have shown.[7–10]

However, although the epidemiological evidence undoubtedly shows that engaging in activity sufficient to improve fitness, including vigorous sports, is associated with low risk, it also shows that activity unlikely to improve fitness may also be effective. For example, some studies have shown a strong, inverse association between some measure of the total amount of energy expended in leisure-time physical activity and cardiovascular[11] or all cause mortality,[11,12] incidence of type II diabetes,[13] hypertension[14] and site-specific cancers.[15,16] In the British regional heart study, the inverse relation between physical activity index and risk of ischaemic heart disease was not reduced by excluding all men who reported doing vigorous sporting activity; thus men who regularly engaged in gardening, do-it-yourself and "pleasure walking" experienced a reduced rate of heart attack.[17]

In many of these studies, the type of activity associated with more favourable health outcomes is likely to have been performed at least partly on an intermittent basis. These include walking, climbing stairs, gardening[12,18,19] and, in one recent Finnish study, repair work.[11] Stair-climbing—surely almost never performed in long continuous sessions—has been associated with a decreased risk of premature death; men who climbed fewer than 20 flights of stairs per week had a 23% higher risk than men who climbed more.[20]

Walking, particularly when undertaken for personal transport, is often performed in rather short sessions at intervals of some hours. The amount of walking has been associated with a lower risk of all cause mortality in middle aged men (21% lower risk as distance increased from less than 5 km (3 miles) to 14 km (9 miles) or more per week),[12] in retired men (59% lower risk for those who walked 3 km (2 miles) or more a day, compared with those who walked less than 1.5 km (1 mile) a day),[21] and in women (~60% lower risk in those expending energy equivalent to walking for about 45 minutes three times a week).[22]

Data from the Harvard alumni show an inverse relation between energy expended in non-vigorous activities and incidence of type II diabetes.[13] This ties in with the finding that glucose intolerance is less common in individuals reporting high total levels of physical activity (expressed as METs per hour per week).[23] In the latter study, most of the activity for men was occupational (and, therefore probably not undertaken in long continuous spells), whereas for women regular walking (not for formal exercise) was the commonest activity. Similarly, in the insulin resistance atherosclerosis study, levels of expenditure in non-vigorous activities (3.5 to 5 METs, typically home maintenance, gardening, indoor household chores, brisk walking) were positively related to insulin sensitivity, independent of vigorous activity.[24]

A high level of physical activity has recently been associated with reduced risk of colon cancer. For example, in Norwegian women, leisure time activity equivalent to walking or cycling for at least 4 hours a week was associated with a 38% decrease in risk.[15] In the United States nurses health study, women active at a level of 3–6 METs (moderate activity) for more than 1 hour a day had a 46%

lower risk than those who participated in these activities at a lower level; walking was the commonest type of leisure activity in these women and therefore a major contributor to the totals of moderate exercise.[25]

Thus aspects of the epidemiological evidence in different populations suggest that physical activity need not be performed in rather long, say 20 minutes or more, sessions to confer a variety (and expanding list) of health gains. Until data are published on the duration of the sessions of activities likely to be performed on an intermittent basis, however, this evidence does not constitute a sufficient rationale for the proposition that physical activity can be accumulated through the day in several short sessions.

Multiple short sessions of activity as a means of improving fitness

The idea that sporadic bouts of activity will be an adequate stimulus to health benefits comes also from studies that have systematically compared the effects of shorter bouts of activity spread throughout the day with those of longer bouts. Two studies are consistently cited in the statements of expert panels[4-6]—namely those of deBusk and colleagues[26] and Ebisu.[27] In the former, 36 sedentary middle aged men performed either one 30 minute session of jogging or three 10 minute sessions on 5 days a week for 8 weeks; the intensity of exercise was 65% to 75% of maximum heart rate (equivalent to 55% to 65% of $\dot{V}O_2MAX$).[26] Men were allocated randomly to the different patterns of exercise but there was no control group. Although both groups of joggers showed similar decreases in heart rate during a standard submaximal

---

Box 17.1 Recommendations for physical activity

- Recent recommendations from the United States Centers for Disease Control and Prevention and the American College of Sports Medicine state that adults who engage in moderate intensity physical activity, enough to expend about 200 kcal a day, can expect many health benefits
- One specific way to achieve this goal is to walk briskly for 30 minutes on most, preferably all, days in the week
- Based mainly on indirect evidence from population studies, it is suggested that the recommended 30 minutes can be accumulated through several short bouts undertaken at intervals during the day

treadmill test, the increase in $\dot{V}O_2MAX$ was significantly greater for the long bout group (4.4 ml/kg/min, 13.9%) than for the short bout group (2.5 ml/kg/min, 7.6%). Decreases in body mass were similar (1.75 kg and 1.79 kg, respectively).

The second frequently cited study compared effects of different running training regimens on endurance fitness and blood lipids.[27] The subjects were 53 young men, randomly assigned to four different groups. Three groups ran equivalent distances on 3 days a week for 10 weeks, in one, two or three separate sessions, and responses were compared with those of a control group who did not train. Runners completing three sessions a day probably exercised for about 8 minutes a session early in the training period, rising to about 16 minutes for the last 3 weeks. $\dot{V}O_2MAX$ increased significantly in all training groups—by 3.9 to 5.6 ml/kg/min (6.9% to 9.8%) from initial values of the order of 55 ml/kg/min. Ebisu also reports a significant increase (pretraining v post-training, within group) in high density lipoprotein (HDL) cholesterol of 0.12 mmol/l (9.6%) in the group training three times a day.[27] It should be noted, however, that HDL cholesterol concentrations increased also in the control group (0.04 mmol/1, 3.4%) and that the investigators do not appear to have compared change in the intervention group with change in controls—that is, the more rigorous test of a change with training.

Recently, three other papers comparing the efficacy of different physical activity patterns have been published. Jakicic and colleagues studied overweight women over 20 weeks.[28] Subjects were randomly assigned to one of two groups: long bout exercise or short bout exercise. All subjects undertook aerobic exercise 5 days a week, "primarily walking". The prescription for long bout walkers was one session of 20 minutes, increasing over 9 weeks to 40 minutes; short bout walkers were prescribed two, progressing to four, 10-minute sessions a day. Predicted $\dot{V}O_2MAX$ increased to a similar degree in both walking groups—that is, by 5.6% and by 5.0% for long and short bout groups respectively. Both groups lost significant amounts of body weight, with a tendency for loss to be greater in the short bout group (8.9 (5.3) kg v 6.4 (4.5) kg, $P < 0.07$). As a consequence of better adherence to the prescription, the short bout group exercised on more days and for a longer total time (224 (70) min/week v 188 (58) min/week) than the long bout group. However, (theoretically) the difference in weight loss between groups was greater than could be attributed to the difference in exercise energy expenditure.

In a longer study, 13 obese women walked briskly (52% of heart rate reserve) for ten minutes, three times per day, 5 days per week for 32 weeks.[29] Fasting blood lipids, insulin and glucose were measured, in addition to peak oxygen uptake and body composition. For the group as a whole, there were no changes in body mass, $\dot{V}O_2PEAK$, or serum concentrations of total, HDL or low density lipoprotein (LDL) cholesterol or triacylglycerol (TAG). However, there were indications that individuals who were older, fatter and particularly unfit at baseline adapted to the exercise regimen with a loss of fat weight, improved $\dot{V}O_2PEAK$, and a decrease in fasting insulin. As in the earlier study from the same group,[28] adherence to the intermittent pattern of moderate exercise was good (~86%) and better than might be expected for prescriptions involving longer, continuous exercise sessions.

A study with a similar design, but incorporating a control group, was undertaken by my research group; sedentary, middle aged women who were, on average, towards the top end of the desirable range of weight for height were studied over 10 weeks.[30] Women following the exercise regimens were randomly assigned to perform on 5 days each week either one 30 minute session of brisk walking or three 10-minute sessions. The intensity of exercise was 70% to 80% of maximum heart rate, 60–70% of $\dot{V}O_2MAX$. $\dot{V}O_2MAX$ increased by the same amount in each of the walking groups (~2.3 ml/kg/min or 8%) but only the short bout group showed a significant decrease in body weight and waist circumference, relative to controls.

Experimental evidence for the recommendation that accumulation of short bouts of activity is one approach to a desirable physical activity goal is thus scanty. Only one of the five studies above compared changes in exercisers with changes in controls in assessing the responses to training; the total number of subjects studied is small (~190); only two studies provide (limited) information on health gains other than changes in aerobic fitness and body weight/fatness.[27,29] However, with patterns of activity based on short sessions—typically 8–15 minutes in duration—of activity per day, four out of five studies found improvements in fitness;[26–28,30] and three found decreases in body weight and/or fatness.[26,28,30] The improvements in fitness and decreases in body weight after multiple short bouts of brisk walking—an activity specifically mentioned in recommendations from expert panels[4,5]— support the suggestion that this activity should be the cornerstone of a generally active lifestyle.[31]

For sedentary middle-aged subjects, gains in fitness with multiple bouts were similar to gains achieved through longer continuous bouts of equivalent duration in the study of Murphy and Hardman.[30] By contrast, deBusk and colleagues found a significantly greater increase in $\dot{V}O_2MAX$ for the men who performed the longer exercise sessions.[26] Training intensity has a direct impact on the magnitude of improvements in fitness so one reason could be that long bout joggers spent a greater proportion of training time above the recommended heart rate range than short-bout joggers (33% v 17%).[26] This may reflect the fact that—in untrained people—heart rate rises progressively during exercise and walkers monitoring heart rate can slow their pace to oppose this rise whereas joggers with low $\dot{V}O_2MAX$ values may not be able to do this without changing their gait to walking.

Until more information is available, the issue of whether there is an interaction of exercise intensity with exercise pattern cannot be resolved. As moderate intensity exercise is recommended for sedentary individuals taking up exercise—because vigorous exercise is hazardous for them[32]—this needs to be done. It can be estimated that the intensity of activity in the studies on accumulation of activity was between 55% and 70% of $\dot{V}O_2MAX$—that is, moderate to moderately vigorous. Many presently sedentary individuals do not exert themselves above 30-35% of their $\dot{V}O_2MAX$,[33] so it may be speculated that exercise below this threshold of intensity could elicit improvements in their fitness. It should be mentioned that, even if the improvements in fitness through short bouts are somewhat less than those acquired through longer bouts, they may be sufficient to confer important, if not optimal, health gains; in at least one data set, the major difference in mortality risk was found between men and women in the lowest fifth for fitness and those in the next highest fifth.[34]

The limited data available show that several short bouts of activity a day are at least as effective as one longer bout as far as weight regulation is concerned,[26, 28, 30] in line with the view that the total energy expenditure of exercise is the most important determinant of exercise induced weight loss.[35] There are indications, however, in two of these studies of more weight loss with short bouts than with equivalent exercise in longer bouts.[28, 30] One possibility is that exercising in short bouts may, for practical reasons, restrict energy intake; subjects performing short bouts of exercise may do so in their lunch hour, restricting the time available for eating.

> ## Box 17.2 Evidence for accumulation of physical activity
>
> - This is, for the most part, indirect
> - Epidemiological studies of physical activity and the risk of morbidity and all cause and disease specific (mainly coronary heart disease) mortality show a reduced risk among men engaging in some specified moderate intensity activities, which are most likely to have been undertaken on an intermittent basis rather than in long continuous sessions; examples include stair climbing, walking, and gardening.
> - A few studies have compared the effects of several short sessions of exercise (walking, jogging, running) a day with those of equivalent exercise performed in one continuous session. Three 10 minute exercise bouts a day, 3 to 5 a week, are sufficient to improve fitness and perhaps decrease fatness
> - There are almost no scientific data from intervention trials on the effect on health related variables of increased physical activity through several short bouts of exercise a day

Importance of energy expenditure

Examination of the way physical activity has been measured and reported in studies such as the Harvard alumni study[12] and the multiple risk factor intervention trial[19] leads to the possibility that benefits were mainly linked to the total amount of energy expended. This does not preclude the possibility of additional benefit from sustained activity; indeed Paffenbarger has been quoted as saying that, among men who expended the same amount of energy weekly, those who performed some form of sustained exercise had significantly lower death and heart attack rates than those who did not[36]—although I am not aware of any published data on this.

It is, however, plausible that at least some of the benefit of activity is achieved through the associated increases in energy expenditure. Recently, the concept of metabolic fitness has been introduced[37] in an attempt to highlight the multiple metabolic benefits of considerable amounts of low intensity exercise taken on an almost daily basis and which have been shown experimentally to be independent of changes in cardiorespiratory fitness as assessed by $\dot{V}O_2\text{MAX}$. The metabolic variables in question include insulin sensitivity, low concentrations of plasma TAG and high plasma concentrations of HDL cholesterol. Changes in these have been closely associated with decreases in body fatness, particularly loss of abdominal fat,[38] but low intensity training in the absence of fat loss can also stimulate changes in lipoprotein metabolism and insulin sensitivity.[39] The latter finding points to a benefit from improved energy turnover per se, and so fits well with recent observations that overweight men who are fit have a lower risk of premature death than those of normal weight who are unfit.[40]

In addition to the study of Ebisu referred to above,[27] one intervention study has shown that exercise induced changes in blood lipids may be related to the energy expenditure of exercise. Three groups of premenopausal women were studied in a randomised trial over 24 weeks; exercisers walked 5 km (3 miles) on 5 days a week at 3, 4, or 5 mph.[41] Improvements in $\dot{V}O_2$MAX were related to the intensity of regular walking but changes in serum concentrations of total cholesterol, LDL cholesterol, HDL cholesterol, and TAG did not differ significantly between the exercise groups. Specifically, women who took 5 hours to walk 24 km (15 miles) regularly experienced the same level of increase in HDL cholesterol as those who took 3 hours.

Plasma HDL concentrations may constitute a "metabolic memory" for ability to degrade TAG rich lipoproteins.[41] The basis of this view is that hydrolysis of TAG by lipoprotein lipase "slims down" these particles, leading to an excess of surface proteins.

Box 17.3 Importance of energy expenditure

- If increased energy expenditure and/or turnover is an important aspect of the health benefits of physical activity then several short bouts of activity may be comparable with one longer bout expending an equivalent amount of energy
- One of the main determinants of an exercise induced loss of body fat is the total energy expended in physical activity
- A session of exercise stimulates short term metabolic changes such as improved insulin/glucose dynamics and lower plasma concentrations of fasting and postprandial triglycerides known to be associated with a reduced risk of cardiovascular disease
- These short term metabolic benefits (which may be important if physical activity is regular and frequent) seem to be linked at least partly to the energy expended in the exercise, suggesting that in this regard accumulating exercise through multiple short bouts may be an effective regimen

Some of these are rapidly acquired by nascent HDL, which become mature spherical particles in the process. Consequently, the concentrations in plasma of HDL and TAG are inversely related. If the capacity to metabolise TAG is low, the residence time in the circulation of TAG rich lipoproteins is increased, enhancing the opportunity for exchange of core lipid with the cholesterol rich lipoproteins, which not only impairs reverse cholesterol transport but also leads to a preponderance of small, dense (atherogenic) LDLs. If the capacity to metabolise TAG is low the postprandial rise in plasma TAG concentration will be high. People spend most of their lives in the postprandial state so repeated episodes of exaggerated postprandial lipaemia may hasten the progression of atherosclerosis, a proposition supported by studies showing higher concentrations of postprandial lipaemia in men with known coronary artery disease than in healthy controls.[42]

Exercise has short-term and possibly long-term effects in reducing postprandial lipaemia.[43-45] There is evidence that energy expenditure per se is an important determinant of the acute decrease in lipaemia evident after exercise. The findings of studies from my laboratory are pertinent. We compared the lipaemic response within subjects to a standard oral fat load consumed 16–18 hours after an exercise session. As might be expected, moderate intensity exercise (60% $\dot{V}O_2MAX$) caused a greater decrease in lipaemia than an equivalent period of low intensity exercise (30% $\dot{V}O_2MAX$).[46] However, when the duration of low intensity exercise was increased so that the energy expended was the same as in the moderate intensity trial—that is, trading intensity for duration (1.5 hours at 60% $\dot{V}O_2MAX$ v 3 hours at 30% $\dot{V}O_2MAX$)—each bout of exercise reduced lipaemia to the same degree.[47] The pattern of prior exercise does not seem to make an important difference to its effect on subsequent lipaemia, at least when a considerable amount of energy is expended. In a recent study young men undertook three oral fat tolerance tests; on the day preceding one test they refrained from exercise; before another they performed 90 minutes of exercise at 60% of $\dot{V}O_2MAX$ in one continuous bout; before another, they performed three separate 30 minute sessions at intervals of several hours, expending the same energy. Exercise reduced postprandial lipaemia to the same degree, irrespective of its pattern.[48]

There does seem to be a relationship between energy expended and the ensuing reduction in lipaemia. When subjects walked at 50% $\dot{V}O_2MAX$ for 1 hour the afternoon before a fat tolerance test their total lipaemic response (assessed as the area under the plasma concentration v time curve over 6 hours) was 12.5% lower than in a control (no-exercise) trial; when the exercise period was extended to 2 hours, the decrease in lipaemia was increased two-fold—that is 23%.[49] Plasma concentrations of heparin-releasable lipoprotein lipase were 27% and 32% higher than control at the end of the fat tolerance tests.[49]

Collectively, these findings suggest that the effect of a session of exercise on postprandial lipaemia is closely linked to energy expenditure, perhaps through some mechanism related to muscle contraction and mediated through changes in the expression of muscle proteins related to substrate acquisition in the exercised muscle. Skeletal muscle lipoprotein lipase, like other proteins critical to the transport and metabolism of energy substrates for muscle, increases rapidly but transiently after exercise.[50]

Aspects of the epidemiological evidence for improved insulin/ glucose dynamics and a lower risk of developing type II diabetes among regular exercisers were referred to above. Experimental studies have shown that enhanced insulin sensitivity is a "genuine response to training but short lived",[51] persisting for only a few days when training is interrupted.[52] Like the effects on postprandial lipoproteins, the short-term effect of exercise on insulin sensitivity appears to be linked to energy expenditure. In one study, indices of insulin sensitivity were measured for eight women with type II diabetes in each of three conditions: after low intensity exercise at 50% $\dot{V}O_2\text{MAX}$; after high intensity exercise at 75% $\dot{V}O_2\text{MAX}$; and after a period without exercise (control).[53] The duration of exercise was adjusted so that energy expenditure was the same for the two exercise conditions. Insulin sensitivity was enhanced in an identical way by each exercise pattern, again suggesting that low intensity exercise can stimulate the same metabolic changes after exercise as high intensity exercise, provided that the same energy is expended.

Thus the energy expenditure of regular exercise appears to be an important determinant of at least some metabolic adaptations which might be expected to confer a reduced risk of cardiovascular and metabolic disease. This is in line with observations that metabolic improvements (decrease in LDL cholesterol, increase in HDL_2 cholesterol, ratio of insulin to glucose areas measured during an oral glucose tolerance test) correlate significantly with losses of total and abdominal visceral fat rather than with the increase in $\dot{V}O_2\text{MAX}$.[38]

Skeletal health

Mechanical loading is an important determinant of bone mass and architecture[54] and the influence of increased physical activity on bone has been much studied. This is one area where the accumulation of exercise throughout the day must, theoretically, be an effective pattern. An osteogenic stimulus arises when bone is exposed to unusual dynamic strain distribution. This effect is quickly "saturated", however, so that there is little extra stimulus to bone formation from high numbers of load cycles. The relevance of this finding is that the structural competence of bone can be maintained by comparatively infrequent loading events and does not require long periods of repetitive activity.[55] This thinking fits well with findings of increased bone mineral density in pre-menopausal women after a daily exercise regimen of 50 vertical jumps.[56] If strain magnitude and strain nature are the determinants of the osteogenic response to exercise, then several brief periods during a day of high impact exercises will in fact be more effective than long periods of endurance-type exercise where the applied loads are typically low.

Walking and cycling as a means of commuting to work

One obvious way to accumulate physical activity regularly is to commute to and from work by bicycle or on foot. A year round commitment to this means at least two exercise sessions, 5 days a week for most weeks of the year. The energy expenditure can be considerable and invariably greater than that achieved through planned exercise.

Researchers in Finland have studied physically active commuting to work. An initial survey showed that walking or bicycling to work offered "basic habitual exercise" to about one-third of the employed urban population. The activity was reported to be "regular, frequent, rather stable year round and brisk in tempo".[57] A randomised, controlled intervention trial was subsequently conducted in healthy men and women who were not regular leisure time exercisers. The mean one way commuting distance was 3 km (2 miles) for walkers and 9.5 km (6 miles) for cyclists. Walkers selected a speed typically equivalent to 53% $\dot{V}O_2MAX$, cyclists closer to 63% $\dot{V}O_2MAX$. On average, 10 weeks of active commuting resulted in a 4.5% net (compared with control) increase in $\dot{V}O_2MAX$ ($P=0.02$) and a 5% net increase in HDL cholesterol

($P = 0.06$). These studies do not provide evidence for the accumulation of bouts of activity as short as 10 minutes, however, because the journeys lasted about 30 minutes.

The regularity and the frequency of physically active commuting to work make it an ideal form of exercise likely to maintain short term metabolic effects afterwards: no special clothing is needed (activities requiring changing are not likely to be undertaken several times a day); the time commitment is minimised because one has in any case to travel to work; and it requires no special skills. The barriers are, of course, bad weather, poor condition of pedestrian and cycling routes and fear of accidents.

Concluding remarks

The argument for accumulation of short bouts of physical activity is predicated largely on the assertion that total energy expenditure is the important determinant of health gains and there is epidemiological evidence for this. A major weakness of this evidence is, however, that there are no data describing the typical duration of sessions of moderate intensity activities likely to have been performed on an intermittent basis on which to assess their contribution to total exercise energy expenditure.

Improvements in fitness probably confer health benefits. Experimental data showing the effectiveness of several short bouts of moderate intensity physical activity in improving fitness are few.[28,30] This is an important gap in the evidence because if activity is to be accumulated through several short sessions it must necessarily be non-sporting and of moderate intensity. On the whole, people will not change into special clothing, travel to a facility and engage in planned, vigorous exercise several times in one day. The debate about the accumulation issue cannot therefore be separated from that about the intensity issue—that is, is moderate intensity exercise (3 to 6 METs) sufficient to confer health gains?[58]

Intuitively, the length of a session of physical activity must influence its potential to confer metabolic adaptations relevant to cardiovascular risk. Indeed aspects of observational studies referred to above make it clear that sustained periods of exercise are probably associated with greater benefits. However, in the absence of data to indicate that, say, three short bouts of activity are equivalent to one longer bout in terms of reducing disease risk, this aspect of current United States recommendations is speculative. Of course, this should not obscure the vital issue of the need to deal with the public health burden in this country attributable to physical inactivity. There is no evidence that adopting a habit of frequent, 10–15 minute bouts of physical activity spread throughout the day will harm a sedentary individual and some evidence that it may be of benefit. Moreover, such a prescription avoids the risks of unaccustomed vigorous exercise by ensuring that activity is moderate in intensity.

1 National Fitness Survey: Main Findings. Sports Council and Health Education Authority, 1992.
2 Morris JN. Exercise in the prevention of coronary heart disease: today's best buy in public health. *Med Sci Sports Exerc* 1994;**26**:807–14.
3 Department of Health. *More people, more active, more often*. Report of Physical Activity Task Force. Department of Health, 1995.
4 Pate RR, Pratt M, Blair SN, *et al*. Physical activity and public health. A recommendation from the Centers for Disease Control and Prevention and the American College of Sports Medicine. *JAMA* 1995;**273**:402–7.
5 Physical activity and health. *A report of the Surgeon General*. Atlanta: US Departments of Health and Human Services. Centers for Disease Control and Prevention, 1996.
6 National Institute of Health Consensus Development Panel. Physical activity and cardiovascular health. *JAMA* 1996;**276**:241–6.
7 Blair SN, Goodyear NN, Gibbons LW, *et al*. Physical fitness and incidence of hypertension in healthy normotensive men and women. *JAMA* 1984;**252**:487–90.
8 Sandvik L, Erikssen J, Thaulow E, *et al*. Physical fitness as a predictor of mortality among healthy, middle-aged Norwegian men. *N Engl J Med* 1993;**328**:533–7.
9 Blair SN, Kampert JB, Kohl HW, *et al*. Influences of cardiorespiratory fitness and other precursors on cardiovascular disease and all-cause mortality in men and women. *JAMA* 1996;**276**:205–10.
10 Lynch J, Helmrich SP, Lakka TA, *et al*. Moderately intense physical activities and high levels of cardiorespiratory fitness reduce the risk of non-insulin-dependent diabetes mellitus in middle-aged men. *Arch Intern Med* 1996;**156**:1307–14.
11 Haapanen N, Miilunpalo S, Vuori I, *et al*. Characteristics of leisure time physical activity associated with decreased risk of premature all-cause and cardiovascular disease mortality in middle-aged men. *Am J Epidemiol* 1996;**143**:870–80.
12 Paffenbarger RS, Hyde RT, Wing AL, *et al*. Physical activity, all-cause mortality, and longevity of college alumni. *N Engl J Med* 1986; **314**:605–13.
13 Helmrich SP, Ragland DR, Leung RW, *et al*. Physical activity and reduced occurrence of non-insulin-dependent diabetes mellitus. *N Engl J Med* 1991;**325**:147–52.
14 Paffenbarger RS, Wing AL, Hyde RT, *et al*. Physical activity and incidence of hypertension in college alumni. *Am J Epidemiol* 1983;**117**:247–57.
15 Thune I, Lund E. Physical activity and risk of colorectal cancer in men and women. *Br J Cancer* 1996;**373**:1134–40.
16 Thune I, Brenn T, Lund E, *et al*. Physical activity and the risk of breast cancer. *N Engl J Med* 1997;**336**:1269–75.
17 Shaper AG, Wannamethee G. Physical activity and ischaemic heart disease in middle-aged British men. *Br Heart J* 1991;**661**:384–94.
18 Magnus K, Matroos A, Strackee J. Walking, cycling, or gardening, with or

without seasonal interruption, in relation to coronary events. *Am J Epidemiol* 1979;**110**:724–33.

19 Leon AS, Connett J, Jacobs DR, *et al.* Leisure-time physical activity levels and risk of coronary heart disease and death: the multiple risk factor intervention trial. *JAMA* 1987;**258**:2388–95.

20 Paffenbarger RS, Hyde RT, Wing AL, *et al.* The association of changes in physical activity level and other lifestyle characteristics with mortality among men. *N Engl J Med* 1993;**328**:538–45.

21 Hakim AA, Petrovitch H, Burchfiel CM, *et al.* Effects of walking on mortality among nonsmoking retired men. *N Engl J Med* 1998;**338**:94–9.

22 Lemaitre RN, Heckbert SR, Psaty BM, *et al.* Leisure-time physical activity and the risk of nonfatal myocardial infarction in postmenopausal women. *Arch Intern Med* 1995;**155**:2302–8.

23 Pereira MA, Kriska AM, Joswiak ML, et al. Physical inactivity and glucose intolerance in the multiethnic island of Mauritius. *Med Sci Sports Exerc* 1995;**27**:1626–34.

24 Mayer-Davis EJ, D'Agostino R, Karter AJ, *et al.* Intensity and amount of physical activity in relation to insulin sensitivity. The insulin resistance atherosclerosis study. *JAMA* 1998;**279**:669–74.

25 Martínez ME, Giovannucci E, Spiegelman D, *et al.* Leisure-time physical activity, body size, and colon cancer in women. *J Nat Cancer Inst* 1997;**89**:948–55.

26 DeBusk RF, Stenestrand U, Sheehan M, *et al.* Training effects of long versus short bouts of exercise in healthy subjects. *Am J Cardiol* 1990;**65**:1010–13.

27 Ebisu T. Splitting the distance of endurance running: on cardiovascular endurance and blood lipids. *Jpn J Phys Exerc* 1985;**30**:37–43.

28 Jakicic JM, Wing RR, Butler BA, *et al.* Prescribing exercise in multiple short bouts versus one continuous bout: effects on adherence, cardiorespiratory fitness, and weight loss in overweight women. *Int J Obes* 1995;**19**:893–901.

29 Snyder KA, Donnelly JE, Jabobsen J, *et al.* The effects of long-term, moderate intensity, intermittent exercise on aerobic capacity, body composition, blood lipids, insulin and glucose in overweight females. *Int J Obes* 1997;**21**:1180–9.

30 Murphy MH, Hardman AE. Training effects of short and long bouts of brisk walking in sedentary women. *Med Sci Sports Exerc* 1998;**30**:152–7.

31 Morris JN, Hardman AE. Walking to health. *Sports Med* 1997;**23**:306–32.

32 Mittleman MA, Maclure M, Tofler GH, *et al.* Triggering of acute myocardial infarction by heavy physical exertion. Protection against triggering by regular exertion. *N Engl J Med* 1993;**329**:1677–83.

33 Haskell WL. Dose-response issues from a biological perspective. In: Bouchard C, Shephard RJ, Stephens T, ed. *Physical activity, fitness and health.* Champaign, Illinois: Human Kinetics, 1994:1030–9.

34 Blair SN, Kohl HW, Paffenbarger RS, *et al.* Physical fitness and all-cause mortality: a prospective study of healthy men and women. *JAMA* 1989;**262**:2395–401.

35 Ballor DL, Keesey RE. A meta-analysis of the factors affecting exercise-induced changes in body mass, fat mass and fat-free mass in males and females. *Int J Obes* 1991;**15**:717–26.

36 Barinaga M. How much pain for cardiac gain? *Science* 1997;**276**:1324–7.

37 Després J-P, Lamarche B. Low-intensity endurance exercise training, plasma lipoproteins and the risk of coronary heart disease. *J Int Med* 1994;**236**:7–22.

38 Després J-P, Pouliot MC, Moorjani S, *et al.* Loss of abdominal fat and metabolic response to exercise training in obese women. *Am J Physiol* 1991;**261**:E159–67.

39 Oshida Y, Yamanouchi K, Haymamizu S, *et al.* Long-term mild jogging increases insulin action despite no influence on body mass index or $\dot{V}O_2$MAX. *J Appl Physiol* 1989;**66**:2206–10.

40 Lee CD, Jackson AS, Blair SN. US weight guidelines: is it also important to

consider cardiorespiratory fitness? *Int J Obes* 1998;**22**(Suppl 2):S2–7.

41 Duncan JJ, Gordon NF, Scott CB. Women walking for health and fitness. How much is enough? *JAMA* 1991;**266**:3295–9.

42 Patsch JR, Miesenböck G, Hopferwieser T, *et al.* Relation of triglyceride metabolism and coronary artery disease. Studies in the postprandial state. *Arteriosclerosis Thrombosis* 1992;**12**:1336–45.

43 Weintraub MS, Rosen Y, Otto R, *et al.* Physical conditioning in the absence of weight loss reduces fasting and postprandial triglyceride-rich lipoprotein levels. *Circulation* 1989;**79**:1007–14.

44 Aldred HE, Perry I, Hardman AE. The effect of a single bout of brisk walking on postprandial lipemia in normolipidemic young adults. *Metabolism* 1994;**43**:836–41.

45 Podl TR, Zmuda JM, Yurgalevitch SM, *et al.* Lipoprotein lipase activity and plasma triglyceride clearance are elevated in endurance-trained women. *Metabolism* 1994;**43**:808–13.

46 Tsetsonis NV, Hardman AE. Effects of low and moderate intensity treadmill walking on postprandial lipaemia in healthy young adults. *Eur J Appl Physiol* 1996;**73**:419–26.

47 Tsetsonis NV, Hardman AE. Reduction in postprandial lipemia after walking: influence of exercise intensity. *Med Sci Sports Exerc* 1996;**28**:1235–42.

48 Gill JMR, Murphy MH, Hardman AE. Postprandial lipemia: effects of intermittent versus continuous exercise. *Med Sci Sports Exerc* 1998;**30**: 1515–20.

49 Herd SL, Hardman AE, Vora V. Influence of brisk walking duration on postprandial lipemia and plasma lipoprotein lipase activity. *Med Sci Sports Exerc* 1997;**29**:S6.

50 Seip RL, Mair D, Cole TG, *et al.* Induction of human skeletal muscle lipoprotein lipase gene expression by short-term exercise is transient. *Am J Physiol* 1997;**272**:E255–61.

51 Dela F, Mikines KJ, von Linstow M, *et al.* Effect of training on insulin-mediated glucose uptake in human muscle. *Am J Physiol* 1992;**263**:E1134–43.

52 King DS, Baldus RJ, Sharp RL, *et al.* Time course for exercise-induced alterations in insulin action and glucose tolerance in middle-aged people. *J Appl Physiol* 1995;**78**:17–22.

53 Braun B, Zimmermann MB, Kretchmer N. Effects of exercise intensity on insulin sensitivity in women with non-insulin-dependent diabetes mellitus. *J Appl Physiol* 1995;**78**:300–6.

54 Lanyon LE. Using functional loading to influence bone mass and architecture: objectives, mechanisms, and relationship with estrogen of the mechanically adaptive process in bone. *Bone* 1996;**18**:37S–43S.

55 Rubin CT, Lanyon LE. Regulation of bone formation by applied dynamic loads. *J Bone Joint Surg* 1984;366-A:397–402.

56 Bassey EJ, Ramsdale SJ. Increase in femoral bone density in young women following high-impact exercise. *Osteoporosis Int* 1994;**4**:72–5.

57 Vuori IM, Oja P, Paronen O. Physically active commuting to work—testing its potential for exercise promotion. *Med Sci Sports Exerc* 1994;**26**:844–50.

58 Blair SN, Connelly JC. How much physical activity should we do? *Res Q Exerc Sport* 1996;**67**:193–205.

Multiple choice questions

1 Which of the following are currently recommended for "health-enhancing" physical activity?

(a) 10 minutes of physical activity a day

(b) 20 to 60 minutes of moderate or high intensity endurance type (aerobic) exercise, three or more times a week

(c) A total energy expenditure in physical activity of about 1400 kcal a week

(d) 30 minutes of physical activity at a moderate level or above on most, preferably all, days of the week

2 Which of the following activities, likely to have been "accumulated" through several short sessions per day are reported in epidemiological studies of physical activity and the risk of cardiovascular and all cause mortality?

(a) Swimming

(b) Vigorous sports

(c) Walking

(d) Stair climbing

3 Many of the metabolic benefits of physical activity are related to:

(a) The size of the muscle mass regularly engaged in exercise

(b) The total energy expended

(c) Associated decreases in stress

(d) Improvements in personal fitness levels

4 Intervention studies have examined the efficacy of several short (about 10 minute) sessions of physical activity (jogging, running, or walking) a day to:

(a) Improve fitness

(b) Decrease body fatness

(c) Modify risk markers for coronary heart disease

(d) Improve sense of wellbeing

5 Higher concentrations of high density lipoproteins in trained people probably reflect:

(a) High carbohydrate diets

(b) Low intake of saturated fat

(c) Enhanced clearance of triglyceride-rich lipoproteins

(d) High energy intake

Answers are on p. 367.

18   Exercise in cardiac rehabilitation

H J N Bethell

Introduction

The notion that exercise is dangerous for patients with heart disease dogged the use of such treatment for the first half of the 20th century. It was a further 30 years before exercise became accepted in rehabilitation. The controversy is made more difficult by the fact that exercise may be dangerous for some patients in some circumstances.[1]

Exercise is now widely believed to benefit a wide variety of patients with heart disease. However, when it is used to treat cardiac patients, exercise should be approached like any other treatment and thought given to the indications, the contra-indications, the mode of action, the type, the dose, the duration of treatment, the expected benefits, and the side effects.

Indications

Acute myocardial infarction

Early mobilisation

Exercise was initially applied to patients recovering from acute myocardial infarction. In the 1940s and 1950s some of the undesirable results of bed rest were being recognised, at least in some quarters; such complications were deconditioning, boredom, depression, venous thrombosis, urinary retention, constipation, and chest infections. In 1952 Levine and Lown described their "armchair treatment of acute coronary thrombosis".[2] The natural progression of this approach was a more rapid increase in mobilisation after the infarction, and by the 1970s several controlled trials of early mobilisation had shown that this was a safe approach and lessened the complications mentioned above.[3,4] The result has been a general acceptance of this regimen, and patients with no complications are now likely to be discharged within 4 to 5 days, when the risk of dangerous arrhythmias is significantly reduced.

Rehabilitation

In 1957 Hellerstein and Ford defined rehabilitation as "the process by which a patient is returned realistically to his greatest physical, mental, social, vocational and economic usefulness and, if employable, is provided an opportunity for gainful employment in a competitive industrial world."[5] In 1968, Hellerstein went on to describe the physical training programme he had devised to improve the fitness of "habitually lazy, hypokinetic, sloppy, endomesomorphic overweight males" who were the usual victims of coronary disease.[6] The perceived wisdom of his multidisciplinary approach to the rehabilitation of coronary patients led to widespread adoption of exercise based programmes to treat patients recovering from acute myocardial infarction programmes in which exercise has been a centrepiece for all the other valuable aspects of rehabilitation such as education, risk factor modification, stress management and relaxation, and job counselling. The spread of such progammes in the United Kingdom has been remarkable. When the members of the British Cardiac Society were surveyed in 1970, only nine of those who replied could offer some form of exercise based rehabilitation to their patients.[7] By 1988 a further survey found 91 programmes[8] and this had risen to 161 by 1992[9] and 274 by 1997.[10] It has also been apparent that only a minority of patients who might benefit from this treatment are currently able to receive it, mainly through lack of adequate resources. In the United Kingdom, cardiac rehabilitation has seldom been commissioned by purchasers, rather it has been initiated by enthusiasts, mainly nurses, who have seen the unmet need. In this they have been supported by the British Heart Foundation who have given start up grants, which have been responsible for the rapid growth of the facility over the past 10 years.

The postinfarction rehabilitation programme has gradually been adapted over the years to accept all the other cardiac patients who may benefit from exercise training; only rarely are specific programmes used to treat other cardiac conditions, which include the following.

Heart surgery

The great majority of surgical patients included in cardiac rehabilitation programmes have had coronary artery bypass grafting. These patients have the same disease as postinfarction patients and benefit from the full rehabilitation package. An increasing number of those who have had coronary angioplasty are now being included. Other surgical conditions such as valve replacements and heart transplants[11] are also treated, and a potential growth area is patients with implanted defribrillators who may become crippled by disabling anxiety.[12]

Angina pectoris

Exercise training may be particularly helpful for anginal patients, particularly when revascularisation is not indicated or is impossible. This indication is discussed further below.

Heart failure

This has traditionally been seen as a contraindication to exercise but over the past 15 years the literature on the benefits of exercise for these patients has been growing. Indeed, it may be these, the most disabled of cardiac patients, who have the most to gain from this treatment.

Contraindications

There are some absolute contraindications, such as unstable angina, worsening heart failure, critical valve stenosis (mainly aortic), malignant arrhythmias, very recent infarction, and any acute intercurrent medical condition such as venous thrombosis or febrile illness.[13] Relative contraindications include severe angina, severe heart failure and non-critical valve lesions, and potentially dangerous arrhythmias.[13] All of the latter may be treated but need much closer supervision than patients with fewer complications.[14] Risk stratification of patients at the onset of an exercise programme takes all these factors and more into account (see below).

Mode of action

Physical fitness

In normal subjects, exercise training increases aerobic fitness by both central and peripheral effects.[15] Centrally, stroke volume, ejection fraction and rate, and force of contraction of the left

341

ventricle increase in response to exercise. The heart beats more slowly and empties more completely with a greater reserve and higher potential cardiac output. There is also a reduction in central sympathetic tone and increase in red cell mass. Peripherally, there is a more efficient distribution of blood to the working muscles, and these muscles extract a greater percentage of the oxygen from their blood supply, so a lower blood flow is required to fuel any level of exertion. The same amount of activity can be performed for a lower blood flow and a lower cardiac output. These peripheral effects are specific to the muscles that have been trained.

The central and peripheral effects of exercise training in normal people contribute about equally to increases in fitness.[15] In patients with heart disease the central effects are less than in normals and take longer to develop. When patients with heart disease undertake physical training, in the short term the resulting decrease in cardiac workload for any given exercise load is due to a reduction in demand from the working muscles.[16,17] It follows that improvements in performance after training are mainly confined to those exercises that have been included in the training programme, and therefore a patient trained on a bicycle ergometer will not necessarily be able to walk any faster. This fact is particularly relevant to most cardiac rehabilitation programmes in the United Kingdom, which typically last 6–12 weeks. However, if exercise training is maintained for a year or more and is sufficiently intense, there will be increases in cardiac performance including increases in stroke volume and ejection fraction and in force of contraction of the left ventricle.[18-20] Studies of these changes, however, have all been performed on low risk younger coronary patients and have not included sicker older patients or those with known poor left ventricular function. One study has measured the results of exercise training on changes in left ventricular function compared with initial left ventricular function; only those with good left ventricular function subjected to intensive exercise showed an improvement in rest peak exercise left ventricular ejection fraction.[21]

Myocardial blood supply

For patients with coronary artery disease, a highly desirable outcome of physical training would be improved blood flow to the heart muscle. Exercise testing of angina patients after exercise training shows that they can achieve a higher heart rate before they develop chest pain[22] and also a higher heart rate at the onset of ischaemic changes shown on the electrocardiogram.[22,23] Myocardial perfusion imaging confirms that improvements in physical fitness are accompanied by improved perfusion,[24] although the exact mechanism is uncertain. Exercise programmes that have been combined with lipid lowering, by either diet or drug treatment, may produce reversal of coronary atheroma for some patients,[25,26] particularly if the training is both vigorous and maintained for many years.[27] The amount of exercise needed to produce reversal of coronary narrowing without the use of other interventions is, however, large, considerably more than is routine in most cardiac rehabilitation programmes.[28] It is proposed that training also increases collateral blood vessels, although this has not been confirmed by angiography.[29] The reason may be that angiography is performed at rest whereas collaterals would be expected to open up during exercise.

Type of exercise

Exercise can be divided into two types: isotonic (often referred to as aerobic), which involves much movement and little strength, and isometric, which involves much force but little movement. Most exercises are mixtures of the two types with one or the other predominating. For many years it was thought that only "aerobic" exercise was suitable for cardiac patients and that isometric training would be dangerous by raising the blood pressure and overloading the heart. Over the past 10 years, however, the value and safety of combining moderate strength training with aerobic training for cardiac patients has been recognised and shown to enhance fitness.[30-32] High resistance training alone also increases fitness but not so rapidly as aerobic training.

Strength training has the advantage of reassuring the patient that he or she is fit to undertake tasks, either at work or at leisure, which need muscular effort, thus enhancing one aspect of quality of life.[33]

Dose

For exercise, the dose involves frequency, intensity, and duration.

Frequency

The American Heart Association recommends for cardiac patients a frequency of between two and four times a week,[34] although there is little evidence to support this figure. Most trials of physical training have used three or four weekly sessions. It has been shown that, for early postinfarction exercise training, a programme of two sessions a week is as effective as three.[35] Increasing from three to five sessions does not seem to produce much further benefit for normal middle aged men.[36]

Intensity

The usual recommendation for exercise intensity for cardiac patients is to reach a target of between 70% and 85% of maximum heart rate, which should be determined from an exercise test.[37] The American Heart Association advises a level of between 50% and 80% of maximum oxygen uptake, also decided from an initial exercise test with the lower end of this range for the higher risk patients.[34] Very low level exercise does not increase physical fitness, with a threshold for benefit of between 40% and 60% of maximum oxygen uptake.[38] The benefit produced by very intense exercise (in excess of 85% of predicted maximum heart rate) is relatively modest and overridden by an increase in the risk of dangerous cardiac arrhythmias.[39] Several recent trials have shown that moderately low level exercise applied to groups of postinfarction patients produces similar increases in aerobic capacity to high intensity exercise.[40,41] However, very intense exercise does produce considerable increases in fitness.[42] and a positive effect on exercise induced ejection fraction increase, which is not found with moderate exercise.[21]

Duration

The duration of exercise shown to increase fitness varies from 20 to 60 minutes.[37] Longer sessions may increase fitness but at the cost of an increase in musculoskeletal injuries.

When patients start on an exercise programme, they may not be able to sustain the necessary intensity and duration of exertion, and therefore these should be increased gradually to the recommended levels.

Duration of treatment

The intention of most exercise based cardiac rehabilitation programmes is to start the patient on a course of exercise, which will continue as long as possible after the period of supervision.

Most cardiac rehabilitation programmes supervise their patients over 6–12 weeks,[8] although some programmes last up to 2 years. These longer term exercise training programmes may have a greater benefit on prognosis than short term programmes.[43] The longer a programme lasts the greater the drop out rate,[44] but long term compliance is imroved by long term supervision and developments in the exercise programme.[45] Certainly those who continue to exercise in the long term gain extra benefits such as greater increase in aerobic capacity and a slowing or reversal in the usual age related decline in performance.

Practical aspects

In the United Kingdom most cardiac rehabilitation programmes are run by nurses or physiotherapists with help from a multi-disciplinary team, which in some cases includes sports scientists or other exercise specialists.[10] The programme is divided into four phases.[13] Phase 1 covers the time in hospital after acute myocardial infarction, and exercise is limited to gradual mobilisation including stair climbing to prepare the patient for discharge. Phase 2 includes the first few weeks at home when the main exercise, usually unsupervised, is a progressive walking programme. Ideally the patient is sent out with clear written guidance, and supplementary support can be given by telephone contact with a primary care team. Phase 3 is the supervised exercise programme which is the centrepiece of a package of care which includes education, dietary instruction, risk factor monitoring, stress management, and relaxation training. Phase 4 is the long term exercise to which it is hoped that most patients will adhere. In practice more than 50% will drop out of regular vigorous exercise once the supervised programme is over. A necessary prerequisite to phase 3 is the exercise test.

Exercise testing

All patients with known heart disease should be exercise tested before entering an exercise programme.[34] The following essential information can be obtained from the test.

The existence of reversible ischaemia

This is common in postinfarction patients and is not rare in patients after a bypass. A substantial proportion of those with exercise induced ischaemia do not suffer pain, so called silent ischaemia. Those who recommend exercise for coronary patients need to know whether their patients are likely to develop ischaemia during a session so that the level of exercise can be modified and prophylactic trinitrate used. Most postinfarction patients with positive exercise tests are referred for coronary angiography.

The level of fitness

This allows an appropriate level of exercise to be prescribed, may contribute to risk stratification, and gives a baseline figure against which future performance can be compared.

The appropriate heart rate response for improving physical fitness

Many cardiac patients will be taking medication, (β blockers, some calcium channel blockers, angiotensin converting enzyme (ACE) inhibitors, antiarrhythmics) which modify resting and exercise heart rates.

Blood pressure response

Patients with very poor left ventricular function and those taking some drugs show a paradoxical fall in blood pressure with exercise and are more susceptible to faintness during sessions.

Rhythm disturbance

Patients who develop arrhythmias during the test, particularly high grade ventricular arrhythmias, demand careful handling[14] and may need a change in medication before the start of the course.

In the United Kingdom most cardiac rehabilitation programmes are performed in hospital gymnasia with circuit training supplemented by "homework", which may be a home based circuit or walking. Sessions are held between one and three times a week and the course usually lasts 6–12 weeks.[47]

Benefits of exercise

Increased physical fitness

Community surveys have shown that the general level of fitness in this country is deplorably low,[48] and patients who suffer coronary problems have even lower levels. The improvements achieved by physical training as described above are of obvious benefit to the daily activities of cardiac patients. The energy costs of a wide variety of activities both at work and leisure have been estimated,[49,50] and can theoretically allow prediction of the ability of cardiac patients to perform such tasks. In the United Kingdom the ability to regain a licence to drive a large goods or passenger carrying vehicle depends on the completion of 9 minutes of the Bruce protocol treadmill test, a feat that may only be possible after exercise training.

One group that may have most to gain is patients with cardiac failure.

Exercise in heart failure

Heart failure was thought to be a contraindication to exercise training, but Conn *et al.* in 1982 showed that an increase in exercise capacity of around 20% could be achieved by patients with ejection fractions of between 13% and 26%.[51] This was confirmed by Sullivan *et al.* in 1989,[52] and since then an increasing literature has added to knowledge of physical training in heart failure.[53,54] Cardiac failure leads to a considerable reduction in physical activity, which produces muscle wasting. This in turn makes exercise harder, further reducing physical efforts and a spiral of deterioration is produced.[55] Exercise, even at relatively low level— that is, about 55% of maximum heart rate[56]—can reverse this process and bring about a useful increase in quality of life.[57] This increase in functional capacity is achieved by a combination of increased muscle metabolism,[58] reduced vascular resistance in the working muscles,[59] reduced sympathetic tone,[57] and perhaps improvements in cardiac performance.[52,57] One possible mechanism is an increase in early diastolic filling after physical training.[60]

Reduced angina

The threshold for angina occurs at a fixed "double product" (the product of heart rate and systolic blood pressure) for any individual.[61] An increase in fitness reduces the heart rate and blood pressure responses to exercise[23] and would therefore be expected to raise angina threshold. Nearly all trials of training for coronary patients have indeed shown a great reduction in angina frequency and an increase in angina threshold.[62,63] Exercise training has been found to be as effective for angina as β blockade[22] and also to reduce the total ischaemic burden.[64]

Enhanced coronary blood flow

This effect, discussed above (myocardial blood supply), may reduce angina, lessen the size of future infarction, and play some part in the mortality reduction which follows exercise based cardiac rehabilitation (see below).

Reduced arrhythmias and heart rate variability

Ventricular ectopic beats are common in normal people but much more common and more frequent in patients recovering from myocardial infarction. Frequent ventricular ectopics are one of the risk factors for sudden death after an infarction.[65] Exercise training increases the cardiac threshold for ventricular ectopic activity, and controlled trials have shown that ectopic beats are less prevalent in trained than untrained postinfarction patients.[66] Increased ventricular ectopic activity is associated with increased sympathetic and decreased parasympathetic tone,[67] which also produces a reduction in heart rate variability,[68] an effect enhanced by β blockade.[69] Reduced heart rate variability is associated with increased mortality after infarction[70] and can be improved by exercise training.[71] A recent trial of exercise training soon after acute myocardial infarction has, however, failed to show a difference in heart rate variability or baroreflex sensitivity between the treated and the control groups.[72]

Improved lipid profiles

Individuals who take regular vigorous exercise have much healthier blood fat profiles than their sedentary peers.[73] Controlled trials of exercise rehabilitation have shown that coronary patients can benefit from this effect with lowering of total cholesterol and a rise in high density lipoprotein cholesterol,[74,75] but the level of exercise needs to be high, equivalent to runing 24 km (15 miles) a week,[76] a much greater exercise load than is used in most cardiac rehabilitation programmes in the United Kingdom. This benefit of exercise is enhanced if the patient can lose weight but is lost if the patient gains weight.[77] Exercise also produces an acute reduction in triglyceride concentration which is maintained for about 48 hours.[73] Those who continue to exercise three or four times a week therefore keep their serum triglyceride concentrations down.

Lowered blood pressure

Treatment of hypertension has a smaller effect on risk of heart attack than on risk of stroke. One reason may be that commonly used hypotensive drugs have adverse effects on blood lipids. Non-pharmacological treatments for hypertension do not have this disadvantage, and exercise training has been shown to lower blood pressure at rest and during exercise in hypertensive coronary patients and may lessen the need for drug therapy.[78]

Improved thrombolysis

A high level of plasma fibrinogen and low fibrinolytic activity are powerful risk factors for coronary disease,[79] and cigarette smoking probably exerts much of its atherogenic effect by this route.[80] Fibrinolytic activity is increased by exercise in normal subjects, and the more vigorous the exercise the greater the response.[81] Patients after infarction[82] and coronary bypass grafting[83] have been shown to respond similarly.

Weight loss

Obesity is a weak independent risk factor for coronary disease but being overweight increases blood pressure and blood cholesterol concentration. The effects of exercise training on weight loss in obese cardiac subjects are disappointing,[84] but some controlled trials of cardiac rehabilitation have shown a weight loss in the treated group.[85] However, a failure to reduce body weight may be due to an increase in lean muscle mass rather than a failure to reduce body fat,[86] and this has also been found in controlled trials.[87] If the patient takes a great deal of exercise, equivalent to runing 24 km (15 miles) or more a week, weight loss is likely. Lesser physical endeavours should be combined with reduced calorie intake.

Psychological benefit and improved quality of life

The psychological state of the coronary patient affects not only the quality of life but also the prognosis, depression being a risk factor for death over the year after myocardial infarction.[88] Cardiac rehabilitation can contribute to the psychological wellbeing of cardiac patients[63,89] but probably not to the extent to which most programme coordinators believe. Controlled trials have shown that exercise is an effective treatment for depression.[90] In postinfarction patients, controlled trials have shown that exercise rehabilitation can produce significant benefits such as increased confidence, wellbeing, and happiness with decreases in anxiety and depression.[91] These benefits, however, are small and relatively short lived if exercise alone is used to treat the patient.[92] A meta-analysis of the effect of controlled trials of exercise on anxiety and depression in coronary patients indicated a small benefit for both of these common problems.[93] The addition of stress management and relaxation treatment significantly enhances the effect of the exercise-only approach.[94] A further meta-analysis by Linden *et al.* concluded that the addition of psychosocial treatments not only reduces psychological distress but also morbidity, risk factors, and mortality.[95] Exercise may also improve the mental activity of elderly demented cardiac patients.[96]

Oldridge has calculated the cost per quality adjusted life year (QALY) gained by cardiac rehabilitation by using a "time trade off" method.[97] In this system, the patient estimates how many years of perfectly healthy life he or she would exchange for a normal life expectancy in the present state of health. The result is added to the life years gained, adjusted for any loss of quality, to give the total QALYs gained. This amounts to 0.071 QALYs per person rehabilitated which, at a cost of £200 gives a figure of £2817. This is similar to the estimated cost per QALY gained by bypass grafting for left mainstem coronary stenosis.

Return to work

Most people in employment before their heart attack will return to work, sometimes in modified form, after 3 to 6 months.[98] For some, however, particularly those nearing retiring age, the attack, or heart surgery, may be a helpful opportunity for the patient to retire from a job that is irksome or even damaging to health. Some controlled trials of rehabilitation have shown an improved return to work for the intervention group[99–101] but many have not.[102] The rehabilitation setting, however, can be used to ensure an earlier return to work for treated patients,[103] and the physical training element can allow recovery of the large goods vehicle or passenger carrying vehicle license, both of which require the patient to perform 9 minutes of the Bruce protocol treadmill test without any changes of ischaemia observed on the electrocardiogram. For a minority of patients disabled either physically or psychologically by their attack, formal rehabilitation has been shown to result in renewed employment.[104]

Improved survival

Regular vigorous exercise provides primary prevention of coronary artery disease.[105,106] None of the randomised controlled trials of exercise based cardiac rehabilitation have been large enough to show a significant decrease in mortality in the treated group, but over the past 10 years there have been several meta-analyses of the combined results of all the randomised controlled trials reported. These have involved up to 4500 patients and all agree that there is a reduction in death rate of between 20% and 25% in the treated groups.[43,107,108] There is a greater advantage to patients treated with a multidisciplinary approach than those taking part in exercise programmes alone.[109]

There are several mechanisms by which exercise may improve the survival of patients with coronary disease as discussed above. They include improved coronary blood flow, decreased ventricular arrhythmias, improved lipid profiles, lowered blood pressure, improved fibrinolysis, weight loss, and reduced depression.

These meta-analyses have also shown no difference in recurrent non-fatal infarction between treated and control groups, but it is interesting to note that the five controlled trials that have followed the patients for 5 years or more have all shown lower reinfarction rates for the treated groups.[100,110-113]

Side effect

Ventricular fibrillation/myocardial infarction

The most serious complications of exercise treatment for cardiac patients are acute infarction and sudden death, usually from ventricular fibrillation. These are most likely in patients with exercise induced ischaemia and those with severe ventricular damage.[114] Ventricular fibrillation is 100 times more likely during exercise than at other times but is still very rare during supervised exercise rehabilitation, between once per 33 000 patient hours[115] and once per 112 000 patient hours of exercise.[116] Myocardial infarction is even rarer during the rehabilitation programme.

Angina pectoris

Angina is an inevitable consequence of exercise training among patients with residual coronary narrowing but can be minimised by careful exercise load prescription, adequate warm up routines, and the use of glyceryl trinitrate before the session. Angina should be kept to a minimum; left ventricular contractility may be impaired not only during an episode of ischaemia but for several hours after, a phenomenon known as myocardial stunning.[117]

Infarct expansion?

After large myocardial infarcts a process of remodelling takes place with myocardial thinning at the site of damage and dilatation of the left ventricle.[118] Jugdutt et al. examined the possibility that infarct expansion may be worsened by exercise in a randomised controlled trial of physical training for 46 patients with anterior Q wave infarcts.[119] Of 22 who were enrolled, 13 completed the programme and six of those showed topographical and functional deterioration. Other studies have claimed to disprove this effect, but the results do not always seem to support this assertion. Jette et al. exercised 10 men with ejection fractions below 30%, two of whom developed left ventricular failure.[120] The remainder showed an increase in work capacity and peak oxygen consumption but an increase in mean pulmonary wedge pressure. Nevertheless they claim that "training did not cause further deterioration in ventricular function". Tavazzi and Ignone found that patients with left ventricular dysfunction and low cardiac output failed to increase their exercise capacity or to show the expected fall in pulmonary artery diastolic pressure with training.[121] The same group, however, went on to randomise 49 patients with anterior Q wave infarcts to training or no exercise at 4 to 8 weeks after the attack and found the degree of remodelling in the two groups to be the same.[122] Further reassurance is provided by the finding that left ventricular mass, volumes, and ejection fraction did not change in either group in a controlled trial of high intensity exercise in men with postinfarction left ventricular dysfunction.[123] It has been shown that reduced left ventricular function can be improved by exercise in patients with chronic coronary disease, perhaps by improving myocardial perfusion.[124] Whether this is also true for patients recovering from a large anterior myocardial infarction is not yet clear, and such patients should certainly be treated with caution.

Others

Other side effects of exercise for cardiac patients include transient arrhythmias and angina pectoris, which are very common, hypotension, which is less common, and musculoskeletal injuries, which should be rare in a well organised programme.

All these exercise induced problems should be kept to a minimum by careful risk assessment of the participants, by appropriate exercise prescription, by a well designed exercise course, and by attention to adequate warming up and cooling down routines.

Conclusion

Ever since the early writings of Hellerstein, exercise has been the centrepiece of most cardiac rehabilitation programmes. It deserves this place as it contributes to both of the two aims of this treatment: to return the patient to good health as rapidly as is safe and to reduce to a minimum the risk of recurrence of the cardiac illness.

However, there are considerable problems in providing exercise based rehabilitation to all who need it or may benefit from it. In the United Kingdom probably less than 20% of eligible patients take part in cardiac rehabilitation programmes.[125,126] A lack of funding is one undoubted reason for this low take up, but patient factors are also important both in the decision to join the programme[127] and, once enrolled, the decision to adhere to the course.[128]

1 Tofler GH, Mittleman MA, Muller JE. Physical activity and the triggering of myocardial infarction: the case for regular exercise. *Heart* 1996;**75**:323–5.
2 Levine SA, Lown B. Armchair treatment of acute coronary thrombosis. *JAMA* 1952;**148**:1365–9.
3 Harpur JE, Kellett RJ, Conner WT, *et al*. Controlled trial of early mobilisation and discharge from hospital in uncomplicated myocardial infarction. *Lancet* 1971;2:1331–4.
4 Hayes MG, Morris GK, Hampton JR. Comparison of mobilisation after two and nine days in uncomplicated myocardial infarction. *BMJ* 1974;2:10–13.
5 Hellerstein HK, Ford AB. Rehabilitation of the cardiac patient. *JAMA* 1957;**164**:225–31.
6 Hellerstein HK. Exercise therapy in coronary disease. *Bull N Y Acad Med* 1968;**44**:1028–47.
7 Groden BM, Semple T, Shaw GB. Cardiac rehabilitation in Britain (1970). *Br Heart J* 1971;**33**:756–8.
8 Horgan J, Bethell H, Carson P, *et al*. British Cardiac Society working party report on cardiac rehabilitation. *Br Heart J* 1992;**67**:412–18.
9 Davidson C, Reval K, Chamberlain DA, *et al*. A report of a working group of the British Cardiac Society: cardiac rehabilitation services in the United Kingdom 1992. *Br Heart J* 1995;**73**:201–2.
10 Lewin RJ, Ingleton R, Thompson D. Adherence to cardiac rehabilitation guidelines: a survey of rehabilitation programmes in the United Kingdom. *BMJ* 1998;**316**:1354–6.
11 Wenger NK, Haskell WL, Kanter K, *et al*. Cardiac rehabilitation services after cardiac transplantation: guidelines for use. *Cardiology* 1991;**20**:4–5.
12 Bourke JP, Turkington D, Thomas G, *et al*. Florid psychopathology in patients receiving shocks from implanted cardioverter-defibrillators. *Heart* 1997;**78**:581–3.
13 Coats A, McGee H, Stokes H, *et al*. *BACR guidelines for cardiac rehabilitation*. Oxford: Blackwell Science, 1995.
14 Kelly TM. Exercise testing and training of patients with malignant ventricular

arrhythmias. *Med Sci Sports Exerc* 1995;**28**:53–61.

15 Astrand PO, Rodahl K. *Textbook of work physiology.* New York: McGraw-Hill, 1986.

16 Rousseau MF, Degre S, Messin R, *et al.* Hemodynamic effects of early physical training after acute myocardial infarction; comparison with a control untrained group. *Eur J Cardiol* 1974;**2**:39–45.

17 Amsterdam E, Laslett L, Dressendorfer R, *et al.* Exercise training in coronary heart disease: is there a cardiac effect? *Am Heart J* 1981;**101**:870–3.

18 Saunamaki K. Feasibility and effect of physical training with maximum intensity in men after acute myocardial infarction. *Scand J Rehabil Med* 1978;**10**:155–62.

19 Ehsani A, Biello D, Schultz J, *et al.* Improvement of left ventricular contractile function by exercise training in patients with coronary artery disease. *Circulation* 1986;**74**:350–5.

20 Hagberg J. Physiologic adaptations to prolonged high intensity exercise training in patients with coronary artery disease. *Med Sci Sports Exerc* 1991;**23**:661–7.

21 Oberman A, Fletcher GF, Lee J, *et al.* Efficacy of high-intensity exercise training on left ventricular ejection fraction in men with coronary artery disease (the training level comparison study). *Am J Cardiol* 1995;**76**:643–7.

22 Todd I, Ballantyne D. Antianginal efficacy of exercise training: a comparison with beta blockade. *Br Heart J* 1990;**64**:14–19.

23 Raffo J, Luksic I, Kappagoda C, *et al.* Effects of physical training on myocardial ischaemia in patients with coronary artery disease. *Br Heart J* 1980;**43**:262–9.

24 Doba N, Shukuya M, Yoshida H, *et al.* Physical training of the patients with coronary heart disease: non-invasive strategies for the evaluation of its effects on the oxygen transport system and myocardial ischaemia. *Jpn Circ J* 1990;**54**:1409–18.

25 Ornish D, Brown S, Scherwitz L, *et al.* Can lifestyle changes reverse coronary heart disease? *Lancet* 1990;**336**:129–33.

26 Schuler G, Hambrecht R, Schierf G, *et al.* Myocardial perfusion and regression of coronary artery disease in patients on a regimen of intensive physical exercise and low fat diet. *J Am Coll Cardiol* 1992;**19**:34–42.

27 Niebauer J, Hambrecht R, Velich T, *et al.* Attenuated progression of coronary artery disease after 6 years of multifactorial risk intervention: role of physical exercise. *Circulation* 1997;**96**:2534–41.

28 Hambrecht R, Niebauer J, Marburger C, *et al.* Various intensities of leisure time physical activity in patients with coronary artery disease: effects on cardiorespiratory fitness and progression of coronary atherosclerotic lesions. *J Am Coll Cardiol* 1993;**22**:468–77.

29 Franklin B. Exercise training and coronary collateral circulation. *Med Sci Sports Exerc* 1991;**23**:648–53.

30 Ghilarducci L, Holly R, Amsterdam E. Effects of high resistance training in coronary artery disease. *Am J Cardiol* 1989;**64**:866–70.

31 McCartney N, McKelvie RS, Haslam DRS, *et al.* Usefulness of weightlifting training in improving strength and maximal power output in coronary artery disease. *Am J Cardiol* 1991;**67**:939–45.

32 McCartney N, McKelvie RS. The role of resistance training in patients with cardiac disease. *J Cardiovasc Risk* 1996;**3**:160–6.

33 Beniamini Y, Rubenstein J, Zaichkowski L, *et al.* Effects of high-intensity strength training on quality-of-life parameters in cardiac rehabilitation patients. *Am J Cardiol* 1997;**80**:841-6.

34 Fletcher GF, Balady G, Froelicher VF, *et al.* Exercise standards. A statement for healthcare professionals from the American Heart Association. *Circulation* 1995;**91**:580–615.

35 Dressendorfer RH, Franklin BA, Cameron JL, *et al.* Exercise training

frequency in early post-infarction cardiac rehabilitation. Influence on aerobic conditioning. *J Cardiopulm Rehab* 1995;**15**:269–76.

36 Pollock ML, Miller HS, Linnerud AC, *et al.* Frequency of training as a determinant for improvement in cardiovascular function and body composition of middle aged men. *Arch Phys Med Rehabil* 1975;**56**:141–5.

37 Wenger NK, Froelicher ES, Smith LK, *et al. Cardiac rehabilitation as secondary prevention.* Rockville, Maryland: Agency for Health Care Policy and Research and National Heart, Lung and Blood Institute, 1995.

38 Franklin BA, Gordon S, Timmis GC. Amount of exercise necessary for the patient with coronary artery disese. *Am J Cardiol* 1992;**69**:1426–32.

39 Hellerstein HK, Franklin BA. Exercise testing and exercise prescription. In: Wenger NK, Hellerstein HK, eds. *Rehabilitation of the coronary patient.* New York: Wiley, 1978.

40 Blumenthal JA, Rejeski WJ, Walsh-Riddle M, *et al.* Comparison of high and low intensity exercise training early after acute myocardial infarction. *Am J Cardiol* 1988;**61**:26–30.

41 Goble AJ, Hare DL, MacDonald PS, *et al.* Effect of early programmes of high and low intensity on physical performance after transmural acute myocardial infarction. *Br Heart J* 1991;**65**:126–31.

42 Martin W, Heath G, Coyle E, *et al.* Effect of prolonged intense endurance training on systolic time intervals in patients with coronary disease. *Am Heart J* 1984;**107**:75.

43 Oldridge N, Guyatt G, Fischer M, *et al.* Cardiac rehabilitation after myocardial infarction. Combined experience of randomised clinical trials. *JAMA* 1988;**260**:945–50.

44 Bruce EH, Frederick R, Bruce RA, *et al.* Comparison of active participants and drop outs in CAPRI cardiopulmonary rehabilitation programs. *Am J Cardiol* 1976;**37**:53–60.

45 Keleman MH, Stewart KJ, Gillilan RE, *et al.* Circuit weight training in cardiac patients. *J Am Coll Cardiol* 1986;**7**:38–42.

46 Rechnitzer PA, Cunningham DA, Andrew GM, *et al.* Relation of exercise to the recurrence rate of myocardial infarction in men. *Am J Cardiol* 1983;**51**:65–9.

47 Thompson DR, Bowman GS, Kitson AL, *et al.* Cardiac rehabilitation services in England and Wales: a national survey. *Int J Cardiol* 1997;**59**:299–304.

48 Allied Dunbar National Fitness Survey. London: Sports Council and the Health Education Authority, 1992.

49 Jette M, Sidney K, Blumchen G. Metabolic equivalents (METS) in exercise testing, exercise prescription and evaluation of functional capacity. *Clin Cardiol* 1990;**13**:555–65.

50 Haskin-Popp C, Nazareno D, Wegner J, *et al.* Aerobic and myocardial demands of lawn mowing in patients with coronary artery disease. *Am J Cardiol* 1998;**81**:1243–5.

51 Conn EH, Williams RS, Wallace AG. Exercise responses before and after physical conditioning in patients with severely depressed left ventricular function. *Am J Cardiol* 1982;**49**:296–300.

52 Sullivan M, Higginbotham M, Cobb F. Exercise training in patients with chronic heart failure delays ventilatory anaerobic threshold and improves submaximal exercise performance. *Circulation* 1989;**79**:324–9.

53 Coats A, Adamopoulos S, Meyer T, *et al.* Effects of physical training in chronic heart failure. *Lancet* 1990;**335**:63–6.

54 Wielenger RP, Coats MS, Mosterd WL, *et al.* The role of exercise training in chronic heart failure. *Heart* 1997;**78**:431–6.

55 Drexler H. Skeletal muscle failure in heart failure. *Circulation* 1992;**85**:1621–3.

56 Bellardinelli R, Georgiou D, Scocco V, *et al.* Low intensity exercise training in patients with chronic heart failure. *J Am Coll Cardiol* 1995;**26**:975–82.

57 Coats AJS, Adamopoulos S, Radaelli A, *et al.* Controlled trial of physical training in chronic heart failure. *Circulation* 1992;**85**:2119–31.

58 Adamopoulos S, Coats AJS, Brunotte F, *et al.* Physical training improves skeletal muscle metabolism in patients with congestive heart failure. *J Am Coll Cardiol* 1993;**21**:1101–6.

59 Hornig B, Maier V, Drexler H. Physical training improves endothelial function in patients with chronic heart failure. *Circulation* 1996;**93**:210–14.

60 Belardinelli R, Demetrios G, Cianci G, *et al.* Effects of exercise training on left ventricular filling at rest and during exercise in patients with ischemic cardiomyopathy and severe left ventricular systolic dysfunction. *Am Heart J* 1996;**132**:61–70.

61 Robinson BF. Relation of heart rate and systolic blood pressure to the onset of pain in angina pectoris. *Circulation* 1967;**35**:1073–83.

62 Dressendorfer R, Smith J, Amsterdam E, *et al.* Reduction of submaximal exercise myocardial oxygen demand post-walk training program in coronary patients due to improved physical work efficiency. *Am Heart J* 1982;**103**:358–62.

63 Bethell H, Mullee M. A controlled trial of community based coronary rehabilitation. *Br Heart J* 1990;**64**:370–5.

64 Todd I, Ballantyne D. Effect of exercise training on the total ischaemic burden: an assessment by 24 hour ambulatory electrocardiographic monitoring. *Br Heart J* 1992;**68**:560–6.

65 Multicentre Post Infarction Research Group. Risk stratification after myocardial infarction. *N Engl J Med* 1983;**309**:331–6.

66 Hertzeanu HL, Shemish J, Aron AL, *et al.* Ventricular arrhythmias in rehabilitated and nonrehabilitated postmyocardial infarction patients with left ventricular dysfunction. *Am J Cardiol* 1993;**71**:24–7.

67 Podrid P, Fuchs T, Candinas R. Role of the sympathetic nervous system in the genesis of ventricular arrhythmia. *Circulation* 1990;**82**(suppl 1):103–13.

68 Malfatto G, Facchini M, Bragato R, *et al.* Short and long term effects of exercise training on the tonic autonomic modulation of heart rate variability after myocardial infarction. *Eur Heart J* 1996;**17**:532–8.

69 Malfatto G, Facchini M, Sala L, *et al.* Effects of cardiac rehabilitation and beta-blocker therapy on heart rate variability after first acute myocardial infarction. *Am J Cardiol* 1998;**81**:834–40.

70 Cripps T, Malik M, Farrell T, *et al.* Prognostic value of reduced heart variability after myocardial infarction: clinical evaluation of a new analysis method. *Br Heart J* 1991;**65**:14–19.

71 La Rovere M, Mortara A, Sandrove G, *et al.* Autonomic nervous system adaptations to short term exercise training. *Chest* 1992;**101** (suppl):299–303.

72 Leitch JW, Newling RP, Basta M, *et al.* Randomized trial of a hospital-based exercise training program after acute myocardial infarction: cardiac autonomic effects. *J Am Coll Cardiol* 1997;**29**:1263–8.

73 Cullinane E, Siconolfi S, Saritelli A, *et al.* Acute decrease in serum triglycerides with exercise: is there a threshold for an exercise effect? *Metabolism* 1982;**31**:844–7.

74 Ballantyne F, Clark R, Simpson H, *et al.* The effect of moderate physical exercise on the plasma lipoprotein subfractions of male survivors of myocardial infarction. *Circulation* 1982;**65**:913–18.

75 Heath G, Ehsani A, Hagberg J, *et al.* Exercise training improves lipoprotein lipid profiles in patients with coronary artery disease. *Am Heart J* 1983;**105**:889–95.

76 Haskell W. The influence of exercise training on plasma lipids and lipoproteins in health and disease. *Acta Med Scand* 1986; suppl 711:25–37.

77 Vu Tran Z, Weltman A. Differential effects of exercise on serum lipid and lipoprotein levels seen with changes in body weight: a meta-analysis. *JAMA*

1985;**254**:919–24.

78 Puddey IB, Beilin LJ. Exercise in the prevention and treatment of hypertension. *Curr Opin Nephrol Hypertens* 1995;**4**:245–50.

79 Meade T, Ruddock V, Stirling Y, *et al.* Fibrinolytic activity, clotting factors and long term incidence of ischaemic heart disease in the Northwick Park heart study. *Lancet* 1993;**343**:1076–9.

80 Meade T, Mellows S, Brozovic M, *et al.* Haemostatic function and ischaemic heart disease: principal results of the Northwick Park heart study. *Lancet* 1986;**ii**:533–7.

81 Ferguson E, Bernier L, Banta G, *et al.* Effects of exercise and conditioning on clotting and fibrinolytic activity in man. *J Appl Physiol* 1987;**62**:1416–21.

82 Estelles A, Aznar J, Tormo G, *et al.* Influence of a rehabilitation sports programme on the fibrinolytic activity of patients after myocardial infarction. *Thromb Res* 1989;**55**:203–12.

83 Wosornu D, Allardyce W, Ballantyne D, *et al.* Influence of power and aerobic exercise training on haemostatic factors after coronary artery surgery. *Br Heart J* 1992;**68**:181–6.

84 Lavie CJ, Milani RV. Effects of cardiac rehabilitation and exercise training in obese patients with coronary artery disease. *Chest* 1996;**109**:52–6.

85 Fletcher G, Cantwell J. Outpatient gym exercise program for patients with recent myocardial infarction. A preliminary report. *Arch Intern Med* 1974;**134**:63–8.

86 Findlay I, Taylor R, Dargie H, *et al.* Cardiovascular effects of training for a marathon run in unfit middle aged men. *BMJ* 1987;**295**:521–4.

87 Hartnung G, Rangel R. Exercise training in post-myocardial infarction patients: comparison of results with high risk coronary and post-bypass patients. *Arch Phys Med Rehabil* 1981;**62**:147–50.

88 Frasure-Smith N, Lesperance F, Talajic M. Depression and 18-month prognosis after myocardial infarction. *Circulation* 1995;**91**:999–1005.

89 Oldridge N, LaSalle D, Jones N. Exercise rehabilitation of female patients with coronary disease. *Am Heart J* 1980;**100**:755–6.

90 Martinsen E, Medhus A, Sandvik L. Effects of exercise on depression: a controlled study. *BMJ* 1985;**291**:109.

91 Taylor C, Houston-Miller N, Ahn D, *et al.* Effects of exercise programs on psychosocial improvement in uncomplicated postmyocardial infarction patients. *J Psychosom Res* 1986;**30**:581–30.

92 Langosch W. Psychological effects of training in coronary patients: a critical review of the literature. *Eur Heart J* 1988; **9**(suppl M):37–42.

93 Kugler J, Seelbach H, Kruskemper GM. Effects of rehabilitation exercise programmes on anxiety and depression in coronary patients: a meta-analysis. *Br J Clin Psychol* 1994;**33**:401–10.

94 Roviaro S, Holmes D, Holmsten R. Influence of a cardiac rehabilitation program on the cardiovascular, psychological and social functioning of cardiac patients. *J Behav Med* 1984;**7**:61–81.

95 Linden W, Stossel C, Maurice J. Psychosocial interventions for patients with coronary artery disease. *Arch Intern Med* 1996;**155**:745–52.

96 Satoh T, Sakurai I, Miyagi K, *et al.* Walking exercise and improved neuropsychological funcioning in elderly patients with cardiac disease. *J Intern Med* 1995;**238**:423–8.

97 Oldridge N. Economic evaluation of cardiac rehabilitation soon after myocardial infarction. In: Broustet J, ed. *Proceedings of the Vth World Congress on Cardiac Rehabilitation.* Andover: Intercept, 1993:519–25.

98 Carson P, Phillips R, Lloyd M, *et al.* Exercise after myocardial infarction: a controlled trial. *J R Coll Physicians Lond* 1982;**16**:147–51.

99 Bertie J, King A, Reed N, *et al.* Benefits and weaknesses of a cardiac rehabilitation programme. *J R Coll Physicians Lond* 1992;**26**:147–51.

357

100 Marra S, Paolilla V, Spadaccina F, *et al.* Long term follow-up after a controlled, randomised post-myocardial infarction rehabilitation programme. *Eur Heart J* 1985;**6**:656–63.

101 Levin L, Perk J, Hedback B. Cardiac rehabilitation: cost analysis. *J Intern Med* 1991;**230**:427–36.

102 Danchin N, Geopfert PC. Exercise training, cardiac rehabilitation and return to work in patients with coronary artery disease. *Eur Heart J* 1988;**9**(suppl M):43–6.

103 Dennis C, Houston-Miller N, Schwartz R, *et al.* Early return to work after uncomplicated myocardial infarction. Results of a randomised trial. *JAMA* 1988;**260**:214–20.

104 Monpere C, Francois G, Brochier M. Effects of a comprehensive rehabilitation programme in patients with three-vessel coronary disease. *Eur Heart J* 1988;**9**(suppl M):28–31.

105 Morris J, Chave S, Adam C, *et al.* Vigorous exercise in leisure-time and the incidence of coronary heart disease. *Lancet* 1973;**i**:333–9.

106 Kannel W, Sorlie P. Some health benefits of physical activity: the Framingham study. *Arch Intern Med* 1979;**139**:857–61.

107 Shephard R. The value of exercise in ischaemic heart disease: accumulative analysis. *J Cardiac Rehab* 1983;**3**:294–8.

108 O'Connor G, Buring J, Yusuf S, *et al.* An overview of randomised trials of rehabilitation with exercise after myocardial infarction. *Circulation* 1989;**80**:234–44.

109 Curfman GD. The health benefits of exercise. A critical reappraisal. *N Engl J Med* 1993;**328**:574–5.

110 Roman O, Gutierrez M, Luksic I, *et al.* Cardiac rehabilitation after myocardial infarction. 9 year controlled follow-up study. *Cardiology* 1983;**70**:223–31.

111 Vermeulen A, Lie KI, Durrer D. Effects of cardiac rehabilitation after myocardial infarction: changes in coronary risk factors and long-term prognosis. *Am Heart J* 1983;**105**:798–801.

112 Hedback B, Perk J, Wodlin P. Long-term reduction of cardiac mortality after myocardial infarction: 10-year results of a comprehensive rehabilitation programme. *Eur Heart J* 1993;**14**:831–5.

113 Bethell HJN, Turner SC, Mulke MA. Unpublished data.

114 Squires RW, Gau GT, Miller TD, *et al.* Cardiac rehabilitation: status 1990. *Mayo Clin Proc* 1990;**65**:731–55.

115 Haskell WL. Cardiovascular complications during exercise training of cardiac patients. *Circulation* 1975;**57**:920–4.

116 Van Camp SP, Peterson RA. Cardiovascular complications of outpatient cardiac rehabilitation programs. *JAMA* 1986;**256**:1160–3.

117 Ambrosia G, Betocchi S, Pace L, *et al.* Prolonged impairment of regional contractile function after resolution of exercise-induced angina. *Circulation* 1996;**94**:2455–64.

118 Pfeffer MA, Braunwald E. Ventricular remodelling after myocardial infarction. *Circulation* 1990;**81**:1161–72.

119 Jugdutt BI, Michorowski BL, Kappagoda CT. Exercise training after anterior Q-wave myocardial infarction: importance of regional left ventricular function and topography. *J Am Coll Cardiol* 1988;**12**:362–72.

120 Jette M, Heller R, Landry F, *et al.* Randomised 4-week exercise program in patients with impaired left ventricular function. *Circulation* 1991;**84**:1561–7.

121 Tavazzi L, Ignone G. Short term haemodynamic evolution and late follow-up of post-infarct patients with left ventricular dysfunction undergoing a physical training programme. *Eur Heart J* 1991;**12**:657–65.

122 Gianuzzi P, Temporelli L, Corra U, *et al.* Attenuation of unfavorable remodelling in postinfarction patients with left ventricular dysfunction. Results of the exercise in left ventricular dysfunction (ELVD) trial. *Circulation*

1997;**96**:1790–7.
123 Dubach P, Myers J, Dziekan G, *et al.* Effect of high intensity exercise training on central haemodynamic responses to exercise in men with reduced left ventricular function. *J Am Coll Cardiol* 1997;**29**:1591–8.
124 Bellardinelli R, Georgiou D, Ginzton L, *et al.* Effects of moderate exercise training on thallium uptake and contractile response to low-dose dobutamine of dysfunctional myocardium in patients with ischemic cardiomyopathy. *Circulation* 1998;**97**:553–61.
125 Campbell NC, Grimshaw JM, Ritchie LD, *et al.* Outpatient cardiac rehabilitation: are the potential benefits being realised? *J R Coll Physicians Lond* 1996;**30**:514–19.
126 Thompson DR, Bowman GS, DeBono DP, *et al.* The development and testing of a cardiac rehabilitation audit tool. *J R Coll Physicians Lond* 1997;**31**:317–20.
127 Harlan WR, Sandler SA, Lee KL, *et al.* The importance of baseline functional and socioeconomic factors for participation in cardiac rehabilitation. *Am J Cardiol* 1995;**76**:36–9.
128 Oldridge N, Wicks J, Hanley C, *et al.* Non-compliance in an exercise rehabilitation program for men who have suffered a myocardial infarction. *Can Med Assoc J* 1978;**118**:361–4.

Multiple choice questions

1 Which of the following are contraindications to exercise based cardiac rehabilitation?
   (a) Stable heart failure
   (b) Unstable angina pectoris
   (c) Malignant arrhythmias
   (d) Chronic obstructive airways disease
   (e) Mitral incompetence

2 Which of the following changes contribute to increases in physical fitness with a three month course of cardiac rehabilitation?
   (a) Increase in stroke volume
   (b) Increase in ejection fraction
   (c) Increase in force of contraction of the left ventricle
   (d) Increase in haemoglobin
   (e) Increase in oxygen extraction by working muscle

3 Which of the following have been shown to lessen angina pectoris after exercise training?
   (a) Improved myocardial perfusion
   (b) Increased coronary collaterals
   (c) Lower double product at a given workload
   (d) Higher haemoglobin level

    (e) Increased respiratory efficiency

4 Which of the following levels of exercise are sufficient to increase physical fitness in cardiac patients?
    (a) Once weekly sessions
    (b) Energy expenditure of 35% of $\dot{V}O_2$ MAX.
    (c) Sessions of 20 minutes duration
    (d) Warm up and stretching sessions
    (e) Heart rate response of 70% maximum

5 Exercise testing is used before cardiac rehabilitation for the following reasons:
    (a) To measure cardiac output
    (b) To detect reversible ischaemia
    (c) To lessen the risk of injury
    (d) To determine appropriate exercise heart rates
    (e) To unmask heart failure

Answers are on p. 368.

Answers to multiple choice questions

Chapter 1

1 (a) false; (b) false; (c) false; (d) true; (e) false
2 (a) true; (b) true; (c) false; (d) true; (e) true
3 (a) true; (b) false; (c) true; (d) true; (e) true
4 (a) false; (b) false; (c) true; (d) true; (e) true
5 (a) true; (b) true; (c) false; (d) true; (e) true

Chapter 2

1 (b)
2 (e)
3 (c)
4 (b)
5 (c)

Chapter 3

1 (a) true; (b) true; (c) false; (d) true; (e) true
2 (a) false; (b) false; (c) false; (d) true; (e) true
3 (a) false; (b) true; (c) true; (d) false
4 (a) true; (b) true; (c) true; (d) false
5 (a) true; (b) true; (c) true; (d) false; (e) false; (f) false

Chapter 4

1 False (exercise and physical activity are complex with multiple determinants).
2 False (many types of physical activity in natural settings are appropriate).

3 False (Marcus *et al.* have demonstrated the efficacy of this model in both worksite and community interventions).

4 False (the answer is adoption, maintenance, relapse, and resumption).

5 True (over 200 studies have examined barriers to adoption or studied dropping out).

6 False (for men exercise adoption was predicted by age and neighbourhood environment; for women adoption of vigorous exercise was predicted by education and social support).

7 True (King *et al.* found that participants in home based activity had significantly higher adherence than those who took part in higher intensity group based programmes).

8 False (few exercise scientists now believe that education alone will increase the proportion of individuals who engage in a programme of either moderate or vigorous physical activity).

9 True (the greatest decrease in mortality risk comes by moving from the no activity category into the moderate activity category).

10 False (the prevalence of those engaging in vigorous activity has not increased since the fitness boom of the 1980s).

11 True (few of these have been evaluated and the author is aware of only one such evaluation at the time of writing).

12 True (interventions may need to be different for men and women, particularly for older men and less educated women).

Chapter 5

1 (a) False – Even though the exact incidence of sudden cardiac death in athletes is unknown, sudden death in young athletes is rare.

(b) False – Premature coronary artery disease is a rare cause of death in young (<25 years) athletes. Large studies from the United States suggest that hypertrophic cardiomyopathy is the commonest cause of exercise related death in young athletes. Coronary artery disease is the commonest cause of exercise related death in older athletes.

(c) True

(d) True

(e) True

2 All true (see box 5.2)

3 All true (see box 5.1) – Cocaine abuse is well recognised among athletes and in some sporting disciplines has reached epidemic

levels. Recognised cardiac complications include myocardial ischaemia or infarction secondary to coronary artery spasm, cardiac arrhythmias, and chemical myocarditis.

4 (a) True – Patients with hypertrophic cardiomyopathy generally have a small left ventricular cavity size. In contrast, athletes have large left ventricular cavity size.

(b) True – Hypertrophic cardiomyopathy is a familiar disease, therefore a family history of premature sudden cardiac death in an individual with left ventricular hypertrophy may be indicative of hypertrophic cardiomyopathy gene inheritance.

(c) False – Isolated Sokolow criteria for left ventricular hypertrophy is common in athletes, however, associated T wave inversion should raise the suspicion of pathological hypertrophy.

(d) False – Physiological hypertrophy regresses after detraining whereas pathological hypertrophy—for example, in hypertrophic cardiomyopathy—persists.

(e) True – Pathological Q waves in a young individual with hypertrophic cardiomyopathy is almost certainly diagnostic of hypertrophic cardiomyopathy. While cardiac amyloid may also cause left ventricular hypertrophy and pathological Q waves, it is very uncommon in fit athletes and is usually confined to older patients with underlying medical disorders such as the paraproteinaemias.

5 (a) True

(b) True

(c) False – Physical examination is a relatively insensitive method of identifying cardiovascular disorders in young athletes. If performed thoroughly, however, it will detect aortic stenosis, hypertrophic cardiomyopathy with the obstructive element, and the Marfinoid appearance.

(d) True

(e) True – It is possible to see the origins of the coronary arteries on short axis views of the aortic root.

Chapter 6

1 (a) false; (b) true; (c) false; (d) false
2 (a) false; (b) false; (c) true; (d) false
3 (a) true; (b) true; (c) false; (d) true
4 (a) true; (b) false; (c) true; (d) true
5 (a) false; (b) false; (c) true; (d) false

Chapter 7

1 (a) true; (b) false; (c) true; (d) false
2 (a) false; (b) false; (c) false; (d) false
3 (a) false; (b) false; (c) false; (d) true
4 (a) true; (b) false; (c) true; (d) true
5 (a) true; (b) false; (c) true; (d) false

Chapter 8

1 (a) false; (b) true; (c) false; (d) true; (e) false
2 (a) false; (b) false; (c) false; (d) false; (e) true
3 (a) true; (b) true; (c) false; (d) false; (e) false
4 (a) false; (b) false; (c) true; (d) true; (e) false

Chapter 9

1 False – Nearly all fatigued athletes are from endurance sports such as swimming, rowing, cycling, and track and field.
2 False – Creatine kinase concentrations are very high after any eccentric work and do not indicate that an athlete will break down with chronic fatigue.
3 True – The controversial question is how important this is in the apparent immunosuppression seen in overtrained athletes.
4 True – If athletes do not overreach they will not get any benefit from training (supercompensation).
5 False – There is no evidence that vitamins offer any protection from chronic fatigue.

Chapter 10

1 (a) false; (b) false; (c) true; (d) true; (e) false
2 (a) true; (b) false; (c) true; (d) true; (e) false

Chapter 11

1 (b)
2 (d)
3 (a)
4 (e)
5 (c)

Chapter 12

1 (e)
2 (a)
3 (b)
4 (b)
5 (c)

Chapter 13

1 (a) false; (b) true; (c) false; (d) false
2 (a) true; (b) false; (c) false; (d) false
3 (a) false; (b) true; (c) false; (d) false
4 (a) false; (b) false; (c) false; (d) true
5 (a) true; (b) true; (c) false; (d) true

Chapter 14

1 (d)
2 (b)
3 (c)
4 (d)
5 (c)

Chapter 15

1 (a) true; (b) false; (c) false; (d) false
2 (a) false; (b) true; (c) false; (d) false
3 (a) false; (b) false; (c) false; (d) true
4 (a) false; (b) false; (c) true; (d) false
5 (a) true; (b) false; (c) false; (d) false
6 (a) false; (b) true; (c) false; (d) false

Chapter 16

1 (a) True
(b) False – They can be adjusted, but not determined, by environmental or exogenous factors—for example, light-dark cycle called "synchronisers".
(c) False – To determine the existence of a rhythmic oscillation in a certain period for a certain biological phenomenon, a great number of accurate measurements and a sophisticated computerised analysis are necessary.

(d) True

2 (a) True

(b) False – Only about 10% of people strictly belong to morning or evening type; the 90% remaining are intermediate.

(c) True

(d) False – No significant differences have been found in athletic performance according to chronotype.

3 (a) False – Rapid air travel across several time zones is necessary to determine a shift in the internal biological clock. Usually, it is said that at least four time zones are required.

(b) True

(c) True

(d) False – About 30% of transmeridian travellers have no symptoms, and another 30% do not adjust well at all.

(e) True

4 (a) True

(b) False – It seems that it is mainly the result of variations in heat loss mechanisms.

(c) True

(d) True

(e) True – Gastric emptying rate is over 50% slower for evening meals.

5 (a) True

(b) True

(c) True

(d) False – Controlled studies on differences in performances have shown, for example, a significant early evening peak for length of jump, vertical jumping performance, and swimming.

6 (a) True

(b) True

(c) True

(d) True

(e) True

(f) False – Short term memory peaks in the morning.

(g) True

(h) False – There is an inverse relation between speed and accuracy, the latter being worse in the afternoon–evening hours. So, sports demanding high accuracy may be favoured in the morning.

7 (a) True

(b) True

(c) False – The simple exposure to a source of light is not

sufficient. When an individual's circadian phase is known, the phase of some circadian rhythms may be advanced or delayed by the exposure to bright light with specific intensity, duration, and timing.

(d) False – Though melatonin undoubtedly has a hypnotic effect, it acts in a highly pleiotropic fashion—for example, eliciting secondary humoral immunological responses or acting as a powerful radical scavenger.

(e) True

(f) True – Evening administration of melatonin advances the body clock, and morning administration delays it.

Chapter 17

1 (a) False – This is insufficient, by majority view.

(b) False – These are the traditional recommendations designed to improve or maintain fitness.

(c) True – Taking an approximation of 100 kcal/mile (about 59 kcal/km), current recommendations are consistent with a daily energy expenditure in physical activity of about 200 kcal or 1400 kcal/week.

(d) True – This is a fair summary of the 1995–96 recommendations of the American College of Sport Medicine, the Centers for Disease Control and Prevention, the United States Surgeon General's Report, and the Health Education Authority's campaign "Active living".

2 (a) False – Seems unlikely most people will travel, change, and swim several times a day.

(b) False – Same reason as (a).

(c) True – In many studies, particularly the landmark Harvard alumni study, walking was scored as "blocks walked", therefore likely to have been mainly walking for commuting and personal transport.

(d) True – Stair climbing is inherently intermittent rather than long continuous periods of exercise.

3 (a) True – Many adaptations are in the muscles that are exercised. Examples include increased glucose transporters, better microcirculation, and enhanced lipoprotein lipase activity.

(b) True – For several metabolic benefits it has been shown that intensity can be "traded" for duration and/or that the effects of several shorter sessions are comparable with those of one longer session expending the same energy.

(c) False – There is no evidence for this.

(d) True – If fitness improves, more energy can be expended in physical activity at a moderate level or above, so that the metabolic benefits are enhanced.

4 (a) True – Several studies have shown that this pattern of exercise is effective in improving fitness.

(b) True – Several studies have shown that this pattern of exercise is effective in decreasing body fatness.

(c) False – There is almost no evidence for this (as of December 1998).

(d) False – There is no evidence for this.

5 (a) False – Trained people do tend to consume high carbohydrate diets but these lower (not raise) high density lipoprotein cholesterol concentrations.

(b) False – The main effect of a low intake of saturated fat is to lower plasma total cholesterol concentration.

(c) True – Degradation of triglyceride-rich lipoproteins is associated with transfer of surface proteins to nascent high density lipoproteins, enabling them to become mature spherical particles.

(d) False – There is no relation between energy intake and high density lipoprotein cholesterol concentration.

Chapter 18

1 (a) false; (b) true; (c) true; (d) false; (e) false
2 (a) false; (b) false; (c) false; (d) false; (e) true
3 (a) true; (b) false; (c) true; (d) false; (e) false
4 (a) false; (b) false; (c) true; (d) false; (e) true
5 (a) false; (b) true; (c) false; (d) true; (e) false

Index

nucleic acid amplification
techniques 187, 194

obesity
see also weight loss
effects of physical activity 26
intermittent exercise 324–5
low intensity exercise
programmes 12
walking 1, 6
obsessive-compulsive personality
traits 214
occupations, physically demanding
cardiovascular protection 4,
6–10
self-selection 4
oestrogen:progesterone ratio 211
oligomenorrhoea 245
orthostatic hypotension
diabetes mellitus 143, 157
overtraining syndrome 174
Oslo diet and exercise study 153
osteopenia 246, 247, 248
osteoporosis 111, 212
benefits of exercise 199
effects of physical activity 25
hypogonadism 242
sedentary lifestyle 45
overreaching 172, 176
overtraining syndrome 171–82
amino acids 178
central fatigue 177–8
clinical investigations 175
hormones 176–7
infections, recurrent 173, 175
management 179–80
pathophysiology 176–8
prevention 174–5
signs 174
symptoms 172–3
underperformance 172–3
oxidative stress 294
2-oxoglutarate 292
oxygen transport 279

PAGE intervention 71
palate, high arched 94
palpitation
arrhythmogenic right ventricular
cardiomyopathy 90
hypertrophic cardiomyopathy 86

Wolff-Parkinson-White
syndrome 92
Paul-Bunnell test 175
Pawtucket heart health programme
76
Pennsylvania County health
improvement project 76
pericardium 86
periodisation 172, 174–5
phototherapy 310–11
physical activity
see also exercise
action stage 71
adherence research 64
cancer risk 25
cardiovascular risk 25
clinical interventions 64
community interventions 64
contemplation stage 71
daily recommendations 11
health benefits *see* health benefits
history 67
hypoglycaemic benefits 137–70
lipid profiles 25, 26
maintenance stage 71
maintenance, predictors 67
minimum intensity for health 3,
11, 12
multiple short sessions 323–6
occupationally-generated 3
optimal 1–24
patterns and psychosocial issues
2–3
precontemplation stage 71
preparation stage 71
psychological wellbeing *see*
psychological wellbeing
stage of change 71
transtheoretical model 71
unsupervised activity 3
physical activity adoption
aspects of physical activity 68–9
barriers to adoption 66, 67, 110,
113
behavioural aspects 70–74
cognitive aspects 70–74
community approaches 75–6
environmental approaches 77
exercise intensity 67–8
family interventions 74